Telepsychiatry and Health Technologies

A Guide for Mental Health Professionals

Edited by

Peter Yellowlees, MBBS, M.D.

Jay H. Shore, M.D., M.P.H.

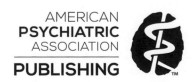

AMERICAN
PSYCHIATRIC
ASSOCIATION
PUBLISHING

Note: The authors have worked to ensure that all information in this book is accurate at the time of publication and consistent with general psychiatric and medical standards, and that information concerning drug dosages, schedules, and routes of administration is accurate at the time of publication and consistent with standards set by the U.S. Food and Drug Administration and the general medical community. As medical research and practice continue to advance, however, therapeutic standards may change. Moreover, specific situations may require a specific therapeutic response not included in this book. For these reasons and because human and mechanical errors sometimes occur, we recommend that readers follow the advice of physicians directly involved in their care or the care of a member of their family.

Books published by American Psychiatric Association Publishing represent the findings, conclusions, and views of the individual authors and do not necessarily represent the policies and opinions of American Psychiatric Association Publishing or the American Psychiatric Association.

If you wish to buy 50 or more copies of the same title, please go to www.appi.org/specialdiscounts for more information.

Manufactured in the United States of America on acid-free paper
21   20   19   18   17   5   4   3   2   1

American Psychiatric Association Publishing
1000 Wilson Boulevard
Arlington, VA 22209-3901
www.appi.org

Library of Congress Cataloging-in-Publication Data
Names: Yellowlees, Peter, editor. | Shore, Jay H., 1970– editor. | American
    Psychiatric Association, issuing body.
Title: Telepsychiatry and health technologies : a guide for mental health
    professionals / edited by Peter Yellowlees, Jay H. Shore.
Description: First edition. | Arlington, Virginia : American Psychiatric Association
    Publishing, [2018] | Includes bibliographical references and index.
Identifiers: LCCN 2017045567 (print) | LCCN 2017046095 (ebook) | ISBN
    9781615371600 (ebook) | ISBN 9781615370856 (pbk. : alk. paper)
Subjects: | MESH: Mental Disorders—therapy | Telemedicine—methods |
    Telemedicine—organization & administration | Mental Health Services—
    organization & administration | Medical Informatics
Classification: LCC RC455.2.D38 (ebook) | LCC RC455.2.D38 (print) | NLM WM
    400 | DDC 616.8900285—dc23
LC record available at https://lccn.loc.gov/2017045567

British Library Cataloguing in Publication Data
A CIP record is available from the British Library.

*This book is dedicated to two modest but highly influential
physicians and leaders in American Psychiatry:*

Robert Hales, M.D., M.B.A.,
*was Editor in Chief at American Psychiatric Publishing, Inc.,
for more than 15 years and has been a long-term invaluable mentor of P.Y.
Dr. Hales has contributed enormously to the discipline of Psychiatry
worldwide, not only through his own remarkable published output
of more than 65 authored and edited books
but also through his encouragement and support
of numerous colleagues to follow in his steps.*

James (Jim) Shore, M.D.,
*was Chancellor of the combined University of Colorado Denver
and Anschutz Medical Campuses; Chairman of the University of Colorado
and University of Oregon Departments of Psychiatry;
and former President of the American Board of Psychiatry and Neurology
and the American College of Psychiatrists. Dr. Shore mentored a generation
of academic leaders and psychiatrists and championed access and service
in public psychiatry for underserved communities.*

Contents

Contributors

Danielle Alexander, M.D.
Psychiatry and Family Medicine Resident, University California Davis, Sacramento, California

Mark Alter, M.D., Ph.D.
Associate Medical Director for On-Demand Services, InSight Telepsychiatry, LLC, Marlton, New Jersey

Daniel J. Balog, M.D.
Medical Director, Clinical Informatics and Telepsychiatry, South Carolina Department of Mental Health, Columbia; and Clinical Assistant Professor, Department of Psychiatry and Behavioral Sciences, Medical University of South Carolina, Charleston

Robert Lee Caudill, M.D.
Associate Professor, Department of Psychiatry and Behavioral Sciences, University of Louisville, School of Medicine, Kentucky

Steven R. Chan, M.D., M.B.A.
Clinical Fellow in Informatics and Psychiatry, Division of Hospital Medicine, University of California at San Francisco School of Medicine

Gregory Evangelatos, M.D.
Resident, Psychiatry & Addiction Medicine, Kaweah Delta Medical Center, Visalia Mental Health, California

Sarina Fazio, Ph.D.(c)., B.S.N., M.S.
Administrative Research Nurse and Doctoral Candidate, Betty Irene School of Nursing, University of California Davis, Sacramento, California

Alvaro D. González, M.A., M.F.T.I.
Mental Health Therapist and Research Assistant, Department of Psychiatry and Behavioral Sciences, University of California Davis, Sacramento, California

Frederick Guggenheim, M.D.
Clinical Professor of Psychiatry and Human Behavior, Alpert Medical School of Brown University, Providence, Rhode Island; and Professor of Psychiatry and Chair Emeritus, University of Arkansas for Medical Sciences, Little Rock, Arkansas

Donald M. Hilty, M.D.
Chief, Behavioral Health Services; Chair, Department of Psychiatry and Addiction Medicine; and Program Director, Kaweah Delta Medical Center, Visalia, California; and Professor, Department of Psychiatry and Behavioral Sciences, Keck School of Medicine at University of Southern California, Los Angeles

Sam Hubley, Ph.D.
Assistant Professor, Helen and Arthur E. Johnson Depression Center, University of Colorado School of Medicine, Aurora

Tiffany Hwang, M.D.
Resident, Department of Psychiatry, University of California at San Diego

Barb Johnston, M.S.N.
Chief Executive Officer, HealthLinkNow Inc., Sacramento, California

Edward Kaftarian, M.D.
Statewide Chief of Telepsychiatry, California Correctional Healthcare Services, and Chief Executive Officer, Orbit Health Telepsychiatry, Los Angeles, California

John Luo, M.D.
Chief Medical Information Officer, Professor of Psychiatry, and Director of Psychiatry Residency Program, University of California, Riverside

Tania Malik, J.D.
Chief Executive Officer, Dagny Diversified, Raleigh, North Carolina; and Board Member, Mindcare Solutions Group, Franklin, Tennessee

Francis Leo McVeigh, O.D., M.S., M.F.T.I.
Chief Scientist, Advanced Technology and Innovation Laboratory, Telemedicine and Advanced Technology Research Center, United States Army Medical Research and Materiel Command, Fort Detrick, Maryland

Matt Mishkind, Ph.D., SPHR, SHRM-SCP
Deputy Director, Helen and Arthur E. Johnson Depression Center, University of Colorado School of Medicine, Aurora, Colorado

Kathleen Myers, M.D., M.P.H., M.S.
Professor, Department of Psychiatry and Behavioral Sciences, and Director, Telemental Health Program, Seattle Children's Hospital, Seattle, Washington

Meera Narasimhan, M.D.
Professor and Chair of Clinical Neuropsychiatry and Behavioral Science, University of South Carolina School of Medicine, Columbia

Michelle Burke Parish, M.A., Ph.D.(c)
Clinical Research Manager and Doctoral Candidate, Department of Psychiatry and Behavioral Sciences, University of California Davis School of Medicine, Sacramento, California

Terry Rabinowitz, M.D.
Professor, Departments of Psychiatry and Family Medicine, Larner College of Medicine at the University of Vermont; Medical Director, Divisions of Consultation Psychiatry and Psychosomatic Medicine; Medical Director, Telemedicine, University of Vermont Medical Center, Burlington, Vermont

Lisa Roberts, Ph.D.
President, Government Market Division, AMC Health, New York, New York

Shazia Shafqat, M.D., M.S.
Graduate student in Health Informatics, University of California Davis, Sacramento, California

Erica Z. Shoemaker, M.D.
Assistant Professor and Director of Child Clinical Services, Department of Psychiatry & Behavioral Sciences, Keck School of Medicine at University of Southern California (USC), Los Angeles, California

Jay H. Shore, M.D., M.P.H.
Professor, Departments of Psychiatry and Family Medicine, School of Medicine, and Centers for American Indian and Alaska Native Health, Colorado School of Public Health; Director of Telemedicine, Helen and Arthur E. Johnson Depression Center, University of Colorado Denver Anschutz Medical Campus, Aurora, Colorado

Peter Shore, Psy.D.
Assistant Professor, Department of Psychiatry, Oregon Health and Science University; and Director of Telehealth, Northwest Veterans Integrated Service Network (VISN 20), U.S. Department of Veterans Affairs, Portland, Oregon

John Torous, M.D.
Staff Psychiatrist and Clinical Fellow in Informatics, Beth Israel Deaconess Medical Center, Harvard University Medical School, Boston, Massachusetts

Carolyn Turvey, Ph.D., M.S.
Professor of Psychology and Research Health Scientist, Department of Psychiatry, University of Iowa and Iowa City VA Health Care, Iowa City, Iowa

Gilbert Andrew Valasquez
Medical Student, American University of Antigua College of Medicine, Coolidge, Antigua

Maryann Waugh, M.Ed.
Grants and Research Director, Behavioral Health, Colorado Access, Aurora, Colorado

Peter Yellowlees, MBBS, M.D.
Professor of Psychiatry and Vice Chair for Faculty Development, University of California Davis School of Medicine, Sacramento, California; President, American Telemedicine Association, Washington, D.C.

DISCLOSURE OF INTERESTS

The following contributors to this book have indicated a financial interest in or other affiliation with a commercial supporter, a manufacturer of a commercial product, a provider of a commercial service, a nongovernmental organization, and/ or a government agency, as listed below:

Steven R. Chan, M.D., M.B.A.   Steven R. Chan is employed by University of California and sees patients as a contracted physician of the HealthLink-Now telepsychiatry firm. Dr. Chan writes for and edits posts on *The Doctor Weighs In* Web site and is allowed to cover conferences with free admission but is not provided financial reimbursement. He has received grant funding from the University of California Davis and the American Psychiatric Association/Substance Abuse and Mental Health Services Administration. Dr. Chan advises—but does not receive financial renumeration from— Whitekoat, Valera Health, and Doximity.

Edward Kaftarian, M.D.   Edward Kaftarian is Chief of Telepsychiatry at California Correctional Healthcare Services, Elk Grove, California, as well as CEO of Orbit Health, Pasadena, California.

Tania Malik, J.D.   Tania S. Malik holds an equity position and is Secretary of the Board of Directors of a telepsychiatry company (Mindcare Solutions Group).

Jay H. Shore, M.D., M.P.H.   Jay H. Shore is the CMO for AccessCare through a contract with the University of Colorado Denver in a part-time capacity, which includes possible equity interest. AccessCare is a for-profit company that provides both telehealth service and technology.

Peter Yellowlees, MBBS, M.D.   Peter Yellowlees is video- editorial writer and presenter for Medscape (2009–present) and is President of the American Telemedicine Association, Washington, DC. Dr. Yellowlees' spouse is CEO of HealthLinkNow Inc, a commercial telepsychiatry company he co-founded with his spouse.

The following contributors stated that they had no competing interests during the year preceding manuscript submission:

Danielle Alexander, M.D.; Gregory Evangelatos, M.D.; Sarina Fazio, B.S.N., M.S.; Alvaro D. González, M.A., M.F.T.I.; Frederick Guggenheim, M.D.; Donald M. Hilty, M.D.; Sam Hubley, Ph.D.; Tiffany Hwang; Barb Johnston, M.S.N.; John Luo, M.D.; Francis Leo McVeigh, O.D., M.S.; Matt Mishkind, Ph.D., SPHR, SHRM-SCP; Kathleen Myers, M.D., M.P.H., M.S.; Michelle Burke Parish, M.A.; Lisa Roberts, Ph.D.; Shazia Shafqat, M.D., M.S.; Erica Z. Shoemaker, M.D.; Peter Shore, Psy.D.; John Torous, M.D.; Carolyn Turvey, Ph.D., M.S.; Gilbert Andrew Valasquez; Maryann Waugh, M.Ed.

Preface

Telepsychiatry and Health Technologies: A Guide for Mental Health Professionals has been written as a practical and clinical guide for psychiatrists and other mental health care professionals in this changing era of health care delivery and technology innovation. The book focuses on the doctor–patient relationship and provides a practical blueprint for how psychiatrists and other mental health care professionals can leverage expanding digital technologies and processes that are currently available, and that are increasingly being used in clinical practice, for the assessment and treatment of patients with psychiatric disorders.

This book was not created using the usual editing process, in that we did not ask individual contributors to write on broad topic areas and produce a chapter for us incorporating content of their own choosing. Instead, as coeditors, we initially mapped out the book down to the section headings of every chapter and then selected colleagues to write various sections of the book based on their individual expertise and knowledge. We have been fortunate in being able to collaborate with more than 30 other practitioners of telepsychiatry across the core mental health care disciplines. These collaborators contributed to both chapters and cases and agreed to work according to our parameters to achieve, we hope, an edited book that flows logically and creates synergy across chapters without duplication.

Our ultimate aim has been to produce a book that is effectively a clinical textbook, and that we hope will become a core resource in the training of mental health care professionals from all disciplines for years to come, as well as a trusted reference for those already trained and adapting to the many new technologies in their workplaces.

This is, importantly, not a technology-centered "health informatics" book for the mental health care field. We have deliberately steered away from trying to describe more than very basic technological issues. Instead, we have emphasized clinical issues and workflows for both individual patients and practitioners, and in the treatment of populations of patients, which is where we believe psychiatrists will increasingly focus in future years. We have tried to be as practical as possible, incorporating more than 30 case examples of patients or programs to highlight clinical techniques and types of patients that can be treated using available technologies in person, online, or in a hybrid form of care combining both. Every chapter concludes with a summary restating the major learning objectives or findings covered. Chapters are broken down into section headings posed as questions based on questions and queries we have been asked over many years of practice.

As practitioners of telepsychiatry, we are well aware that telepsychiatry is not a new medical practice, with the first video psychiatric consultations having taken place at the University of Nebraska in 1959, 58 years ago. In the course of writing this book, we have come across many people who have contributed to the field of telepsychiatry, including Frederick Guggenheim, M.D., who in 1969 began working with Thomas Dwyer, who coined the term "telepsychiatry,"[1] and with Kenneth Bird, M.D., of the Massachusetts General Hospital (MGH) Department of Medicine. Dr. Bird was the initiator of a feasibility study using microwave interactive video conferencing between MGH and Boston's Logan Airport as well as with the Bedford VA hospital. Dr. Guggenheim described his experiences as follows:

> What was so good about the Telepsychiatry project was that there were no instructions to follow: I could just find my own way. What was not so good, was any lack of supervision or any feedback from either end of the interactive dyad. This was the era of: "See one. Do one. Teach one."
>
> At Logan's Medical Station, I saw scheduled patients one afternoon a week, typically doing Employee Assistance Program–type counseling. One case was a forty-year-old married African American baggage handler at Logan, with no prior psychiatric history. His marriage was crumbling, resulting in a brief reactive depression. A nurse there then prepared him for our interview, which seemed to be like any other psychiatric interview, except that we were three miles apart. We got along

---

[1] Dwyer TF: "Telepsychiatry: Psychiatric Consultation by Interactive Television." *American Journal of Psychiatry* 130(8):865–869, 1973.

well, and I continued to see him for about three sessions, over as many weeks. I then went on vacation for a week. To my surprise, after returning from vacation, I learned from the MGH Psychiatric Emergency Service that Mr. A had been brought by his family to MGH after a suicide gesture. He talked to one of the MGH psychiatric residents there who offered him a psychotherapy appointment right away with a clinic psychiatrist, "a real doctor." "No thank you," said Mr. A. "I want to see my TV doctor." We continued to meet weekly, he at Logan Airport Medical Station, and I in the television studio in the basement at MGH, until he achieved a satisfactory resolution of his marital crisis and his mild–moderate depression.

One challenge to video conferencing was making the equipment adapt to our clinical needs. I found that paranoid patients became more comfortable if we could diminish the size of my body image on the monitor in the patient's interview room. We also learned to have the camera turned towards the door when the patient entered so that I could welcome them and study their gait and movements before they sat down. Another challenge was establishing a working relationship with the medical-surgical nursing service at Bedford VA hospital, twenty miles north of MGH. There were no guidelines or goals for what types of patients would be most suitable for an interactive format and the initial patients offered to me as interviewees turned out to be complicated. The first patient I saw was partially deaf. We were both frustrated. The second patient had known Huntington's dementia, with few social skills and little ability to concentrate in an interview. I was able to handle these situations with tact and grace, and eventually the nurses began to see me as an asset and started to send some of their lonely, long-term patients to interview, allowing me to focus on existential issues for individual patients.

After our early period of adjustment, the nurse at the VA studio suggested that I start doing group therapy for patients on the substance abuse unit. I started weekly group therapy with eight to ten heroin-addicted patients, hospitalized for six months of detox and supportive therapy. The group members continued for many months to attend on a volunteer basis and both the patients and I thought it was a clinically useful way to spend our time.

In summary, with structured goals and some inventive camera work, telepsychiatry proved to be a very satisfactory modality both for clinical evaluation and for individual and group psychotherapy. The only component in the usual doctor-patient relationship missing was the ability to shake hands.

It is fascinating to read about Dr. Guggenheim's experiences in 1969 and how similar they were to experiences that we have both encountered and still occur commonly in many ways today. So while this book is being written 48 years after Dr. Guggenheim started seeing patients using videoconferencing, the conclusions that he reached around the ability to treat patients and preserve the doctor–patient relationship are a relevant and excellent starting point for this book.

The first four chapters are the foundation of the book and describe the current status and use of communications technologies, primarily video, text/Internet, e-mail, and telephony, in mental health care. We start in Chapter 1 by reviewing the current status of mental health care practice; the clinical, policy-related, and financial pressures on practitioners and patients; the types of technologies available; and the importance of the doctor–patient relationship and how to maintain this relationship in the hybrid (online and in-person) treatment settings of the future. We then cover the history of and the evidence base for the use of technology in mental health care in Chapter 2, before moving to the business side of clinical practice in Chapter 3, including how to set up and manage a telepsychiatry practice and overcome the barriers of licensing, reimbursement, and the many administrative issues involved. We finish this section by reviewing the many work practices, settings, and models of care influenced by technology, from private practice to emergency departments, and from primary integrated care and the patient's medical home to care in the home and community, which are examined in Chapter 4.

The core clinical practice section of the book comes next and is structured for maximum usefulness to practicing psychiatrists and other mental health care professionals. Chapter 5 is focused on the patient and how to use technology to collect information and develop relationships. It includes sections on media skills for video and ethical guidelines and advice on how to effectively interact with patients using health technologies. Chapter 6 is about collecting data from nonpatient sources, including social media, apps, smartphones, tablets, and search engines, as well as examining data that can be collected through remote monitoring in home and community environments. Chapter 7 discusses writing notes and clinical documentation in electronic health record environments where data integration and health information exchange occurs. Here we also cover policies of importance, as well as the use of clinical templates and automated dictation systems and tips for good practice, self-care, and avoiding burnout—topics that lead into Chapter 8, which is about the use of indirect consultations in a hybrid care environment, working with patients both in person and online, which is how we believe most psychiatrists will be practicing within a few years. We provide specific advice on how to conduct asynchronous telepsychiatry video consultations and how to work with patients using e-mail and messaging, both of which we believe will be of great future importance.

The final section of the book is about the management of data to provide quality care to specific populations of patients (defined geographically, culturally, or diagnostically) as well as to individuals. Chapter 9 explores the use of big data and decision support, and addresses why technology is so important when providing care to numerous different populations of patients, while Chapter 10 concentrates on quality and competencies and the importance of applying the evidence base, guidelines, and knowledge described throughout this book to support ongoing professional development.

This book is intended to provide psychiatrists and mental health care professionals from all other disciplines with practical guidance and advice on how best to make use of telepsychiatry and a range of health technologies in their practices now and in the future. We are in the midst of a revolution in Western society, transitioning from an industrial age to an information age. Western medicine is being transformed by technology that is simultaneously improving care while imposing challenges on the existing health care structures and processes. All providers are being forced to adapt to the now-continuous changes in health care systems created by technology-driven innovation. We hope this book can be a tool that helps providers to keep pace with and adapt to their changing workplace environments. The practice of mental health care is changing rapidly in the face of increasing needs from larger numbers of patients, and we believe that the sensible use of health technologies will lead to substantial reductions in the current gap in health care supply and demand, will improve models of care delivery, and ultimately will result in better health for more patients than our traditional systems of care have been able to provide.

Peter Yellowlees, MBBS, M.D.
Sacramento, California

Jay H. Shore, M.D., M.P.H.
Aurora, Colorado

Acknowledgments

We have been friends and colleagues for twenty years, and during that time there have been many people that we both know who have positively influenced us, particularly the many colleagues in America and around that world that we have met through our membership in the American Telemedicine Association, quite a few of whom have assisted in the writing of this book. These include Barb Johnston, M.S.N., Don Hilty, M.D., Carolyn Turvey, Ph.D., Robert Caudill, M.D., Terry Rabinowitz, M.D., Lisa Roberts, Ph.D., Peter Shore, Ph.D., Ed Kaftarian, M.D., and Kathleen Myers, M.D.

At University of California Davis, PY would like to acknowledge the long-standing support and collaboration of numerous psychiatric colleagues, including Robert Hales, M.D., M.B.A., James Bourgeois, M.D., Glen Xiong, M.D., Steven Chan, M.D., Lorin Scher, M.D., Robert McCarron, D.O., and Andres Sciolla, M.D. These have all contributed to the work of the UCD telepsychiatry research team, which has produced and validated many of the ideas and concepts discussed in this book and which currently includes Michelle Parrish, M.A., Alberto Odor, M.D., Ana-Maria Iosif, Ph.D., Jennifer Bannister, and Alvaro Gonzalez.

At University of Colorado, Jay Shore would like to acknowledge the ongoing support, mentorship, and collaboration in telehealth of friends and colleagues, including Spero Manson, Ph.D., Douglas Novins, M.D., Marshall Thomas, M.D., Matthew Mishkind, Ph.D., Christopher Schneck, M.D., Alexis Giese, M.D., Rachel Dixon, Maryann Waugh, M.S., Frank Degruy, M.D., Byron Bair, M.D., Nancy Dailey, R.N., William "Buck" Richardson, Gary Hoggan, M.D., Jeff Lowe, M.S.W., Laura Martin, M.D., Jacqueline Calderone, M.D., Karl Friedl, Ph.D., Ron Poropatich, M.D., and Francis McVeigh, O.D., M.S.

Finally, we both wish to acknowledge the amazing support and love we receive from our families, and our wives in particular, Barb and Jessica, as well as Jay's children, Fiona and Nola, who keep Jay young at heart and informed on social media trends and apps.

1

Psychiatric Practice in the Information Age

Peter Yellowlees, MBBS, M.D.

Jay H. Shore, M.D., M.P.H.

This is both an exciting and a challenging time to be working in mental health care. In this introductory chapter, we explore many of the complex issues affecting psychiatrists and other mental health care professionals, and the country as a whole, as they strive to change and provide the most effective form of care for all patients. We begin by reviewing the current status of the practice of psychiatry, noting immediately a severe deficit in the number of psychiatrists in the United States that will progressively get worse over the next decade. We then examine how technology is being leveraged to address these current and impending workforce changes, especially as they relate to access and patient care issues; the technologies currently available; and the broad social, environmental, political, and technical influences affecting providers and patients. All of this will influence the doctor–patient relationship, which will increasingly exist both in-person and online in a hybrid form. This changed relationship, in which technology provides much of the infrastructure for mental health care in the future, will mainly be positive for patients and providers, but may also have unintended consequences. Psychiatrists and other mental health care professionals will need to protect themselves and their own health as the practice environment evolves.

1

WHAT IS THE CURRENT STATUS OF PSYCHIATRISTS AND THE PRACTICE OF PSYCHIATRY IN THE UNITED STATES?

There is a severe deficit of psychiatrists in the United States, and this shortage is likely to get significantly worse over the next decade. There are also shortages of practitioners in other groups of mental health care professionals, especially in rural regions, as well as of practitioners with subspecialist expertise, especially in treating children and the elderly.

As of April 2017, there were about 45,000 psychiatrists in the United States, with an estimated shortfall of about 6,000, which is projected to increase to 15,000 by 2025 (National Council Medical Director Institute 2017). There are even more serious shortages of physicians specializing in child/adolescent and geriatric psychiatry. The average age of the current cohort of psychiatrists is about 56 years, and approximately 65% of this cohort is male. The psychiatrists in this cohort are being only partially replaced by newly trained psychiatrists, 55% of whom are female, and female psychiatrists are known to work about 20% less on average than males over the course of their careers, primarily because of women's historically much larger share of responsibility for parenting and family caregiving. Over the next decade, large numbers of the aging (mainly male) cohort will retire at a time when 10% fewer (mainly female) replacements nationally are being trained. These further reductions will inevitably lead to an increasing shortage of available clinical time from the current pool of psychiatric expertise, which we have calculated could be reduced by up to 20% of total available hours in the next decade.

In addition, the demand for mental health care services in the United States is constantly rising, accelerated by the Affordable Care Act of 2010, which, while positively increasing the size of the insured population, has also increased the imbalance between the number of individuals who require mental health care and the number of psychiatrists available to help those individuals. In this setting, the knowledge that by 2030, 20% of the population will be older than 65 years makes increasing supply-and-demand imbalances inevitable.

Physician shortages are also occurring in primary care, where most patients with mental illness are treated. Fortunately, other mental health care professionals, such as psychologists, nurse practitioners, and psychiatric social workers, are not in such short supply. These groups are increasingly assuming primary treatment roles, either independently or as physician extenders in a team. Having other mental health professionals provide traditional psychiatric care generally works well, although there are a number of areas in which the scope of practice is changing, such as where psychologists or nurse practitioners are being granted defined prescribing rights, leading to substantial rivalries and controversies that remain to be resolved.

The treatment of mental disorders also has changed dramatically over the past several decades, with the potential impact of improved prevention and early intervention, increased treatment in the community rather than in psychiatric hospitals, and reduction of stigma associated with such disorders. The mainstreaming of mental illness back into the general health system, including the passage of mental health care parity laws (requiring health insurers to provide the same level of benefits for mental health care and substance abuse services as they provide for treatment of other medical disorders) and the development of new pharmacotherapies and psychotherapies, have also led to substantial changes in care. Not surprisingly, although most of these factors are very positive, they have had unintended consequences and have led to the situation where most outpatient psychiatric care in the United States is now provided in the local community in a primary care setting, whereas inpatient psychiatric care is now provided in highly institutionalized or correctional settings (Bashshur et al. 2016).

In 2008, 13.4% of U.S. adults received professional treatment for a mental disorder, although only 58% of those with a serious mental illness and about half of children with a diagnosable psychiatric disorder did so. Nearly 25% of all patients seen in primary care have a psychiatric disorder, and increasing numbers of psychiatrists and other mental health care providers are starting to be involved in collaborative or integrated care programs with primary care providers (PCPs). Still, only 10% of mentally ill patients are treated by a psychiatrist, and only an estimated 50% of the patients seen by PCPs are accurately diagnosed (Moyer 2010). Yet, the primary care setting has become the de facto mental health care outpatient system in the United States (Katon 2011), where PCPs, without specialist support and advice, tend to miss diagnoses and underprescribe appropriate medications. The national move to support patients being seen in primary care in a more effective manner as part of a "patient-centered medical home"—wherein the PCP becomes the primary coordinator of care—is occurring partially in response to this situation. The patient-centered medical home model has led to increasing numbers of psychiatrists working alongside PCPs in collaborative integrated care programs, as will be discussed in Chapter 4 ("Clinical Settings and Models of Care in Telepsychiatry: Implications for Work Practices and Culturally Informed Treatment"), often supported by a variety of technologies.

Simultaneously, industry and commercial pharmacy chains, in particular, have started to support what is becoming a provider value coordination chain of care. This chain of care increasingly originates in patients' homes, or their PCPs' offices, linked to retail pharmacies containing virtual telemedicine clinics incorporating enterprise electronic record systems, such as at CVS and Walgreens, or to similar clinics being developed in "big box" stores such as Target and Walmart, and often connected to other urgent care community clinics or to large health systems that use the clinics as outreach services to maintain or increase their market shares. The number of these retail health environments in the United States doubled between 2012 and 2015, and the overall effect is intended to keep care in the community and to reduce the need for hospitalizations or emergency department visits. The retail stores are, of course, not providing these health services for philosophical reasons but because they see a potentially profitable market if they can become the new "one-stop shop" for health care provision and for the sale of the many health care-related goods, from prescriptions to glasses to wound-care materials.

Unfortunately, the increasing prevalence of mental disorders, with their serious social and economic consequences, has not been matched by a commensurate overall expansion of resources for treatment. The number of inpatient psychiatric beds has decreased dramatically throughout the country, a trend that started in the 1960s. For example, from 1995 through 2012, California lost 30%, or more than 2,800, of its mental health care beds, while its population increased by more than 5 million (Bashshur et al. 2016). Many patients, especially those with psychoses, have ended up incarcerated in jails or prisons, which have become America's "new asylums." Bashshur et al. (2016) quoted figures demonstrating that in 2012 there were an estimated 356,268 inmates with severe mental illness in prisons and jails compared with an estimated 35,000 patients with severe mental illness housed in state psychiatric hospitals. It is indeed likely that the number of mentally ill persons in correctional institutions is currently 10 times the number of residents in state hospitals.

The costs of mental illness are enormous; Bashshur et al. (2016) quoted estimates from 2007 of almost $200 billion in lost earnings per year, with mood disorders such as depression being the third most common cause of hospitalization in the United States. The total costs associated with mental illness are usually calculated on the basis of direct expenditures for mental health care services and treatment (direct costs) as well as productivity losses due to disability caused by these disorders (indirect costs) (Insel 2008). In 2015 the National Institute of Mental Health estimated the total costs associated with serious mental illnesses, such as schizophrenia and bipolar disorders, to be in excess of $300 billion per year. In addition, the care of patients with comorbid medical and behavioral conditions accounts for up to one-half of all health care spending, and patients with comorbid psychiatric disorders, such as depression, and chronic medical disorders, such as heart failure, chronic obstructive pulmonary disease, and diabetes, are less likely than others to adhere to prescribed medication regimens and health advice, such as diet, exercise, and smoking cessation. As a result, such patients carry greatly increased risks for functional impairment, medical complications, and mortality. In 2010, mental and behavioral disorders were estimated to be responsible for 7.4% of the global burden of disease, with unipolar major depressive disorder, anxiety disorders, and drug and alcohol use disorders accounting for 76% of the burden of this category of disorders. The global cost of mental disorders alone was estimated by the World Health Organization at $2.5 trillion in 2010, with a projected increase to over $6 trillion by 2020 (Bashshur et al. 2016).

In summary, it is clear where the majority of patients with significant mental disorders are presenting for treatment. They either are outpatients in primary care settings or have become inpatients in the correctional system. In both settings, treatment of patients with psychiatric disorders is extremely costly and has an added substantial negative impact on the outcomes and costs of patients' other medical conditions that are commonly associated with them. General hospital emergency departments and acute care clinics are acting as overburdened and reluctant intermediaries as they attempt to shuffle patients between these environments in order to avoid becoming the primary treatment sites themselves. These services are victims of the law of unintended consequences associated with the partial implementation of the community mental health care movement and the closing of mental hospitals from 1963 onward.

So if the patients are either in primary care or in the correctional system, where are the psychiatrists? Access to expert mental health care in both primary care and correctional environments can be difficult, because the majority of psychiatrists and therapists work in other settings, with many still in small-group private practices, and many others working for increasingly consolidated large health systems. This situation has to change, or at least the practice of tomorrow's psychiatrists needs to change, to permit adoption of communications technologies with the potential to reach those populations of patients whose clinical needs are the greatest.

How Is Technology Being Leveraged to Address Workforce, Access, and Care Issues in Psychiatry?

Technological changes, be they digital, nano, genomic, or cloud based, or some combination thereof, are one of the most obvious trends currently transforming the U.S. health care market. Not surprisingly, one partial solution to the problem of access to psychiatrists needed in primary care and corrections, as well as in emergency departments, is the expansion of telemedicine programs that are increasingly being used to support patients within those environments. This move expands on the original aim of most telepsychiatry programs, which was largely to serve patients in geographically remote and medically underserved areas. Today's programs are almost all employing real-time, or *synchronous,* telepsychiatry and are essentially providing the same type of psychiatric care traditionally provided in person, just removed at a distance. So, while they do not make care much more efficient (except in saving psychiatrist travel time), they do reduce the problem of access to psychiatrists in many cases.

The problem of lack of access to psychiatric care, however, is not only about the number of psychiatrists available but also about how they work, and much of this book focuses on that. The way that most psychiatrists currently work with patients is inefficient. Psychiatrists, wherever they work, typically see only one patient at a time in traditional office-practice direct-consultation mode, and many patients are "no shows," with studies suggesting overall no-show rates of between 10% and 30%. Although psychiatrists have for many years offered occasional "curbside consultations" (usually consisting of brief telephone conversations about patients seen by referring providers), increasing numbers of psychiatrists are starting to conduct indirect consultations routinely as part of their core work. To do this, they usually collaborate in person with mental health care and primary care teams or use asynchronous technologies such as telephony, e-mail, messaging, and videoconferencing to manage individuals and panels of patients while being paid by the hour rather than by the patient seen. There is evidence that psychiatrists performing indirect consultations spread their skills and knowledge more effectively and are able to manage larger numbers of patients, up to 50% more, while collaborating with other mental health care and primary care professionals. So, the increase in indirect consultations is not only solving the perennial problem of psychiatrist access, but also increasing psychiatrists' efficiency.

The bottom line is that we need both better access to and more efficient use of existing psychiatrist resources in order to address the widening gap between supply and demand in mental health care services. For psychiatrists to change their work practices and increasingly incorporate both direct and indirect technology–enabled consultations is a tall order. For this to happen widely, considerable change management is required. Many psychiatrists will need retraining to enable them to incorporate the necessary range of technologies into their practices to support a move to increased electronic direct and indirect consultations. Furthermore, major changes must occur in the way psychiatrists are paid, with a move away from "fee for service" to time-based or population-based (i.e., capitation) payments, in which value and outcomes are measured and rewarded.

WHAT TECHNOLOGIES ARE BEING USED ROUTINELY IN CURRENT PSYCHIATRIC PRACTICE?

Technologies currently being used in psychiatry can be divided into those that have become a standard part of daily practice—referred to here as *base* technologies—and *emergent* technologies—those that are not yet in widespread use or deployment (Figure 1–1).

This book's major focus will be on base technologies, which consist of the following:

1. *E-mail.* E-mail was initially used solely for administrative purposes in medicine but is increasingly also being used for communication

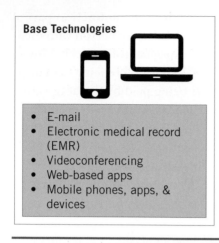

Base Technologies

- E-mail
- Electronic medical record (EMR)
- Videoconferencing
- Web-based apps
- Mobile phones, apps, & devices

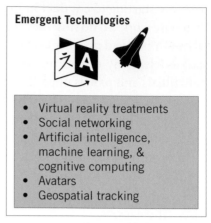

Emergent Technologies

- Virtual reality treatments
- Social networking
- Artificial intelligence, machine learning, & cognitive computing
- Avatars
- Geospatial tracking

FIGURE 1–1.   Technologies used in psychiatric practice.

Source.   Diagram by Steven Chan, M.D., M.B.A. Used with permission. Icons are open source under SIL International's open font license (OFL) 1.1. Font Awesome, by Dave Gandy (http://fontawesome.io).

about patients (between providers) and direct communication with patients. Recent pilots have also looked at structured e-mail behavioral health interventions.

2. *Electronic medical records (EMRs).* With the mandates for meaningful use (i.e., the Centers for Medicare & Medicaid Services financial incentive program to increase EMR use) and the potential gains from better documentation, coordination, and information flow and a decrease in medical errors, there is now widespread adoption of EMRs in American medicine. Psychiatrists working in health systems and organizations were among the first to use EMRs, while those in private practice settings are being coerced and incentivized to adopt this practice as they are drawn into larger systems of care. Nearly 80% of physicians in outpatient practices are now using EMRs (Furukawa et al. 2014). In addition to medical documentation and billing, EMRs hold the potential, through data mining, patient registries, and artificial intelligence, to enhance patient care by supporting real-time population health outcomes and treatment and decision support guidance.

3. *Videoconferencing.* Live interactive videoconferencing has rapidly matured as a field over the past three decades, initially germinating in

large health care systems and more widely diffusing into a broader range of care settings, populations, and clinical activities.

4. *Web-based applications.* Initially used in mental health care for administrative purposes, education, and information retrieval and dissemination, Web-based applications are currently being widely deployed as structured and semistructured interventions.

5. *Mobile devices.* Mobile phones are the ubiquitous mental health care technology of the 21st century. Encompassing the traditional functions of phone systems along with texting and "apps," mobile smartphones also now incorporate and allow untethered use of the other base technologies described here.

Emergent technologies are those technologies that are not in widespread and consistent use in the practice of psychiatry but are being currently piloted or used in limited settings. Examples include virtual reality treatments, social networking, artificial intelligence, avatars, and geospatial tracking. Factors that have favored and promoted widespread use of base technologies include timing (how long they have been in use), wider adoption by the medical community, and wider adoption and use by society with diffusion into psychiatry, as well as mandated adoptions (e.g., EMRs). Although scientific evidence has helped support diffusion of some of the base technologies, the body of supporting scientific evidence is highly variable across these technologies.

CASE EXAMPLE 1: ASSESSMENT FOR ADHD CONDUCTED VIA TELEPSYCHIATRY[1]

A 14-year-old boy, Jacob, and his mother were seen together via videoconferencing from their PCP's office to evaluate Jacob for possible attention-deficit/hyperactivity disorder (ADHD). The patient and mother were each interviewed separately and then interviewed together, with their PCP joining the interview at the end. Jacob was a freshman in high school, and despite excelling in his tribal language, he had been in special education classes since the fourth grade. Neither Jacob nor his mother knew why this was, but the mother wondered whether it was related to a hearing defect diagnosed at birth that had required intensive speech lessons. In the past year, Jacob had frequently been truant and was failing most courses; he stated that he was bored, that "my teachers

---

[1]Case provided by Danielle Alexander, M.D.

teach too slow," and that "it's the same thing over and over." There was considerable conflict at home, and Jacob was now living with his aunt. His mother was unemployed, and his father has been in jail and unavailable for most of his childhood. Jacob said he thought his parents were using drugs, because he "found syringes" in a first-aid kit at home, and he himself had recently started smoking marijuana. On mental status examination, Jacob sat calmly for nearly an hour and answered questions thoughtfully and fully. There was no significant hyperactivity. He was mildly dysphoric, but he brightened later in the interview. A diagnosis of adjustment disorder was made, and Jacob and his mother were told that special education was likely not needed. Formal IQ testing and assessment to evaluate for specific learning disorders such as dyslexia was recommended, as was obtaining a tutor to assist Jacob with reading and writing and enrolling Jacob in summer school to help him catch up with his age group before joining a regular class. At follow-up via the family PCP 1 year later, Jacob had successfully integrated into age-appropriate classes at the local public high school.

❙ KEY CONCEPT

Children and families can be accurately assessed through video-conferencing using the same techniques as are used in office practice.

WHAT ARE THE BROAD SOCIAL, ENVIRONMENTAL, POLITICAL, AND TECHNICAL INFLUENCES AFFECTING TODAY'S PROVIDERS AND PATIENTS?

Psychiatry, medicine, and society are undergoing a radical transformation driven by advances in technology, particularly over the past three decades. The structure and organization of a medical system derives from the society in which it is practiced. Traditional cultures in which healers live in the community where they provide care arguably are the original "patient-centered and holistic" medical systems. Western medicine has been on a trajectory of increasing urbanization, centralization, and industrialization over the course of the past millennia. Peak industrialization of Western medicine was achieved at the end of the 20th century as health care systems became organized along a production plan model adopting quality improvement models from other industries. This transformation coincided with a technology revolution driven by the development and continuing optimization of the microprocessor leading to the personal computer, Internet, and mobile technologies (Shore 2015).

This technology revolution is changing the organization and structure of society at large, and of medicine and psychiatry specifically, in predictable and unpredictable ways. Psychiatry's theoretical models of brain function have adapted the new metaphors of technology, with concepts such as "networking," "processing," and "binary memory storage" shaping current neuroscience research. The administration and practice of psychiatry in all settings has transformed over the past two decades. Unfortunately, the promises made of the enhancements of technology to society and Western medicine have yet to be achieved. Patients and providers have been told, and many expect, that technology will make medicine more efficient, personalized, convenient, connected, and data driven. While technology has propelled medicine toward these laudable goals, it has also contributed to often equally unpredicted issues of increasing inefficiency, depersonalization, inconvenience, disconnection, and amplified misinformation. Take the case of electronic medical records whose promises included increased efficiency of care and improved communication and coordination along with better information management. Unintended real-world consequences of EMRs have included increased workloads for physicians, contributing to burnout, and patients experiencing decreased personalized attention from distracted providers managing EMRs during sessions, as well as information overload for all.

The promise of these technologies has fallen short as we continue to use technology to build on the industrial model of medicine rather than using it to transform structures of care and delivery into information-age medicine. Drs. Yellowlees and Nafiz (2010) captured this well in their article on the future of patient–provider relationships:

> Computers do well what humans do badly and vice versa…. Computers never forget and are excellent at scheduling, reminding, and remembering, but humans are still much, much better at data analysis and decision making…. We need to make sure that we use computers…for what they are best at, and that we do not forget or set aside the honed human skills in pattern recognition and data interpretation that are essential to the diagnostic process and that make psychiatrists such sensitive and broadly trained physicians. (p. 100)

The authors urged that business process redesign be carried out before implementation of technological innovations.

Another impact of the revolution in technology is how the timing of exposure to technology influences individuals and their subsequent experiences with technology in health care. A useful emerging framework is that of *digital natives* and *digital immigrants,* terms coined by Marc Prensky in 2001 (Prensky 2001). *Digital natives* refers to individuals born after the 1990s who have grown up with technology (video games, cell phones, Internet, social networking platforms) as part of their daily lives. *Digital immigrants* refers to individuals born and raised prior to this time period who have been exposed to technology much later over the course of their lives. Figure 1–2 summarizes the differing perspectives of these groups.

Prensky, writing more than a decade and a half ago, predicted that digital natives would become the majority and, compared with digital immigrants, would have the expectation that technology would be present in all aspects of their daily lives. There is evidence that patients' willingness and desire to engage with technologies can be linked to generational attitudes, as found in one study in which younger age was correlated with a greater desire for and acceptance of videoconferencing (Gardner et al. 2015). As the population of digital natives increases, we anticipate both an increasing demand for technology in mental health care and a change in expectations about how and when those technologies will be deployed. For example, digital natives who have grown up with social networking seem to have a more liberal perspective on the sharing of medical information and technologies and fewer concerns about the boundaries of personal privacy.

For patients, providers, and health care systems, the pace of change and adjustment needed to keep up with technologies continues to increase. Predigital modes of diffusion of innovation across systems are unable to keep pace with current changes in society. The old lore that it took 20 years for an innovation in medicine to be created, validated, and then widely adapted to a field was slow then, and this timeline now appears glacial, with some digital innovations diffusing within weeks to months in a consumer marketplace (Morris et al. 2011). Scientific methodologies and systems used to vet, validate, and diffuse medical innovations have not kept up with the pace of the current age. This imbalance presents challenges to the individual mental health care provider when he or she is trying to assess new treatments and treatment modalities, and the difficulty is compounded by the explosion in information, both reliable and unreliable, currently available online. Although the expression is somewhat clichéd, technology has truly become disruptive. Facebook was

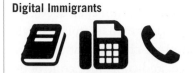

Digital Immigrants	Digital Natives
• Use Internet for information second rather than first • Print out e-mail • Prefer to share computer content in-person • Learn slowly, step by step, one thing at a time	• Enjoy parallel processing & multitasking • Prefer graphics & visuals before text • Thrive on instant gratification & rewards • Work best when networked • Learn quickly, easily processing information presented in a random manner

FIGURE 1–2. Differences between digital immigrants and digital natives.

Source.   Content based on Prensky 2001. Diagram by Steven Chan, M.D., M.B.A. Used with permission. Icons are open source under SIL International's open font license (OFL) 1.1. Font Awesome, by Dave Gandy (http://fontawesomc.io).

founded a little over a decade ago and has already been used in revolutions that have overthrown governments. The rapidity of change for this technology is in contrast to another disruptive technology, the printing press, which also changed the world but took decades to centuries to begin to reach its full impact. New paradigms are needed to vet and exploit emerging technologies as well as to better understand their speed and pace and the impact of their implementation and dissemination.

WHAT TECHNOLOGIES ARE NOW BEING USED ROUTINELY IN PSYCHIATRIC PRACTICE?

The American health care system has seen the simultaneous commodification of health care, calls for more universal health care availability, and, for some, the consideration of health care as a fundamental right within U.S. society. The conceptualization of the patient as "consumer" of health care arose from the managed care of the 1990s. This term implies a different relationship between the patient/consumer and his or her provider(s) of care, with increasing emphasis on consumer needs, demands, and satisfaction with care provided (Buntin et al. 2006). This perspective turns the psychiatrist into a provider of marketplace services or products to consumers (i.e., patients)—a change that creates increased accountability, consumer choice, and consumer control over medical care while at the same time weakening the primary obligation of a "healer" to care for the sick, to a large extent replacing this with a producer's obligation to provide a viable product for the marketplace.

In parallel, the past two decades have witnessed a changing emphasis on the structure of health care funding and organization in the United States. The U.S. health care system has shifted during this time to a greater focus on population-based health care, starting with the rise and expansion of health maintenance organizations (HMOs) in the 1990s and progressing to accountable care organizations (ACOs) in the 2010s. National recognition of the growing burden of health care costs to the U.S. economy and acknowledgment that increased spending on health care does not guarantee a better health care system have triggered an ongoing national debate about health policy and legislation. It is well recognized that national levels of health care spending are high and do not correlate with improved life expectancy outcomes in the United States compared with similar industrialized nations (Figure 1–3).

In 2001 the Institute of Medicine's Committee on Quality of Health Care in America issued one of the decade's most influential reports on the quality of U.S. health care, *Crossing the Quality Chasm: A New Health System for the 21st Century,* calling for a revamping of the U.S. health care system. The report focused on six guiding principles—that health care be *safe, effective, patient-centered, timely, efficient,* and *equitable.* This report introduced the concept of "patient-centered" care to the nation, defining it as "providing care that is respectful of and responsive to individual patient preferences, needs, and values, and ensuring that patient values guide all clinical decisions" (Institute of Medicine 2001, p. 6). Patient-centered care is now often the battle cry and justification for the use of many technologies in medical treatments (Shore 2015).

An equally influential concept introduced in 2007 by the Institute for Healthcare Improvement was the Triple Aim, which has had an enormous impact on discussions involving health care restructuring and reform (Figure 1–4; Institute for Healthcare Improvement 2017). According to this framework, innovations designed to optimize health

Life expectancy in years

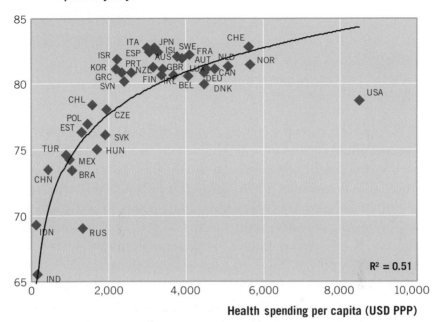

Health spending per capita (USD PPP)

FIGURE 1–3. Life expectancy at birth and health spending per capita, 2011 (or nearest year).

AUS = Australia; AUT = Austria; BEL = Belgium; BRA = Brazil; CAN = Canada; CHE = Switzerland; CHL = Chile; CHN = China; CZE = Czech Republic; DEU = Germany; DNK = Denmark; ESP = Spain; EST = Estonia; FIN = Finland; FRA = France; GBR = United Kingdom; GRC = Greece; HUN = Hungary; IDN = Indonesia; IND = India; IRL = Ireland; ISL = Iceland; ISR = Israel; ITA = Italy; JPN – Japan; KOR = Korea; LUX = Luxembourg; MEX = Mexico; NLD = Netherlands; NOR = Norway; NZL = New Zealand; POL = Poland; PRT = Portugal; RUS = Russian Federation; SVK = Slovak Republic; SVN = Slovenia; SWE = Sweden; TUR = Turkey; USA = United States; USD PPP = U.S. dollar purchasing power parity.

Source. Reprinted from Organisation for Economic Co-operation and Development (OECD): "Life expectancy at birth and health spending per capita, 2011" (Figure 1.1.2, p. 25), in *Health at a Glance 2013: OECD Indicators* (DOI: http://dx.doi.org/10.1787/health_glance-2013-5-en). Paris, OECD Publishing, November 21, 2013. Copyright © 2013, OECD. Used with permission.

care system performance must simultaneously address the following goals:

- Improving the patient experience of care (including quality and satisfaction)
- Improving the health of populations
- Reducing the per capita cost of health care

The Triple Aim brings together concepts of patient experience in the context of population health and cost, moving to a value-based discussion, one that looks at cost as a function of quality (defined as improved individual and population health). It overlays and builds on the concepts put forth in the Institute of Medicine's (2001) report. Recently, a fourth aim—Improving provider experience and satisfaction (resulting in the Quadruple Aim)—has been added to emphasize that the health and perspectives of the provider workforce have a direct impact on how care is provided (Bodenheimer and Sinsky 2014). How achievable these goals are within the structure of the U.S. health care system has yet to be determined, but these goals/markers have become the current guiding principles of health care reform.

The Affordable Care Act of 2010 (ACA), the largest piece of health legislation to date for the 21st century, expanded the debate regarding the extent and appropriate level of government/public funding compared with private funding of care. The Triple Aim movement, along with the ACA, is driving large health care systems, including the Centers for Medicare & Medicaid Services (CMS), to look at different health care payment models, including capitated payments, at-risk models, and shared medical and mental health care payment structures. These have led to the recent introduction of the Medicare Access and CHIP [Children's Health Insurance Program] Reauthorization Act of 2015 (MACRA) as well as merit-based incentive payment systems and a number of alternative payment models by CMS, all of which are novel systems of payment designed to lead to payment for quality and value. These, when aligned with future payment penalties, are intended to change the long-standing disincentives inherent in the fee-for-service system. What these payment changes will do is to encourage efficient medical practice, notably practice supported by the technologies and changed clinical processes discussed in this book. It is evident that if, by

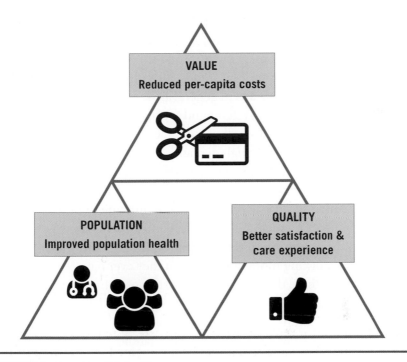

FIGURE 1–4.　The Triple Aim.

Source.　Content based on Triple Aim concept by the Institute for Healthcare Improvement (http://www.ihi.org/Engage/Initiatives/TripleAim/Pages/default.aspx). Diagram and illustrations by Steven Chan, M.D., M.B.A. Used with permission. Icons are open source under SIL International's open font license (OFL) 1.1. Font Awesome, by Dave Gandy (http://fontawesome.io).

using technology, more patients can be treated over a set period of time with better clinical outcomes, everyone gains—patients with good care, providers with professional and financial rewards, and payers with reduced per capita costs across populations. Increasingly, stakeholders in the U.S. health care system are seeing the various payment changes, which have been supported by other federal actions, such as the 2009 Health Information Technology for Economic and Clinical Health (HITECH) Act, that strongly encourage the use of more information technologies in daily clinical practice.

It is interesting how in the past two decades the role of government as an influencer, through the use of federal regulations, has had an increasingly substantial impact on daily mental health care practice. This proliferation of government directives, with their heightened emphasis on value, quality, transparency, and evidence-based practice and their progressively greater focus on population-based preventive care, has become one of the most important trends currently transforming the U.S. health care market. Physicians in general are increasingly becoming employees of large health care systems and organizations, with a decrease in the number of private and small-group practitioners. This trend applies to psychiatrists as well, although demand, workforce needs, and current health care funding still allow psychiatrists to "opt out" of the general health care environment by entering "boutique" practices. However, even psychiatrists in private practice are not immune to the technological penetration of medicine. Both billers and patients increasingly demand the use of technologies in these settings. Mental health care providers are working more in teams than they ever have.

Psychiatrists these days have a wide variety of options, including the ability to choose not only their workforce settings but also their organizational configurations, team approaches, and preferred patient populations. At the same time, because of the national shortage of psychiatrists, compensation has been rising, in some places rapidly, so that in 2016 in California, for example, newly trained psychiatrists straight out of residency are being offered salaries of around $300,000, with start-up bonuses of $100,000 (often described as "golden handcuffs") to help pay off student debt, as well as generous retirement plans.

Medical and psychiatric training has not kept pace with the technological and health care structural changes. A 2014 survey of 183 U.S. residency training programs found that only 21 offered any training and experience in telepsychiatry, and often just as an elective (Hoffman and Kane 2015). Data are not available for other technology training given or offered to trainees. Table 1–1 (adapted from Shore 2015) describes emerging trends in technology and their implications for clinical practice.

CASE EXAMPLE 2: FAMILY THERAPY DELIVERED VIA TELEPSYCHIATRY[2]

April, a 16-year-old girl with anorexia who lived with her family in a rural town (population of 5,000) approximately 3 hours away from the nearest metropolitan area academic health center, began to deteriorate,

---

[2]Case provided by Donald M. Hilty, M.D., and Erica Z. Shoemaker, M.D.

TABLE 1–1. Emerging trends in telepsychiatry and implications for clinical practice

Major trends	Implications/recommendations
Increasing consumer demand for technology in mental health care	Psychiatrists need to be educated on the administrative and clinic issues in technology use.
	Psychiatrists need to be comfortable in deploying technology in clinic care.
Increasingly mobile and flexible technology platforms (e.g., Web-based videoconferencing, mobile access to records)	Will increase flexibility of structuring clinical practice for psychiatrists in terms of provider and patient location. May enrich and diversify practices.
Technology being applied to new models of psychiatric care (e.g., integrated care, store-and-forward telepsychiatry)	Psychiatrists need to keep abreast of new models and seek training and experience providing these.
	Will increase relevance of psychiatry and practice opportunities
Change in reimbursement models for mental health care services	Psychiatrists need to stay up to date on progress in this area, but likely they will see an expansion of clinical service opportunities.

Source. Adapted from Shore 2015.

and her illness became so severe that she required hospitalization. Telepsychiatry enabled the addition of family therapy—an evidence-based intervention for anorexia—to the inpatient care of this young woman. Six weekly 1.5-hour sessions were conducted by a therapist and a child psychiatry fellow, both overseen by a board-certified child and adolescent psychiatrist, with a focus on trust, honesty, and communication. By the end of her hospitalization, April felt emotionally closer to her parents, understood the severity of her eating disorder, and was better able to take charge of her illness. Key dimensions emphasized in her treatment were to refrain from isolating herself and to more openly ask for help. She was discharged with a body mass index (BMI) of 19.5 (up from 17.3) and a hemoglobin value of 12.2 (up from 10.8). The staff of the inpatient unit felt that the family therapy had been key for April's recovery and empowered her.

▌ KEY CONCEPTS

Treatment with family therapy can be successfully conducted via telepsychiatry.

Telemedicine allows efficient use of provider skill sets, enables scarce treatment interventions, and connects health professionals across geographic boundaries.

How Are Doctor–Patient Relationships Changing?

The integration of communications technologies into practice allows psychiatrists to practice routinely in a hybrid manner with patients, seeing individuals both in person and online, depending on the practitioner's and patient's mutual convenience and wishes (Yellowlees et al. 2015). In the future, instead of telemedicine facing its own stigma of being inferior to in-person care and only worth using where access for patients is difficult, telemedicine will increasingly be considered to be a best practice that improves, augments, and replaces traditional in-person practices. There are already some patients who, one could argue, are better seen either online or with the aid of a range of technologies—especially children, and adults who are avoidant, such as those with post-traumatic stress disorder (PTSD), for whom the current standard of practice should be a hybrid model involving both in-person and online care. Use of hybrid care models will become more widespread as we increasingly customize our patient care, moving toward an era of what has been called "precision medicine"—an emerging approach to disease treatment and prevention that takes into account individual variability in genes, environments, and lifestyles for each person—a time when your genetic code is combined with your postal code.

While the in-person relationship will undoubtedly remain the core of medical and psychiatric practice for years to come, it is fascinating how the strengths of the online approach to care can serve to improve the overall doctor–patient relationship. The addition of the online component increases the ability of both doctor and patient to empathize with each other and form a meaningful, trusting therapeutic dyad and interaction through their therapeutic relationship, which is now a hybrid relationship. The addition of interactions via videoconferencing, e-mail, text messaging, and telephony leads to improved access and interactions at times and places that were previously not possible and is exciting and rewarding for both patient and psychiatrist. The incorporation of a "virtual environment" between doctors and patients should increase patients' trust in their providers by enabling them to interact more intimately, how, when, and where they feel safe, while at the same time allowing providers to observe patients more objectively using the extra electronic distance and "virtual space" within the consultations. The clinical use of this "virtual space" is discussed in more detail in Chapter 5 ("Media Communication Skills and the Ethical Doctor–Patient Relationship"). Of course, all of this can potentially be undertaken across languages and cultures as geographic access barriers are dramatically reduced through the use of technology. In this environment, both patients and physicians gain more choice and a more equal power relationship in which either may reserve the right to decide whether to have the next component of the relationship play out in person or online, immediately or in the future.

What will all this mean for the psychiatrist–patient relationship of the future? It is worthwhile taking a brief look at the current process of that relationship using an informatics perspective. As we dissect typical doctor–patient consultations, it is evident that there are three core components: 1) *data collection*—obtaining the history, conducting the physical examination, and gathering information; 2) *data analysis*—formulating a diagnosis from this information; and 3) *project implementation*—creating a treatment plan. What we are doing now, and what will happen in the future as psychiatrists increasingly adopt multiple communications technologies, is breaking up these three components. Other medical specialties, such as pathology and radiology, in which data collection is no longer routinely done by the specialists, have already gone down this path. We are seeing this same process occurring in asynchronous telepsychiatry, examined in detail in Chapter 8 ("Indirect Consultation and Hybrid Care"), in which the physician extender undertakes a recorded interview with the patient, the psychiatrist analyzes that interview, and the PCP subsequently implements the psychiatrist's plan. Similar changes will increasingly occur as we move to more mobile and asynchronous environments and clinical processes that inevitably will accelerate the breakup of the traditional consultation processes as described earlier; this, in turn, will lead to much better prevention, assessment, and treatment opportunities for patients than are available today, with more and more indirect care occurring via many technologies, as described in Chapter 8. Customized hybrid care will be without a doubt tomorrow's gold standard in psychiatric treatment.

We believe that the future psychiatrist–patient relationship in most instances will be a hybrid form of relationship, both in person and online. This relationship will include the core strengths of the traditional in-person medical consultation, which has long been the gold standard for practice, where there is immediacy and trust in the personal interaction, and where use of the relationship, through transference and counter-transference, can lead to healing and support. This traditional, primarily provider-focused relationship will be supplemented and improved by on-line interactions through multiple technological modalities—phone, video, e-mail, messaging, apps, and text. These technologies are more patient focused in that they provide patients with improved convenience and access to their providers, potentially anytime and anywhere, as well as immediacy, and in many cases, more intimacy than can be found in direct in-person consultations, as we discuss in Chapter 5. From the provider's perspective, there are major advantages in the online relationship, through the provider's capacity to use the virtual space within the clinical interaction and ability to be both an intimate participant and an objective observer. For providers, the online component may also be more convenient, allowing them to work from home at preferred times and freeing them from the typical business week practice while also enhancing their safety on occasions with certain patient groups.

The only caveat about moving to this future hybrid relationship style of practice concerns the need for physicians to ensure that appropriate professional boundaries—ethical, physical, technical, and time-related—are maintained. We all are familiar with the disinhibition that can accompany e-mail interactions and how easy it is to regret pressing "send"—or, even worse, "send to all"—when we have written an emotion-charged response to some issue. Spontaneous and unguarded emotional responses can also occur in practice within the doctor–patient relationship, with potentially either positive or negative impacts. Physicians need to think about the sort of practice they wish to have and should write into their policies, available to their patients, some simple "rules" of communication and engagement for all of the technologies that they use to interact directly with patients (we describe possible templates for such guidelines in Chapter 8). Having "rules of engagement" for interactions ensures that both physicians and patients truly understand the expectations regarding this area of the relationship and that the rights of both to privacy are protected (Freeman 2014). The hybrid relationship is certainly beneficial for patients and, with a few qualifications, is also likely to be beneficial for psychiatrists. One thing we are certain about is that the practice of psychiatry, and mental health care more generally, is changing in an exciting way and will be very different in future decades.

HOW WILL CHANGING HYBRID DOCTOR–PATIENT RELATIONSHIPS AFFECT PROVIDERS?

Physicians work best when they themselves are cared for (Thomas et al. 2007), and it is widely acknowledged that maintaining the health of physicians is essential to maintaining high-quality patient care. Physicians are the most essential and most vulnerable group of providers within the health system, and ensuring that they are fit to practice is core to the provision of any form of high-quality health care. While there are relatively few studies of psychiatrists specifically, those studies that have been done do not indicate that as a group they are particularly different from practitioners from most other medical specialties (Yellowlees et al. 2014).

Overall, approximately 15% of physicians during their professional lifetimes will develop a substance abuse and/or mental health–related condition that may potentially impair their ability to practice medicine to the best of their ability. Related concerns are those of physician burnout, depression, neurocognitive impairment, disruptive behavior, and suicide (McLellan et al. 2008).

The demands on a psychiatrist come from both professional and personal venues—hence, the need to focus on work–life balance that is now taught to all physicians at medical school and throughout residency. Admittedly this balance is not necessarily straightforward to implement, and the current often-quoted rates of up to 40% for physician burnout in most major health systems are a continuing indicator of a systemic incapacity to address this need. A recent study of pediatricians evaluated the balance between personal and professional commitments, levels of current burnout in work, and career and life satisfaction (Starmer et al. 2016). Having good health, support from physician colleagues, and adequate resources for patient care were all found to be associated with a lower prevalence of burnout and a higher likelihood of work–life balance and career and life satisfaction. These results give us some leads as to how we can use communication technologies to improve our own mental states, find a satisfactory work–life balance, and avoid burnout.

How Can Clinicians Use Technology to Stay Well and Better Manage Their Practices?

One of the hidden advantages of using technological tools in your practice, and in your life, is that these tools can assist you in keeping well and happy and remaining fit to practice. First, it is important to make sure that these technologies, and the better access that patients have to you as a result, do not interfere adversely with your life (Figure 1–5).

You need to control these communications and have a clear policy that patients understand. The obvious way that interference happens is via the smartphone—through texting, e-mail, or telephony. We all carry smartphones, and the tendency is to be looking at them constantly, checking and responding, so we literally never get away from work, even for a few minutes. You need to decide how much access your patients can have to you and to make sure that they know this. You may grant different levels of access to some patients for various clinical or personal reasons, and if you do this, make sure that you tell the patients and have a specific discussion about when, and how—phone, text, or e-mail—they can access you. Keep your work phone numbers and e-mail addresses separate from your personal ones. In many work settings, patients are given a secure work e-mail address to use or can send messages through a tethered EMR, for instance, and are encouraged to use that ahead of the

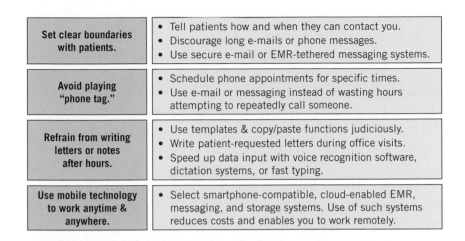

Set clear boundaries with patients.	• Tell patients how and when they can contact you. • Discourage long e-mails or phone messages. • Use secure e-mail or EMR-tethered messaging systems.
Avoid playing "phone tag."	• Schedule phone appointments for specific times. • Use e-mail or messaging instead of wasting hours attempting to repeatedly call someone.
Refrain from writing letters or notes after hours.	• Use templates & copy/paste functions judiciously. • Write patient-requested letters during office visits. • Speed up data input with voice recognition software, dictation systems, or fast typing.
Use mobile technology to work anytime & anywhere.	• Select smartphone-compatible, cloud-enabled EMR, messaging, and storage systems. Use of such systems reduces costs and enables you to work remotely.

FIGURE 1–5. How to use technology to stay sane.

EMR= electronic medical record.
Source. Diagram by Steven Chan, M.D., M.B.A. Used with permission.

phone or text for all nonurgent communications. They are told to expect a response generally within a fixed period of time, say 24–72 hours. It is important to strongly discourage long e-mails or messages and to avoid getting into the habit of writing long letters with patients. If patients want a long discussion, they need to set up a time and consult on the phone, by video, or in person. Urgent communications should go to a phone cover service. When clinicians are away, they must place an "out of office" response on their work e-mails, providing alternative sources for cover, both urgent and nonurgent.

Technologies themselves are simply a communication tool that if leveraged appropriately can enhance relationships, communication, and connections. On the other hand, technologies can also create distance and miscommunication and create barriers in relationships. Psychiatrists need to think through how best to deploy and use technologies within their doctor–patient relationships and must educate their patients regarding expectations for technology use.

The other potentially negative component of these technologies relates to the added countertransference, and potentially transference, that occurs during online interactions (discussed in detail in Chapter 8).

So much for the negative side of technologies—what about the positive effects they can have for clinicians as they practice psychiatry? It all really comes down to clinicians managing their technologies efficiently. There are many benefits that these technologies can bring.

The two biggest reinforcements in life for most of us are time and money. The real advantage of most communications technologies, if we manage them carefully and do not let them manage us, is that we free up a lot of time. This is an important benefit that allows us to avoid burnout and reduces the stresses upon us. We can also make more money if we are prepared, or able, to charge for asynchronous or indirect consultations, as discussed in Chapter 8, especially when working in integrated primary care systems. Yet, time is the real saver as far as preventing stress and burnout is concerned. Let's examine some of the ways that this can occur.

Everyone has played "phone tag"—that awful experience in which it takes several attempts to finally talk to someone. Phone tag can waste hours per week, is hard to control, and is stressful, and the calls may end up being at very inconvenient times. If you insist on patients contacting you by e-mail or messaging, you will hardly ever have to waste time on playing phone tag. If patients need to speak to you on the phone, simply set up phone appointments at specific times as necessary, and tell patients in advance how long you have available. In the future, many of these phone appointments will be done by video and will be chargeable. So, stop playing phone tag.

Most psychiatrists have to write numerous letters about their patients and are used to dictating these after clinic hours several times per week. Use the technologies available to minimize or make such letter-writing sessions a thing of the past. Make sure that you keep good template-driven notes in the patient's electronic medical record and that you complete these at the time of your patient consultation—whether by typing or by dictation. It is vital to avoid getting into the habit of writing your notes after clinic hours or waiting a day or so before you complete them. It will take a lot longer to write notes when the patient is not fresh in your mind, and more importantly, you will forget important issues that you should be mentioning. It is very worthwhile to develop templates for all of the typical consultations that you undertake and to automate your notes as much as possible. Remember that there are two good reasons for keeping high-quality documentation—for yourself and your colleagues, to help you manage your patient to the best of your ability, and for others, to make sure that you are appropriately paid by being able to demonstrate collection of the required data elements. While making good notes in the EMR may not in itself save time, having good EMR documentation will save time and stand you in good stead in the future when you are asked to provide information about patients or to write letters about them. Such requests occur frequently and are the reason that you need to have well-prepared documentation easily accessible and in electronic form. If a patient needs a brief letter, write it in front of him or her during your consultation, using templates and cutting and pasting from your notes, whether you are seeing the patient in person or on video. The patient then can walk out of the room at the end of the consultation with a newly signed letter fresh off the printer, or—if the patient is elsewhere—can receive the letter via fax or secure e-mail attachment after the consultation (assuming that this process does not involve your working after hours). If referring physicians want to see your notes, find out if they can be given access to your EMR system for their own patients if they are not part of your health system, or automatically send them your notes in pdf. The notes should be written in a format that can be easily understood by other doctors, because many notes end up being sent to additional personnel and departments. At the end of the day, if you use your computerized systems and templates properly and have skills (e.g., rapid and accurate touch-typing) or technology (e.g., a good voice-recognition dictation system) that allow you to efficiently enter your notes, you should have no letters to dictate or sign and several extra hours available each week that used to be spent on patient-related administrative tasks. Chapter 7 ("Clinical Documentation in the Era of Electronic Health Records and Information Technology") further elaborates on the details of charting and EMRs.

Finally, the biggest saver of stress is the ability to choose when, where, and how much you work. There is nothing magical about the 40-hour workweek, such that patients must be seen between 8 A.M. and 5 P.M. Monday to Friday. The single most useful component of a hybrid practice is the greater number of choices you have about when and how many hours you work, especially hours that fit in with your lifestyle. If you are a young parent, you can choose to work from home with a babysitter looking after your children in another room. You not only work more conveniently and can check on your children easily, but you don't have to travel to work and to drop off your children, thus saving time and, if you want, opening up more time for practice. If you have a hobby or interest that is best pursued during the traditional work week, you can work at night or on weekends. Your patients will appreciate your being available then, because they can see you without taking time away from their work, reducing the huge hidden cost of patient work absence caused by health care needs. We know that increased flexibility and choice are really important in avoiding burnout, and this is something that younger generations of practitioners in particular are going to take advantage of. Working from home is likely also to be cheaper and more convenient, with no travel costs and no need to rent clinic space and pay for all the other costs of a traditional office practice. You can potentially ultimately live in the place you have always dreamed of, perhaps by the beach, while still running a practice remotely in an area of high need, either full time or on holidays and breaks.

SUMMARY

We are in the midst of a great and challenging transformation from an industrial society to a technology-based society. This change is, in turn, transforming the way we in mental health care practice across the board, from the structure of our practices and the modes of reimbursement to the style of relationships we have with our patients. The speed and visibility of these changes are disruptive and disorienting at the individual and system levels. At the same time, we are lucky to live in a time of incredible medical and scientific advances with seemingly limitless potential, at times constrained only by the narrowness of our vision.

In this chapter, we have discussed several important themes:

- We are in an era of ongoing change and adaptation such as has not been previously experienced, with changes in health care systems, globalization, climate, financing, clinical processes, and social movement across borders and around the world.
- Fortunately, there is an increasing number of tools, technologies, and processes and a better understanding of history that can be employed to support psychiatrists in managing such changes, especially through the use of the core technologies we discuss in this book— video, e-mail, EMRs, and Web-based and mobile tools.
- The changing hybrid doctor–patient relationship will have a significant impact on providers.

- Providers will have to learn to use technologies to maintain their own health and to better manage their practices and professional lives.

Individual psychiatrists need to develop their own processes and perspectives to enable them to take a systematic approach to change the way they practice clinically using technology and communications systems. The way we all work in the future will be different and will have a strong digital underpinning. We are convinced that future generations of psychiatrists will deliver better care in more accountable ways than has been the case in the past and that the processes that future generations use will be different from the ones that are used now. They will be working in a world where video is data, where augmented reality is reality, and where automated, algorithmically driven care pathways will complement clinical experience. We believe that the roles of psychiatrists, in particular, will change as they increasingly take on roles as clinical leaders, teachers, and mentors for teams of providers, both seeing individual patients and managing populations of patients while using mobile, easily accessible systems that are patient centered and flexible.

REFERENCES

Bashshur RL, Shannon GW, Bashshur N, Yellowlees PM: The empirical evidence for telemedicine interventions in mental disorders. Telemed J E Health 22(2):87–113, 2016 26624248

Bodenheimer T, Sinsky C: From triple to quadruple aim: care of the patient requires care of the provider. Ann Fam Med 12(6):573–576, 2014 25384822

Buntin MB, Damberg C, Haviland A, et al: Consumer-directed health care: early evidence about effects on cost and quality. Health Aff (Millwood) 25(6):w516–w530, 2006 17062591

Freeman N: Telemedicine privacy, security considerations for providers. Health IT Security, January 23, 2014. Available at: http://healthitsecurity.com/2014/01/23/telemedicine-privacy-security-considerations-for-providers/. Accessed June 22, 2017.

Furukawa MF, King J, Patel V, et al: Despite substantial progress in EHR adoption, health information exchange and patient engagement remain low in office settings. Health Aff (Millwood) 33(9):1672–1679, 2014 25104827

Gardner MR, Jenkins SM, O'Neil DA, et al: Perceptions of video-based appointments from the patient's home: a patient survey. Telemed J E Health 21(4):281–285, 2015 25166260

Hoffman P, Kane JM: Telepsychiatry education and curriculum development in residency training. Acad Psychiatry 39(1):108–109, 2015 24477901

Insel TR: Assessing the economic costs of serious mental illness. Am J Psychiatry 165(6):663–665, 2008 18519528

Institute for Healthcare Improvement: IHI Triple Aim Initiative: Better Care for Individuals, Better Health for Populations, and Lower Per Capita Costs. Cambridge, MA, IHI, 2017. Available at: http://www.ihi.org/Engage/ Initiatives/TripleAim/Pages/default.aspx. Accessed August 17, 2017.

Institute of Medicine, Committee on Quality of Health Care in America: Crossing the Quality Chasm: A New Health System for the 21st Century. Washington, DC, National Academy Press, 2001. 25057539

Katon WJ: Epidemiology and treatment of depression in patients with chronic medical illness. Dialogues Clin Neurosci 13(1):7–23, 2011 21485743

McLellan AT, Skipper GS, Campbell M, DuPont RL: Five year outcomes in a cohort study of physicians treated for substance use disorders in the United States. BMJ 337(7679):1154–1156, 2008 18984632

Morris ZS, Wooding S, Grant J: The answer is 17 years, what is the question: understanding time lags in translational research. J R Soc Med 104(12):510–520, 2011 22179294

Moyer K: Primary care doctors carrying heavier mental health load. American Medical News, October 25, 2010. Available at: www.amednews.com/article/ 20101025/profession/310259962/2/. Accessed August 29, 2015.

National Council Medical Director Institute: The Psychiatric Shortage: Causes and Solutions, March 28, 2017. Washington, DC, National Council for Behavioral Health, 2017. Available at: https://www.thenationalcouncil.org/wp-content/uploads/2017/03/Psychiatric-Shortage_National-Council-.pdf. Accessed August 22, 2017.

Prensky M: Digital natives, digital immigrants, part 1. On the Horizon 9(5):1–6, 2001. Available at: http://www.marcprensky.com/writing/Prensky%20-%20Digital%20Natives,%20Digital%20Immigrants%20-%20Part1.pdf. Accessed December 30, 2016.

Shore J: The evolution and history of telepsychiatry and its impact on psychiatric care: current implications for psychiatrists and psychiatric organizations. Int Rev Psychiatry 27(6):469–475, 2015 26397182

Starmer J, Magnuson T, Freed GL: Work-life balance, burnout, and satisfaction of early career pediatricians. Pediatrics 137(4): e20153183, 2016 27020792

Thomas MR, Dyrbye LN, Huntington JL, et al: How do distress and well-being relate to medical student empathy? A multicenter study. J Gen Intern Med 22(2):177–183, 2007 17356983

Yellowlees P, Nafiz N: The psychiatrist-patient relationship of the future: anytime, anywhere? Harv Rev Psychiatry 18(2):96–102, 2010 20235774

Yellowlees PM, Campbell MD, Rose JS, et al: Psychiatrists with substance use disorders: positive treatment outcomes from physician health programs. Psychiatr Serv 65(12):1492–1495, 2014 25270988

Yellowlees P, Richard Chan S, Burke Parish M: The hybrid doctor–patient relationship in the age of technology—telepsychiatry consultations and the use of virtual space. Int Rev Psychiatry 27(6):476–489, 2015 26493089

2

Evidence Base for Use of Videoconferencing and Other Technologies in Mental Health Care

Matt Mishkind, Ph.D., SPHR, SHRM-SCP

Maryann Waugh, M.Ed.

Sam Hubley, Ph.D.

The new information age in which we live is an exciting time to be a part of psychiatric care, as advances in telecommunications technologies have made it increasingly possible to provide and receive a range of safe and effective mental health care services that reach beyond traditional clinical settings. As discussed below, delivering health care from a distance is not a new concept; however, technological advances over the past few decades have allowed providers, patients, and systems to reconceptualize human–technology interactions in health care. These interactions have led to the development of a health care discipline commonly known as *telemedicine* or *telehealth.*

This chapter is intended to provide a historical perspective on the development of health care delivered at a distance, including a review of the evidence supporting its effectiveness. The preponderance of the evidence supporting telemedicine for use in mental health care, known as *telemental health care* or *telepsychiatry,* is based on the use of synchronous audio- and visual-telecommunications technologies. Accordingly, these technologies have become synonymous with telemedicine. However, other technologies, such as e-mail, the Internet, and electronic health records (EHRs), are increasingly being used during telemedicine encounters. Much of the discussion concerning efficacy focuses on these synchronous technologies, although we present various technologies throughout the chapter and differentiate between them.

What Is the History of Medicine Delivered at a Distance?

Communicating over distances is not new to the history of humans; people have been using audio signals such as drums and horns and visual signals such as smoke to send messages for thousands of years. It has been suggested that information about the bubonic plague was spread across Europe using heliographs and bonfires, the same modes of communication used to spread information about war and famine (Zundel 1996). We know that many of these early communications were unidirectional or had significant gaps in time between responses. In today's terms, we would label these early communications as *asynchronous*. As human society has evolved, so too have communication formats to include petroglyphs, pictograms, ideograms, and alphabets to the point where today we can have almost instant communication with anyone in the world and even, in the case of astronauts, in space.

The introduction of alphabets allowed humans to communicate more intricate concepts through written language. Letter writing has long been an important part of medical practice, and research shows that it was an important part of medical communication in the 18th century when doctors and patients were geographically separate (Wannell 2007). Letter writing was often used as a way to gain more information about the human side of patients, including their family lives. One of the most notable uses of letter writing for psychiatric care comes from the York Retreat, an asylum where doctors and families used letter writing as a way to stay connected about issues ranging from routine, administrative information to more complex details about care and treatment. Less research into medical letter writing is available for the 19th and 20th centuries, perhaps due to advances in other forms of more synchronous communications during those periods.

The expansion of synchronous (or near synchronous) communications and technologies in the United States began with the first intercity telegraph services between Washington, D.C., and Baltimore in 1844. During the American Civil War, telegraph was used to order medical supplies and even transmit casualty lists (Zundel 1996), suggesting one of the first examples of telemedicine. Alexander Graham Bell patented the telephone in 1876, and long-distance telephone links appeared in the 1880s. The telephone, or what is commonly referred to now as the "Plain Old Telephone Service," or "POTS," has been in use for transmitting medical information since its development, and it remains an important component of our telecommunications infrastructure. We are fortunate now to live in a society where calling a doctor's office for advice, and even making 911 calls in an emergency, are ubiquitous. Many telephone medical advice programs, which are staffed largely by nurses, are designed to provide patients with information, assessments, and recommendations for routine medical problems without requiring a physician office or an emergency department visit. The 911 system, which got its start in 1957 when the National Association of Fire Chiefs recommended the use of a single number for reporting fires, now works from almost any telephone in the United States. It connects people with dispatchers who are trained to assess the nature of an emergency, send medical or other assistance as indicated, and even provide some level of medical instruction.

The telephone has also been used to provide medical monitoring, with one of the oldest telephone-based monitoring programs for pacemaker surveillance being operated by Veterans Affairs Medical Centers in San Francisco and Washington, D.C. Other monitoring systems rely on radio-based technologies to raise an alarm if a patient does not check in on a regular basis or if a patient triggers the alarm following an emergency such as a fall. Additionally, the use of interactive voice response systems allows individuals to initiate telephone calls and respond to recorded questions using a touch-tone keypad. Radio has been around since World War I and was being used to dispatch medical teams by the time of the Korean conflict (Zundel 1996).

The National Aeronautics and Space Administration (NASA) helped pioneer telemedicine applications because it was necessary to monitor astronaut health for the manned space program (Cermack 2006). The problem that NASA needed to solve was how to allow physicians on Earth to continuously monitor the physiological functions of astronauts in space. Ultimately, NASA was able to develop telemetry and telecommunications equipment and systems that allowed physicians to monitor astronauts' heart rate, blood pressure, respiration rate, and temperature during short-term flights. As manned space travel evolved into extended flight times, so also did the development of NASA's telemedicine capacity; as a result, systems that can diagnose and help treat in-flight emergencies are now in place.

The 1950s saw an expansion in the use of televisions, most notably the development of closed-circuit television. One of the first medical uses of television occurred in Nebraska in 1964 (discussed later in the chapter), and in 1967, a television-based telemedicine system was developed that linked the medical station at Boston's Logan Airport with Massachusetts General Hospital. These initial programs were not sustainable because of the technological and administrative maintenance costs. However, they successfully demonstrated that technology could be used to monitor patients and provide medical services from a distance and also that patients and providers were willing to participate in long-distance health care. Nevertheless, it may be argued that it was not until home computing and telecommunications technologies such as the Internet achieved widespread use that telemedicine really started to expand.

In 1965, Gordon Moore, cofounder of Intel Corporation, predicted that computing capacity would double every 18–24 months, while costs would decrease. This prediction has largely held true through today. Similarly, fixed network transfer capacity grows an order of magnitude every 3 years, wireless network transfer capacity every 5–10 years, and mass storage every 3 years. All of this has allowed for advances in both hardware and software such that today's smartphones are more powerful, and obviously smaller, than the computers NASA first used to send humans into space. The advent of digital communications, especially in the 1990s, brought consumer technology to a tipping point where telemedicine became a reality not just for larger systems but also for private practitioners. It seems evident that this advancement is continuing and telecommunications applications are quickly increasing in prevalence, with computers, tablets, smartphones, and other mobile devices being leveraged for virtual in-person interaction.

How Have Regulations Developed to Support and Hinder Telemedicine Expansion?

History provides an interesting look at how telemedicine in general has advanced. However, regulatory history has also proven to be one of the main barriers to the broad expansion of telemedicine. In the United States, this constraint dates back to the signing of the Constitution. The U.S. Constitution provides certain powers to the states, and one of those powers is the regulation of licensure requirements for a wide range of health care professionals (Kramer et al. 2015). State licensing boards focus primarily on protecting the health care services received in their state and have historically viewed the delivery of health care services as occurring where the patient is located. Prior to the expansion of telemedicine services, almost all clinical health care encounters occurred in person, and the issue of delivering care into another state was rarely encountered. However, the expanding delivery of telemedicine services now raises issues about cross-state licensure and how to legally provide care across state lines. The general solution, for now, is for most telemedicine providers to obtain a license in each state where their patients are located.

The federal government has been able to allow some categories of health care providers to provide clinical services in any state, as long as the provider is licensed to practice in one state. This preemption of state licensure requirements is not absolute and typically requires that the provider be delivering care as part of his or her federal duties and that the provider and patient locations be on federal property. While limited, Section 713 of the National Defense Authorization Act for Fiscal Year 2012 amended Title 10, U.S. Code §1094(d) to clarify these licensure requirements. This legislative change provided a precedent for expanding the use of telemedicine through regulatory change.

Solutions have been recommended to ease the regulatory burden of obtaining multiple licenses and to more readily capitalize on the advantages that telemedicine technologies provide to patients seeking accessible, quality health care. A 2015 article provided a history of the Association of State and Provincial Psychology Boards (ASPPB) Principles and Standards for Telepsychology with potential solutions to cross-jurisdictional care provision (Webb and Orwig 2015). The authors noted five possible models put forth by the ASPPB Telepsychology Task Force. Model one argues that telepsychology occurs in cyberspace and therefore requires no jurisdictional authority. Model two is essentially the current model, in which providers are required to have a license in every jurisdiction where they provide care. Model three allows the provider to be licensed in his or her home jurisdiction, with regulatory authority falling where the patient is located. Model four requires a license only in the home jurisdiction, similar to the requirements for many federal providers. Finally, model five expands the fourth model by requiring the provider to be certified to practice telepsychology. This last model was deemed most appropriate for the delivery of telepsychology. Other regulatory bodies, including the Federation of State Medical Boards and the National Council of State Boards of Nursing, are undertaking efforts to address the cross-jurisdictional licensure issue, without consensus on the best approach.

Other regulatory issues, such as malpractice insurance and credentialing and privileging, are also evolving as technology increases opportunities to provide health care from a distance. In the United States, individual states have the authority to regulate malpractice insurance within their borders (similar to licensure). Currently there is no standard for malpractice coverage of telemedicine services, and insurance companies are adjusting their policies to meet current marketplace demands. One of the historical questions related to malpractice is how and when a patient–provider relationship is established, especially given the different modalities used to provide care.

Hospitals have a duty of care to their patients, and ensuring that only those individuals with appropriate credentials are allowed the privilege to provide health care services is one way to fulfill that duty. The credentialing and privileging process traditionally required a health care provider to present documentation and the hospital to verify the documents before granting privileges to practice. This process was often burdensome, if not impossible, for some telemedicine providers because some hospitals required a provider to be physically present to "present" his or her documents. The Centers for Medicare & Medicaid Services (CMS) released new regulations on telemedicine credentialing and privileging in 2011 that allowed for the originating hospital (patient site) to rely on the credentialing and privileging decision of the distant hospital (provider site) if certain conditions were met. The Joint Commission and other accrediting institutions, such as the Accreditation Association for Ambulatory Health Care, have issued similar guidance.

As telemedicine advances, so also does the need for new and modified regulations. One example is for mobile health, often known as *mHealth*. Views as to how best to protect patients who may use apps (applications) continue to evolve. The process of proving that a health care application is effective before it is published lacks full standardization, and as a consequence, consumers (providers and patients) need to evaluate apps before use. Several articles are now available to help guide the development and selection of mobile applications for health care (Boudreaux et al. 2014). Understanding how to provide safe and effective care over distances remains critically important as the speed at which technological innovations occur continues to outpace the speed at which regulations are developed. Examples where progress has been made but standards continue to evolve include Health Insurance Portability and Accountability Act (HIPAA) standards for the use of mobile applications, guidelines when social media and health care collide, and the privacy of storing and sending health care data over public networks. Some of these issues can be managed through hardware and software developments; however, many others will rely on both provider and patient vigilance in following regulations.

The American Telemedicine Association (ATA) was established in 1993 to promote medical care for health professionals and consumers that is delivered via telemedicine. The ATA has done a a a great deal to advance standardization across telemedicine through the development and publication of guidelines. There are currently 18 available guidelines, of which the first—"Home Telemedicine Clinical Guidelines"—was published in 2003 and the most recent—"Practice Guidelines for Telemental Health With Children and Adolescents"—was published in March 2017. Additional guidelines are in development.

Other associations have also released practice guidelines as telemedicine continues to expand. Organizations releasing guidance for telemedicine include the American College of Radiology, the Federation of State Medical Boards, the National Institute of Standards and Technology, and the American Psychological Association, among others.

How Did Telepsychiatry Evolve?

Telepsychiatry—psychiatry-focused telemedicine—originated with institutionally based videoconferencing (Shore 2015). In other words, telepsychiatry has its roots in providing psychiatric care from one institution (e.g., hospital or university) to another using synchronous two-way audio and video connections. While some health care advances originate from individual clinicians, the required infrastructure of early telepsychiatry programs required the resources of large institutions to be effective. Moreover, as we have seen from the general history of the development of telemedicine, even large institutions often did not have the resources to sustain their own programs. Fortunately, telepsychiatry has expanded rapidly over the past two decades concurrently with revolutions in technology and devices such as smartphones and telecommunications, including the Internet, as well as overall changes in the health care landscape focused on improving care and access while reducing costs. While it may seem intuitive to anchor the birth of telepsychiatry within this period, it has been argued that current telepsychiatry programs and devices represent at least the third generation of telemedicine.

The *first generation* of telemedicine dates back to the 1950s, with many citing a project in 1959 as the birth of telepsychiatry (Shore 2015). In that year, clinicians at the University of Nebraska used two-way interactive television to transmit neurological examinations across campus to medical students, which evolved into evaluating the use of interactive television for group therapy consultations. In 1964, a telemedicine link was established with the Norfolk State Hospital (112 miles away) to provide speech therapy, neurological examinations, diagnosis of difficult psychiatric cases, case consultations, research seminars, and education and training. In 1968 a pilot project was established and shown to be successful delivering telepsychiatry services in Boston and New Hampshire. The next 20 years continued the trend of small, yet successful pilot programs demonstrating overall effectiveness.

The *second generation* could be considered to date from 1989, when the Secretary of the U.S. Department of Health and Human Services directed the Health Resources and Services Administration and CMS to fund the MEDNET project (now HealthNet) at Texas Tech University. This project prompted users to demand a greater ability to integrate systems and devices, which gave manufacturers incentives to develop multiapplication systems. Successful first-generation telepsychiatry applications, such as video consultations, were integrated with other applications for specialties such as dermatology. These changes led to broader implementation, as devices could be used for more than one specialty or type of health care delivery. It was during this second generation that the body of telepsychiatry research began to develop and larger, systems-based programs, such as those in the U.S. Department of Veterans Affairs (VA) and the U.S. Department of Defense, began to demonstrate sustainability.

The late 1990s saw an expansion in telecommunications technologies, most notably the Internet. These advances and the ability to take, store, and send ever-advancing digital images have placed us well into the *third generation* of telepsychiatry. Several factors account for the faster pace of innovation in these technologies and their attendant applications: 1) the underlying technologies are multiuse, 2) the broadcast infrastructure is stable, 3) cost effectiveness is more evident, and 4) the markets are much broader than simply health care. For example, many smartphones now come with built-in capability to video chat with any other person in the world with a similar app. This feature was not built specifically for telepsychiatry, but given its familiarity, many are using these features to provide telepsychiatry services to people in a variety of settings. One of the other notable factors with the current generation of telepsychiatry is the collaboration between the public and private sectors. Whereas previous generations saw many programs develop through large, often governmental organizations, the reductions in cost and administrative burdens are opening the doors for a broader segment of providers to enter the discipline.

It is not clear what will constitute the *fourth generation* of telepsychiatry. There are a number of evolving trends, including, as in previous generations, the combining of different technologies. For example, one possible candidate for next-generation telepsychiatry is the use of augmented reality to support health care provision. The first head-to-head research study comparing virtual reality exposure therapy (VRET) with prolonged exposure in the treatment of combat-related posttraumatic stress disorder (PTSD) was recently published (Reger et al. 2016). Although VRET was not as efficacious as prolonged exposure, it was better than no treatment and did produce significant reductions in symptoms, suggesting that augmented reality may be one of the next advances in health care delivery.

HOW DID THE EVIDENCE BASE FOR TELEPSYCHIATRY DEVELOP?

The foundational question regarding telepsychiatry is whether mental health care services delivered via the various telemedicine platforms produce outcomes similar to those of mental health care services delivered in person. As seen in the previous sections, this empirical question has been fundamental to the development and expansion of technology in mental health care as successful pilot projects have started to blossom into longer-term and sustainable programs. The use of two-way audio and visual technologies to treat mental illnesses synchronously has been most widely researched and therefore has the most robust evidence base supporting its efficacy. The evidence base for other technologies (e.g., electronic medical records or text messaging) is smaller but accumulating rapidly as the ubiquity of personal and other technologies continues to grow.

Baer and colleagues conducted a thorough review of the telepsychiatry literature, looking for historical trends through 1996 (Baer et al. 1997). They organized the results into five categories of publications:

1. Reports describing synchronous technologies used for continuing provider medical education
2. Descriptive reports of clinical demonstration pilot projects with no control group or condition
3. Clinical demonstrations with a control condition
4. Studies of tools and assessment psychometric reliability over synchronous telemedicine
5. Cost-effectiveness studies

Baer et al. (1997) found that reports of educational and consultative uses were predominant, with experimental rigor lacking in some studies. Unfortunately, early telemedicine implementations used to treat all medical specialties were limited by pilot funding and were not associated with many outcome publications. As previously noted, NASA was conducting research and development in telemedicine as early as the 1960s, and by the 1980s NASA required its astronauts to receive continuous monitoring of not just physical but also behavioral health and performance, to track physiological indicators of spaceflight- and microgravity-related stress as an uncharted and unknown frontier. These data were collected via devices built into the crew members' space suits and were communicated via satellite to the distal NASA team, but the data appear never to have been aggregated or published and have been rumored to be distributed across multiple NASA sites (Cermack 2006).

A review spanning the years 2003 through 2013 returned 755 telepsychiatry-related articles, indicating a significant recent growth in this arena of research (Hilty et al. 2013). However, the review revealed few studies that documented changes in health- or cost-related outcomes. The authors of this review concluded with recommendations that future research include randomized trials with well-defined comparison conditions and measures of return on investment—as well as research aimed specifically at underresearched diagnoses such as anxiety, substance use, and psychosis (Hilty et al. 2013). A 2015 review more broadly analyzed the state of the evidence for telemental health care, using a range of 2005 through 2015 (Bashshur et al. 2016). Much as in Hilty et al.'s (2013) review, results showed a growing number of studies looking at feasibility, treatment adherence, satisfaction, and even health outcomes and costs. Twenty-three randomized controlled trials (RCTs) met or exceeded a sample size of 150 and had similarly positive findings related to health and quality-of-life outcomes across patient groups. Five cost-related studies, all with adequate sample sizes, yielded results that favored telemental health care over in-person care costs (Bashshur et al. 2016).

In recognition of the remaining need to address persistent research limitations, the ATA convened field experts to recommend consistent and meaningful assessment and outcome measures for telepsychiatry research. While there was strong consensus that measures of provider and patient satisfaction are still important, there was also a clear message that the additional measures of care quality, symptom reduction, and value on investment are needed—and they are needed in conjunction with RCTs with appropriate comparison groups (i.e., in-person care or treatment as usual). There was also a call for further rigorous research of populations with specific diagnostic and cultural characteristics in order to address generalizability limitations (Shore et al. 2014b). It is hoped that building a common lexicon of evaluation and research measures will help unify the fields of telemedicine and telemental health care, improve the ability of researchers and evaluators to obtain grants and other funding for this important work, and assist advocates and policy leaders in making sound policy decisions related to care access, reimbursement, and regulation.

WHAT IS THE EVIDENCE BASE FOR THE INDICATIONS FOR AND CONTRAINDICATIONS TO TELEPSYCHIATRY DELIVERY?

Various approaches exist for assessing whether one type of clinical treatment is similar or inferior to another type of treatment. Telepsychiatry researchers often employ what is known as *noninferiority designs,* in which treatments delivered via telemedicine are compared with treatments delivered in person or with "treatment as usual." This type of design is not intended to show that telepsychiatry is the exact equivalent of in-person care; rather, it aims to demonstrate that telepsychiatry is not inferior to traditional treatment methods. In the following section, we review briefly the data on the feasibility, efficacy, and effectiveness of technology in mental health care and draw comparisons to in-person delivery of mental health care services.

INDICATIONS FOR TELEPSYCHIATRY

A large body of research demonstrates that mental health treatment via real-time audio and video telecommunications technology has clinical outcomes and user satisfaction very similar to those for in-person care for depression, anxiety, PTSD, substance use disorders, panic disorder, and attention-deficit/hyperactivity disorder and additionally has demonstrated utility in supporting care plans for persons with developmental disabilities or dementia (Hilty et al. 2013). One exception to this finding is that for the treatment of depression in primary care settings using collaborative care models, telepsychiatry appears more efficacious than care as usual but less efficacious than in-person services (Hilty et al. 2013).

Most studies suggest that both patients and mental health care professionals endorse telepsychiatry as an acceptable delivery method; however, telepsychiatry is not universally heralded. In contrast to mental health care providers, who report lower satisfaction with telepsychiatry and greater concerns about potential adverse effects of telepsychiatry on the therapeutic alliance, allied health providers and patients (especially parents of child and adolescent patients) report higher satisfaction with telepsychiatry and fewer concerns about potential adverse effects of telepsychiatry on the therapeutic alliance. The few studies that were designed rigorously enough to evaluate telepsychiatry versus in-person care supported the claim that telepsychiatry and in-person care are statistically equivalent in terms of efficacy. All in all, experts generally agree that mental health care services delivered via telepsychiatry are as efficacious as those delivered in person.

Researchers and health care leaders are now shifting attention to best practices for implementing and sustaining telepsychiatry services. One of the most impressive large-scale efforts to implement telepsychiatry has occurred within the VA. The VA conducts several hundred thousand mental health care encounters via telemedicine each year, and the literature is replete with examples of telepsychiatry in the VA and a diverse portfolio of demonstration projects documenting the successful use of telepsychiatry in various settings. Some of the lessons learned from these projects have been distilled into a set of recommendations for assessment and outcome measures for evaluating telepsychiatry implementation initiatives (Shore et al. 2014b). Similarly, the ATA has published practical guidelines for clinical, technical, and administrative issues that offer valuable information for those seeking to establish telepsychiatry practices (see ATA Web site: www.americantelemed.org).

There is a particularly large gap between the need for psychiatric services and the numbers of psychiatric providers available in the health care industry. Telepsychiatry is used to maximize the ability of a relatively small number of psychiatrists to support the needs of a large and dispersed population by leveraging technology to save travel and time. Studies assessing the efficacy of telepsychiatry show that its treatment outcomes are equal to those of in-person psychiatric care across the previously noted diagnoses. And perhaps most critically (because treatment outcomes rely on providing the right treatment for each condition), telepsychiatry has led to improved diagnostic and treatment accuracy. In fact, diagnostic and medication changes are the most frequent outcomes of telepsychiatry encounters (Hilty et al. 2013). Psychiatric access alone is not sufficient for treatment success. Adherence to prescribed medication dosages and regimens is also critical. Text-messaging applications to remind patients to take medications as prescribed have been linked to higher rates of medication adherence in general. Text-messaging interventions aimed at medication adherence have been shown to be effective in patients taking psychotropic medications to manage schizophrenia (DeKoekkoek et al. 2015).

CONTRAINDICATIONS TO TELEPSYCHIATRY

Overall, the bulk of the telemental health care literature points to the conclusion that use of two-way audio and visual technologies to deliver mental health treatment is no less effective than in-person care delivery for a broad range of mental disorders. There are, however, some studies that suggest lower efficacy levels. While one trial demonstrated worse outcomes and higher costs for adult outpatient services delivered via telepsychiatry compared with those delivered in-person (Hilty et al. 2013), most of the research showing lower levels of efficacy has focused on overall satisfaction, and more specifically on frustrations with technology. These frustrations are typically related to instability of broadband connections or poor quality of audio (Hilty et al. 2013). Technological advances are continuing to reduce these concerns. However, it is still important to take all reasonable measures to ensure appropriate broadband or wireless connection when patients and providers are using technology to access and provide mental health treatment.

To further ensure good satisfaction levels, practitioners must remain aware of cultural differences in comfort with and access to technology. Such differences include those related to age-based culture, with literature noting that older patients have increasing need and motivation to access health care but struggle with technology-related anxiety and resistance to change relative to younger patients, who have grown up with technology. While mental health care technology has been used successfully across all age groups and a wide range of cultural groups, it is important to note that because of this technology, providers are more frequently treating patients from unfamiliar backgrounds and cultures. It is important for providers to practice cultural humility and seek opportunities to learn about each individual patient and family's interpretation of mental illness, treatment, and comfort with technology. While these issues are not new to mental health treatment, the technology may create increased risk for culturally based misinterpretations (Shore et al. 2012).

In addition, more research is needed for technology-enabled treatment for psychotic disorders (Hilty et al. 2013). The impact of technology on paranoid ideation requires further attention and may need evaluation on a case-by-case basis. There are additional cautions for the use of Web-based interventions with youth. These asynchronous strategies, which are typically designed for self-guided use with adult patients, are being shown to have efficacy with adolescents, albeit with certain caveats. Based on current research, Web-based programs are a better match than traditional in-person treatment for adolescents with mild mood disorder symptoms, although it has been recommended that such technology-based interventions be used with adult supervision and be used to supplement—rather than replace—in-person treatment (Myers and Comer 2016).

WHAT IS THE EVIDENCE BASE FOR USE OF OTHER TECHNOLOGIES IN MENTAL HEALTH CARE?

Mental health care quality and mental health care access are improved through the use of EHRs, POTS and mobile phones, e-mail, Web-based applications, and both synchronous and asynchronous audio-video connections. Web-based and synchronous technology treatments in particular are well supported by the telemental health care research, as described previously.

TELEPHONE

Phone-specific interventions have documented efficacy. Behavioral health care interventions typically delivered via in-person formats have been successfully conducted distally via telephone, with better symptom reduction in comparison with care as usual. For example, the "Strongest Families" program for families of children with behavioral health symptoms uses a participant handbook, instructional videos, and weekly telephone contacts from a health coach to deliver educational and personalized behavioral training. This intervention was designed to overcome barriers to accessing care by eliminating the need for travel, making appointment times convenient for patients and families, situating telephone interventions in the comfort of families' homes, and allowing flexible make-up times for missed appointments (McGrath et al. 2011). Phone-based solutions such as these allow for distally delivered/supported, individualized care in rural and other settings and in populations of patients who may not have access to synchronous telecommunications equipment or connectivity. Interactive voice response (IVR) technology also makes use of phone contacts to solicit, collect, and facilitate patient–provider interaction—for example, by presenting automated, prerecorded questions or instructions to which patients can respond using the phone keypad or voice recognition. IVR technology is used to reach patients in their own homes and to support care provision for hard-to-reach groups such as the homeless. The privacy afforded by IVR systems appears to facilitate honest and accurate reporting; the automation eliminates interviewer bias and patient stigma, and the verbal nature of the technology-based interaction benefits patients with low literacy skill. Despite these advantages, IVR systems—in common with other forms of technology-enabled care delivery—are not routinely used in mental health care settings, likely because of limitations imposed by regulatory constraints (Strizke and Page 2010).

One well-known example of telephone-based behavioral health care is the Massachusetts Child Psychiatry Access Program (MCPAP), which has revolutionized psychiatric care access and support for Massachusetts youth and primary care providers. MCPAP includes regional consultation teams that include psychiatrists, advanced practice registered nurses, therapists, care coordinators, and administrative support. MCPAP teams provide a telephone consultation within 30 minutes of the primary care physician's (PCP's) request, regardless of a patient's insurance status. More than 95% of pediatric PCPs in Massachusetts are enrolled in MCPAP, and through their participation have reported a 56% improvement in their ability to effectively support their patients' psychiatric needs. As mobile phone technology has advanced to include text, e-mail, Web browsers, and even streaming audio/video applications, smartphones have become ubiquitous handheld and convenient tools used to access more robust Web-based and synchronous telecommunications–based interventions as well as provide a supplemental means of psychiatric consultation and communication.

MOBILE HEALTH

Mobile applications (apps) are developed using software and operating language that is specifically designed for mobile devices, most commonly smartphones and tablets. Sometimes referred to as mHealth, mobile apps are growing exponentially, with a recent review by the World Health Organization reporting that depression apps were the second most common type of health condition mobile app (Martínez-Pérez et al. 2013). Common functions for mental health care mobile applications include targeted educational content, structured mental health assessments, symptom or behavior logs, and context sensing or unobtrusive monitoring. While the value proposition for mobile apps is that they are presumably with patients and available at all times, thus providing real-time support, the research has yet to catch up to the proposition. One of the primary reasons for this lag in research is the rapid proliferation of mobile apps; there are so many to choose from that it is difficult to pick one to evaluate. There have been few good RCTs involving mental health–related mobile apps; however, given the rapidly expanding mobile health marketplace, it is arguable whether evaluations that take several years to complete would be of great use. The current emphasis in the field appears to be education of app developers about best practices to help ensure that key components of apps are evidence based. For example, one study (Morrison et al. 2012) reported that social context and support, messaging contact, and self-management were the most helpful functions in apps, as discussed in Chapter 6 ("Data Collection From Novel Sources"), and it could thus be argued that development that focuses on these components has the greatest potential to enhance overall effectiveness of these tools.

WEB-BASED TREATMENTS

The Internet has been a powerful platform for education and information dissemination for both providers and patients. For providers, it has changed the availability of access to scientific evidence and data, making such information available in real time for clinical use. Patients now use the Internet as part of their treatment process to obtain information before the clinical encounter, to independently manage their own conditions, and to decide whether to seek help; and they use the Internet after the clinical encounter to enhance their understanding of or verify information received during the encounter or even, at times, to obtain second or additional opinions about this information. This behavior has shifted the patient–provider relationship and roles from passive help-seeker to active consumer, necessitating more collaborative relationships and more guidance to patients regarding reliable Internet information. Essentially the provider becomes a "prescriber" of Internet information (McMullan 2006). The Web has also been leveraged as a platform for communication between patients and providers around administrative aspects of treatment in a continuum of scheduling and billing functions to full patient portals.

INTERNET-BASED PSYCHOTHERAPY

Internet-based psychotherapy (IBP)—the use of Web sites to augment care—is still in its infancy. The first published report on IBP appeared in the late 1990s, the same era that witnessed the surge in widespread Internet usage. While many IBP programs involve some level of interaction and guidance from a licensed psychotherapist, and thus are similar to synchronous services, other IBP programs do not involve this component. A systematic review and meta-analysis addressed the critical question, "Does IBP perform similarly to in-person psychotherapy?" (Andersson et al. 2014). The results from this meta-analysis of 13 RCTs evaluating psychotherapies for anxiety disorders, depression, and somatic symptom disorders indicated that differences in effect sizes for therapist-guided IBPs versus in-person psychotherapies were nonsignificant.

There are no published reports of large-scale implementation of IBPs in the United States. Abroad, the United Kingdom has formally included IBPs in its systematic national reform effort titled "Improving Access to Psychological Therapies" (Clark 2011). In this stepped-care model, IBPs are heavily recommended in "Step 2: Low-Intensity Service," which is sandwiched between "Step 1: Primary Care" (i.e., collaborative care model) and "Step 3: Intensity Service" (which includes weekly, one-on-one, in-person, evidence-based psychotherapy) (Clark 2011). Although this program represents the only large-scale, systematic implementation of IBP, there are several IBP programs that are in widespread use.

IBP has received some criticism regarding the modified role of the therapist and potential threats to the therapeutic alliance. In addition to concerns about privacy and security of information stored on the Internet, several studies have demonstrated lower alliance ratings by patients and providers for IBP compared with in-person psychotherapy. However, findings from most studies suggest that patients receiving IBP give high ratings to the therapeutic alliance with the program, the psychotherapist providing guidance, or both (Barack et al. 2008).

Internet-based cognitive-behavioral therapy (ICBT) is another model leveraging mental health care technology to increase access to well-established, evidence-based behavioral health care. ICBT implements the core tenets of conventional cognitive-behavioral therapy (CBT) using Web-based patient access to psychoeducational materials, lessons, and activities; ongoing Web-based patient assessments to monitor progress; and patient–provider messaging primarily using e-mail-like texts instead of real-time communication (Hedman et al. 2012). A large body of RCTs shows that the efficacy of ICBT is well established for depression, panic disorder, and social phobia. ICBT is considered probably efficacious for a large number of additional diagnoses, including generalized anxiety disorder, obsessive-compulsive disorder, severe health anxiety (hypochondriasis), and specific spider phobia, as well as functional disorders. Functional disorders that are conceptualized as having a large mental health component through behavioral and emotional factors, for which there is growing evidence for ICBT treatment's effectiveness, include chronic pain, tinnitus, irritable bowel syndrome, sexual dysfunctions, chronic fatigue, and eating disorders. Across this large body of RCTs, there was diversity in the ICBT model, with both behavioral health specialist–guided and –unguided versions, some with telephonic support, some with individualized e-mail contact, and some with online problem-solving therapy. The overall conclusion was that ICBT generally works for any disorder for which CBT works (Hedman et al. 2012). There are increasing numbers of applications specifically designed for youth—for example, a self-directed CBT gaming intervention for adolescents with depression and an adolescent anxiety app developed to empower youth through exposure and response prevention (Myers and Comer 2016).

E-MAIL

E-mail is a way to electronically send messages over a communications network. It may be argued that e-mail provides for similar interactions as letter writing and thus serves many of the same purposes. However, because of its electronic nature, e-mail allows for communication to occur almost synchronously and therefore is more conducive to intervention therapies. Although there is limited research for e-mail therapies, there is some evidence to support the use of e-mail as a way to augment treatment. For example, one study used a social cognitive theory–based e-mail intervention to influence the physical activity of breast cancer survivors (Hatchett et al. 2013). Results indicated that participants receiving e-mail messages targeting physical activity showed significantly increased self-reports of physical activity. Some evidence suggests that follow-up contact with individuals, typically in letter format, following a suicide attempt can significantly reduce future attempts. A pilot study using both postal mail and e-mail contact modalities showed that 63% of participants preferred to receive e-mail rather than postal mail contacts, suggesting that electronic contacts may better engage participants (Luxton et al. 2012).

ELECTRONIC HEALTH RECORDS

The increasing use of EHRs is also improving the ability of patients and providers to document and share details related to patients' past mental health treatment histories and the efficacy of various medications and therapeutic interventions. Documenting this information allows patients and providers more flexibility in moving forward with ongoing or new treatment plans, regardless of changes in providers and locations. Because mental health care centers were not eligible for the meaningful use incentives of federal funding to support the costly transition to electronic records, EHRs are still developing as a way to improve care across mental health care agencies. For this reason, their impact on mental health care outcomes is not well established in the literature. EHRs are, however, common components of Web-based and telecommunications-based applications. Integrated care is an excellent example of how shared EHRs have been used to support team-based, whole-person care. Within these team-based models, psychiatric providers document each patient encounter directly into the medical record of the originating primary care site. This innovative approach replaces the historic model of separate and difficult-to-share physical and mental health care records and allows a primary care provider to have a comprehensive account of a patient's complex and interacting physical and mental health care needs. The move to EHRs is also patient centered and allows patients to access and track their own medical records, enabling them to be better-educated self-advocates in their own care. EHR use and development are addressed in more detail in Chapter 7 ("Clinical Documentation in the Era of Electronic Health Records and Information Technology").

WHAT ARE SOME OF THE SPECIFIC MODELS AND USE CASES FOR TECHNOLOGY, AND HOW HAVE THESE BEEN APPLIED AND DEVELOPED?

Mental health care technology is being used in increasingly diverse organizations by providers ranging from psychiatrists and behavioral health specialists to primary care and pediatric physicians. While traditional behavioral health settings such as community mental health care centers and inpatient psychiatric centers certainly benefit from technology to increase care access and quality, a variety of community-based, general care, school, military, native, and long-term care organizations are also using technology to improve the mental health of their members. The number of providers and organizations delivering telepsychiatry services is growing, and it would be nearly impossible to provide a comprehensive list. The following section provides a brief overview of the broad range of telepsychiatry service options currently available (see

Chapter 4, "Clinical Settings and Models of Care in Telepsychiatry: Implications for Work Practices and Culturally Informed Treatment," for more detailed discussion of telepsychiatry models).

PRIMARY CARE

Collaborative care models—in which behavioral health specialists are integrated into primary care settings—are particularly promising. These models typically include virtual psychiatric consultation with primary care providers within a care team that includes general and specialist providers as well as care management. Collaborative, primary care–based models increase patient access to mental health care by delivering services within a familiar primary care setting, reduce stigma associated with traditional mental health treatment locations, and increase primary care providers' capacity to manage patients' psychiatric needs and medications within the general practice setting. Over the past decade, there has been a growing body of evidence for technology-enabled and -supported collaborative care models, including specific telepsychiatry-based, integrated care services (Hilty et al. 2013). Patients with chronic behavioral health disorders often have comorbid physical diseases, and integrating care of these comorbid diseases with care of the mental disorders improves outcomes across both health domains. Improvements in health information technology are also supporting the efficacy of collaborative care models. Health information technology includes the methods that allow physical and mental health care providers and patients to store and share health care information for communication and team-based decision making. Critical components of true collaborative care are patient engagement in treatment and patient self-management. Web-based portals are increasingly providing patients with access to educational tools and ongoing assessments for team review, and patient registries are supporting care managers in their efforts to engage and follow up with patients and remind them about appointments and treatment regimens, as well as to conduct systematic reviews of individual and population-level patient outcomes (Bauer et al. 2014).

CHILD AND ADOLESCENT PROVIDERS

Children and adolescents are increasingly able to access technology-enabled mental health care services in familiar, nonclinical settings, including schools and homes (Myers and Comer 2016). School-based health centers are a natural fit to support team-based collaborative care with a telepsychiatry component, and school-based behavioral health professionals are also resources for supervising youth who are using Web-based and possibly self-guided telepsychiatry applications. Child and adolescent care providers are also beginning to leverage synchronous technologies to provide in-home, family-based behavioral health care. Without the assistance of technology, access to such evidence-based treatment is largely restricted to major metropolitan communities. With telepsychiatry applications, however, families with personal hardware and connectivity have participated in virtual treatment for youth with obsessive-compulsive disorder and early conduct disorder (Myers and Comer 2016).

NURSING HOMES

There is some evidence that telepsychiatry has been effective and efficient for psychiatric evaluation and assessment of depressed patients with dementia. Patients referred for virtual psychiatric evaluation for possible cognitive impairment may subsequently receive a diagnosis of Alzheimer's disease, psychiatric illness, or (to a lesser extent) mild cognitive impairment. Improved diagnostic accuracy improves treatment efforts, and patient satisfaction and outcomes for virtual assessment are similar to those for in-person assessment (Hilty et al. 2013). This use of technology allows patients to receive much-needed assessment and care without requiring either provider travel (which is often time-inefficient and cost-prohibitive) or patient travel (which is often impractical because of physical and mental risks).

VETERANS AND MILITARY SERVICE MEMBERS

Mobile health care, or *mHealth,* is a particular focus for mental health care delivery to military service members who have returned to civilian settings. mHealth applications give end users a high degree of anonymity during use, and because users typically have their mobile devices on and nearby most of the time, these apps allow ongoing communication and automated treatment reminders from therapists to patients. The military offers a variety of mHealth applications, including self-guided CBT, guided anger-management therapy, therapist text/e-mail messaging options, and even mobile access to EHRs (Shore et al. 2014a). Some mHealth applications not only provide support to service members but also collect information from these users. Utilizing data such as geographic location (which is already collected by standard mobile technology [e.g., smartphones]) and physiological measures (e.g., heart rate, which can be collected via mobile applications and small peripheral devices), mHealth is also being leveraged by military personnel to improve overall population care quality and to identify ongoing need by location (Shore et al. 2014a).

MINORITY AND UNDERSERVED POPULATIONS

Telepsychiatry historically has been seen as a tool to improve access to care, especially for rural and underserved populations. A number of specific services have demonstrated the ability of telepsychiatry to build programs for ethnic/minority populations that increase both access and quality of care. Examples include programs for Hispanic populations (Hilty et al. 2013) and African American communities as well as longstanding programs for rural Native American veterans (described in a case example in Chapter 9, "Management of Patient Populations") (Shore et al. 2012).

WHAT HAS BEEN THE HISTORY OF AND EVIDENCE BASE FOR PATIENT COMFORT WITH TECHNOLOGY-ENABLED PSYCHIATRIC CARE?

Numerous studies have demonstrated patient satisfaction with telepsychiatry and other technologies. While there are measurable differences in exposure to and comfort with technology related to patient socioeconomic status and culture, patient age has consistently been found to play an important role in patient comfort. As discussed in Chapter 1 ("Psychiatric Practice in the Information Age"), younger patients who are "digital natives" are very comfortable with virtually all applications and models of technology supported in mental health care and in fact may find it wasteful and antiquated to have to travel to access services that can be more conveniently accessed online. In addition, digital natives typically have very minimal concerns about the digital exchange and storage of personal health information (Yellowlees et al. 2015). Older patients, on the other hand, may be less comfortable with digital applications. Those termed "young elderly," patients between 60 and 75 years old, are specifically lagging behind in technology adoption and comfort. Researchers who have studied the use of online and mobile applications for this age group recommend evaluating individual perceptions toward technology, levels of technology anxiety, and resistance to change, as well as perceptions about the advantages to be gained from, and barriers to, technology use. These factors are likely to be influenced not just by patients' prior technology experience but also by the level of support available to help them orient to and practice the technology use, as well as the usability of the technology interface. Applications that are easy to navigate, do not have an overwhelming number of functions, can accommodate potential physical limitations (i.e., eyesight limiting text size options), and offer obvious advantages over in-person care for this older age group are much more likely to be met with acceptance. As was previously noted for adolescent users of online mental health care applications, a hybrid treatment plan that involves both in-person and digital care may be a good way to optimize patient comfort and engagement while still making efficient use of patient and provider time.

Patients who do participate in technology-supported mental health care generally report that they are satisfied with their experiences using technology to support their mental health care. This finding is consistent across a variety of patient age groups, patient ethnicities and cultures, and provider organizations (Hilty et al. 2013). As a general rule, however, it is important to carefully match specific technologies with specific patients who have the technological skills and comfort level to benefit from the care delivered via the technologies. This approach maximizes patient-centeredness, which is a core tenet of care across all delivery modes.

SUMMARY

In this chapter, we began by tracing the development of technology, especially as it relates to health care delivery. Early examples of technology-enabled communication in health care include telegraph messaging in the 1840s, long-distance telephone communication since the 1880s, radio-based monitoring since the early 1900s, emergency (911) and nurse advice lines since the 1950s, and even telemetry and telecommunications used to monitor astronaut physiology during flights in the 1970s.

The advent of closed-circuit television technology in the 1950s was associated with significant advances in distance-based medical services delivery, representing the birth of real-time audio and visual communications and setting the stage for many of today's synchronous telemedicine service delivery systems. This long and varied history shows that telemedicine and telepsychiatry encompass a much longer historical trajectory than is widely recognized and have a strong foundation on which to grow and expand.

The evidence base is substantial, with an exponential growth in telepsychiatry-related studies in the past decade.

- The use and efficacy of telepsychiatry has been documented across a variety of populations receiving service in a variety of settings and using a continuum of technology-enabled service delivery options.
- Audio and visual telecommunications technologies still have the largest literature base, while phone, e-mail, and other mHealth solutions have less platform-specific evidence.
- These platforms are often used as part of overall telesolutions but have received less research attention as stand-alone applications. A larger body of high-quality research is still needed across all technology types, and future research will likely include larger numbers of RCTs with well-defined comparison conditions and measures of return on investment. Future research will likely also address specific populations and technology-enabled interventions for currently underresearched diagnoses.
- Recent advances in technology have led to ubiquitous and affordable technology options. Telepsychiatry, once limited by technology and cost, is now limited primarily by policy and payment regulations.

As evaluations of patient and provider risk, credentialing limitations and needs, and other regulatory issues evolve, a variety of telemedicine and mHealth solutions and guidelines are beginning to appear. Furthermore, as continually rising health care costs intensify demands to maximize provider efficiencies, to deliver care using more efficient venues, and to better engage and retain patients in effective treatment, policies will likely shift to accommodate increased use of technology. Already legislation is expanding to improve the ability of behavioral health care providers to fund technology implementation with new access to meaningful use incentive dollars. It is likely that telemedicine will continue to grow rapidly and that new combinations of technology will lead to ongoing improvements in care access and quality as well as in patient experiences and outcomes.

REFERENCES

Andersson G, Cuijpers P, Carlbring P, et al: Guided Internet-based vs. face-to-face cognitive behavior therapy for psychiatric and somatic disorders: a systematic review and meta-analysis. World Psychiatry 13(3):288–295, 2014 25273302

Baer L, Elford DR, Cukor P: Telepsychiatry at forty: what have we learned? Harv Rev Psychiatry 5(1):7–17, 1997 9385015

Barack A, Hen L, Boniel-Nissim M, Shapira N: A comprehensive review and a meta-analysis of the effectiveness of Internet-based psychotherapeutic interventions. J Technol Hum Serv 26(2–4):109–160, 2008. Available at: http://www.tandfonline.com/doi/abs/10.1080/15228830802094429. Accessed April 5, 2017.

Bashshur RL, Shannon GW, Bashshur N, Yellowlees PM: The empirical evidence for telemedicine interventions in mental disorders. Telemed J E Health 22(2):87–113, 2016 26624248

Bauer AM, Thielke SM, Katon W, et al: Aligning health information technologies with effective service delivery models to improve chronic disease care. Prev Med 66:167–172, 2014 24963895

Boudreaux ED, Waring ME, Hayes RB, et al: Evaluating and selecting mobile health apps: strategies for healthcare providers and healthcare organizations. Transl Behav Med 4(4):363–371, 2014 25584085

Cermack M: Monitoring and telemedicine support in remote environments and in human space flight. Br J Anaesth 97(1):107–114, 2006 16731572

Clark DM: Implementing NICE guidelines for the psychological treatment of depression and anxiety disorders: the IAPT experience. Int Rev Psychiatry 23(4):318–327, 2011 22026487

DeKoekkoek T, Given B, Given CW, et al: mHealth SMS text messaging interventions and to promote medication adherence: an integrative review. J Clin Nurs 24(19–20):2722–2735, 2015 26216256

Hatchett A, Hallam JS, Ford MA: Evaluation of a social cognitive theory-based e-mail intervention designed to influence the physical activity of survivors of breast cancer. Psychooncology 22(4):829–836, 2013 22573338

Hedman E, Ljótsson B, Lindefors N: Cognitive behavior therapy via the Internet: a systematic review of applications, clinical efficacy and cost-effectiveness. Expert Rev Pharmacoecon Outcomes Res 12(6):745–764, 2012 23252357

Hilty DM, Ferrer DC, Parish MB, et al: The effectiveness of telemental health: a 2013 review. Telemed J E Health 19(6):444–454, 2013 23697504

Kramer GM, Kinn JT, Mishkind MC: Legal, regulatory, and risk management issues in the use of technology to deliver mental health care. Cogn Behav Pract 22(3):258–268, 2015. Available at: http://www.sciencedirect.com/science/article/pii/S1077722914000807. Accessed April 5, 2017.

Luxton DD, Kinn JT, June JD, et al: Caring Letters Project: a military suicide-prevention pilot program. Crisis 33(1):5–12, 2012 21940244

Martínez-Pérez B, de la Torre-Díez I, López-Coronado M: Mobile health applications for the most prevalent conditions by the World Health Organization: review and analysis. J Med Internet Res 15(6):e120, 2013 23770578

McGrath PJ, Lingley-Pottie P, Thurston C, et al: Telephone-based mental health interventions for child disruptive behavior or anxiety disorders: randomized trials and overall analysis. J Am Acad Child Adolesc Psychiatry 50(11):1162–1172, 2011 22024004

McMullan M: Patients using the Internet to obtain health information: how this affects the patient-health professional relationship. Patient Educ Couns 63(1–2):24–28, 2006 16406474

Morrison LG, Yardley L, Powell J, et al: What design features are used in effective e-health interventions? A review using techniques from Critical Interpretive Synthesis. Telemed J E Health 18(2):137–144, 2012 22381060

Myers K, Comer JS: The case for telemental health for improving the accessibility and quality of children's mental health services. J Child Adolesc Psychopharmacol 26(3):186–191, 2016 26859537

Reger GM, Koenen-Woods P, Zetocha K, et al: Randomized controlled trial of prolonged exposure using imaginal exposure vs. virtual reality exposure in active duty soldiers with deployment-related posttraumatic stress disorder (PTSD). J Consult Clin Psychol 84(11):946–959, 2016 27606699

Shore J: The evolution and history of telepsychiatry and its impact on psychiatric care: current implications for psychiatrists and psychiatric organizations. Int Rev Psychiatry 27(6):469–475, 2015 26397182

Shore J, Kaufmann LJ, Brooks E, et al: Review of American Indian veteran telemental health. Telemed J E Health 18(2):87–94, 2012 22283396

Shore JH, Aldag M, McVeigh FL, et al: Review of mobile health technology for military mental health. Mil Med 179(8):865–878, 2014a 25102529

Shore JH, Mishkind MC, Bernard J, et al: A lexicon of assessment and outcome measures for telemental health. Telemed J E Health 20(3):282–292, 2014b 24476192

Strizke WG, Page A: Electronic patient monitoring in mental health services, in Health Information Systems: Concepts, Methodologies, Tools, and Applications. Edited by Rodrigues JJPC. Hershey, PA, IGI Global, 2010, pp 871–888

Wannell L: Patients' relatives and psychiatric doctors: letter writing in the York Retreat, 1875–1910. Soc Hist Med 20(2):297–313, 2007 18605330

Webb C, Orwig J: Expanding our reach: telehealth and licensure implications for psychologists. J Clin Psychol Med Settings 22(4):243–250, 2015 26621557

Yellowlees P, Richard Chan S, Burke Parish M: The hybrid doctor–patient relationship in the age of technology—telepsychiatry consultations and the use of virtual space. Int Rev Psychiatry 27(6):476–489, 2015 26493089

Zundel KM: Telemedicine: history, applications, and impact on librarianship. Bull Med Libr Assoc 84(1):71–79, 1996 8938332

3

The Business of Telepsychiatry

How to Set Up a New Practice or Integrate Technology Into an Existing Practice

Edward Kaftarian, M.D.

Robert Lee Caudill, M.D.

Tania Malik, J.D.

Peter Yellowlees, MBBS, M.D.

The global market for telemedicine is expected to be greater than $34 billion by the end of 2020 (Monegain 2015). The drivers of this growing market include an aging population and a growing health economy, the increased prevalence of chronic disease, changes in government regulations, a demand for value and evidence-based care, and a growing acceptance of innovative approaches to deliver care via rapidly evolving technologies. These factors are covered primarily in Chapter 1 ("Psychiatric Practice in the Information Age").

Telepsychiatry, in particular, promises to be one of the largest areas of growth in the telemedicine market. A large segment of mentally ill people live in areas that have inadequate access to mental health care services. Bringing doctors and patients together via technology represents a great business opportunity to either expand a current practice or start an entirely new one. More importantly, it offers a chance to improve countless lives.

In this chapter, we explore some of the most important factors clinicians must consider when launching a telepsychiatry business, whether they are integrating technologies into their current practices or starting afresh with a new business. We begin with a brief review of how communications technologies have evolved. We then discuss how these technologies might further change and mature over time and how they can be integrated into a telepsychiatry practice. This information will help clinicians to choose appropriate technologies according to the nature of the business.

We then provide an overview of how the business rules and regulations of telemedicine should be conceptualized and consider various funding models for practice. Finally, we examine the salient elements of a thoughtful business plan.

WHAT ARE THE BARRIERS TO IMPLEMENTING TELEPSYCHIATRY?

Many studies have examined why clinicians often reject new information systems. Treister, in 1998, proffered 11 reasons, all of which are still relevant today (Table 3–1).

Thankfully, all of these issues can be addressed and overcome. Physicians frequently complain about "change toxicity," which is usually defined as too many workplace changes going on at the same time. This appears to be the most significant barrier to physician adoption of new technology. Nowadays, implementations of electronic medical record (EMR) systems and telemedicine technologies often occur simultaneously, thus multiplying the unsettling effects of rapid change.

When telepsychiatry is being implemented in large systems, it is harmful to exclude physicians from the planning and implementation process. Physicians who feel a sense of ownership of the process will be more likely to embrace change. In single-practice environments, a lack of training and the use of less user-friendly interfaces can be significant obstacles to adopting new technologies.

WHAT PRINCIPLES UNDERLIE SUCCESS IN IMPLEMENTING A TELEPSYCHIATRY PRACTICE?

Many papers have been written describing the business of telemedicine, but relatively few have attempted to describe the underlying principles

TABLE 3–1.   Reasons why physicians fail to accept new information systems

1. Too much change ("change toxicity")

2. Failure to begin with an adequate physician base of support

3. Lack of user-friendly interface

4. Concern regarding the information collected

5. Failure to collect the most important information

6. Physician technophobia

7. Excluding physician involvement from the financial analysis

8. Failure to include marketing to physicians in the implementation plan

9. Inadequate training of physicians to use the system

10. Lack of strong, centralized information systems leadership respected by physicians

11. Lack of control by the organization over physician practices

Source.   Based on Treister 1998.

that lead to the successful development of such businesses. In 2005, Yellowlees described seven such principles that apply well to any form of telepsychiatry (Table 3–2). He later expanded these principles to include factors that may be important to the consumer. For example, consumers may prefer to choose their own online physicians or therapists. Also, telepsychiatry systems and programs ought to be culturally and ethnically appropriate for the patients served (Yellowlees 2008).

The principles listed in Table 3–2 are well served by seeking the input and involvement of providers at every point in the implementation process. Sharing telemedicine system information is regrettably one of the least frequently applied principles. Despite the abundance of telepsychiatry clinical guidelines and outcome studies, there is a scarcity of guidance on how to assemble telepsychiatry programs in a variety of environments. We hope that this book will help address this deficiency in the literature.

TABLE 3–2.   Principles for successful development of telemedicine systems

---

1. Telemedicine applications and sites should be selected pragmatically, rather than philosophically.

2. Clinician drivers and telemedicine users must own the systems.

3. Telemedicine management and support should follow best-practice principles.

4. The technology should be as user-friendly as possible.

5. Telemedicine users must be well trained and well supported, both technically and professionally.

6. Telemedicine applications should be evaluated and sustained in a clinically appropriate and user-friendly manner.

7. Information about the development of telemedicine must be shared.

Source.   Yellowlees 2005.

WHAT FACTORS INFLUENCE PROVIDERS' ACCEPTANCE AND ADOPTION OF TECHNOLOGY?

The most significant barrier to telepsychiatry adoption is providers themselves. Patient satisfaction surveys and empirical evidence demonstrate that patients tend to embrace telepsychiatry as a treatment modality. Providers, on the other hand, may be less likely to see telepsychiatry as a positive development. Providers, particularly those who began practicing before the tech boom of the 1990s, may be more reluctant to depart from the long-established and time-honored tradition of face-to-face clinical encounters. Naturally, the older generations of providers, by virtue of their greater experience and seniority, are typically the health care leaders and decision makers. Therefore, they have a disproportionate power to either support and drive innovation, or stifle it.

The process of technology innovation, diffusion, and implementation has been described by Everett Rogers (2003). This process typically involves a diffusion curve with five well-defined categories of adopters: innovators (typically 2.5% of all technology adopters), early adopters (13.5%), early majority adopters (34%), late majority adopters (34%), and laggards (16%). Rogers's fascinating research in *Diffusion of Innovations* shows that innovators and early adopters are those most likely to make a leap of faith and adopt a new technology or an innovative process. Early majority adopters, by contrast, have to be convinced by evidence that an innovation works well before they will use it.

So how do we apply this theory to the implementation of a telepsychiatry system? One can assign providers to one of the five Rogers categories. It is prudent to choose innovators or early adopters for the pilot phase of the program. These individuals are more likely to embrace the ups and downs of a startup while maintaining a positive, can-do attitude. Once they have succeeded, they can then assist as trainers and educators for the second group of providers: the early and late majority adopters. Those in this second group of providers are likely to accept innovations if they are convinced that the effort is worthwhile and can improve patient care. The key is not to waste much time with the laggards. It is tempting to try to convince the most defensive and disinterested individuals in any group to change. One might hypothesize that if those individuals can be changed and accept the new process, surely all others will follow. However, such efforts are often futile. Laggards, where technology is concerned, tend to consume significant time and energy that could be better spent on the much larger numbers of providers who are early or late majority adopters. One should pay attention to laggards only after the great majority of other providers are involved in using telepsychiatry. At that stage, probably about half of the laggards will finally and reluctantly change and join their colleagues, whereas anecdotal experience suggests that the remaining half will literally either resign or move on to different roles.

A BRIEF HISTORY OF COMMUNICATIONS TECHNOLOGY

The ability to speak and share audio data at a distance has long existed. Although interactive synchronous videoconferencing was widely predicted in science fiction, early attempts at adding a visual dimension to telephones were not widely adopted. Many ambitious attempts to implement clinical care by use of such technology were made before the infrastructure was in place to support sustainable programs, as described in Chapter 2 ("Evidence Base for Use of Videoconferencing and Other Technologies in Mental Health Care").

Early vehicles of videoconferencing came in three basic forms: dedicated video teleconferencing (VTC) units, Internet-based "free" videoconferencing programs, and videocalling features that were packaged with smartphones. Each form had pros and cons regarding its application to the delivery of health care. All remain in use.

Nowadays, cloud-based meeting space is available and can provide a secure videoconferencing platform on a subscription basis. The convenience of cloud-based videoconferencing may prove to be the key to tapping into the direct-to-consumer market, as these programs are typically compatible with most operating systems and most hardware platforms. Historically, telemedicine professionals seeking to acquire gear had to choose from competing technologies using protocols that were often incompatible with each other. Fortunately, most of these protocol skirmishes are becoming historical footnotes.

The earliest units worked with only one protocol or the other. Next came units that supported both. Over time, protocol compatibility has become less of a concern, as cloud-based virtual meeting spaces can be reached by a wide variety of devices that seamlessly integrate the connections.

HOW TECHNOLOGY IMPLEMENTATION HAS EVOLVED

Advancement of the science driving the technology is only one way telemedicine is evolving. People and organizations are picking and choosing the technologies that are most relevant and useful. This form of "natural selection" has eliminated features of technology that did not meaningfully advance clinical care. In addition, application of technologies has changed and evolved in creative ways in order to optimize their efficacy. The following are some examples of areas in which this evolution has occurred (see Chapter 5, "Media Communication Skills and the Ethical Doctor–Patient Relationship," for additional examples).

Use of VTC Units

There has been recent movement away from the use of large, dedicated VTC units toward more portable and flexible arrangements. While the older and larger units were often equipped with features such as pan, tilt, and zoom cameras, such features were rarely necessary, especially at the clinician's end.

Size of Image

Early work in videoconferencing postulated the desirability of a "representational silhouette" whereby both the clinician and the patient appeared on the screen in dimensions roughly equivalent to those that would have been experienced had the meeting taken place in person. Larger monitors were seen as more desirable. The smaller personal computer (PC) displays and tiny images now seen so clearly on tablets and smartphones would have generated skepticism. Nevertheless, as familiarity with videoconferencing grows and the practice of speaking with friends as well as professionals over videoconferencing platforms comes to be seen as commonplace, the artificiality of seeing a reduced size image of a conversational partner increasingly appears to be less of an impediment.

Access to the Medical Record

Easy access to the electronic health care records is a necessity for most medical encounters. It is advantageous to use a technology that can grant access to the medical record while simultaneously providing the videoconferencing platform. VTC units had difficulty accomplishing this dual purpose and would sometimes require additional data drops into an office space designed with only a PC and Voice Over Internet Protocol (VoIP) telephony in mind. A dual-monitor PC with a strategically mounted high-definition universal serial bus (USB) webcam solves this problem by allowing the provider to access the medical record while seeing the patient in real time.

Parallax Angle Issues

Lack of eye contact was often an issue when clinicians took notes on a clipboard held in their hands. It became an even greater challenge when the clinician's attention became directed to a monitor screen for data review and entry while simultaneously attempting to establish eye contact with the patient. Telemedicine setups can either reduce this problem or worsen it, depending on the placement of the camera. Placement of a webcam on a dual-monitor PC system tends to reduce the gaze angle and improve the sense of eye contact between patient and clinician. To simulate eye contact, the camera must be placed as close as possible to the image of the person on the screen. As technology evolves, the camera will likely one day be integrated into the direct center of the screen. Until then, camera placement remains an important determinant of whether participants of a videoconferencing session experience virtual eye contact.

Availability of the Technology

Digital camera resolution has increased, while the physical size of these devices has decreased, and the webcams preinstalled on the lids of laptops and on most tablets now offer high-definition resolution. Many clinicians have come to prefer the dual-monitor solution most easily achieved by using a desktop PC equipped with a high-definition webcam, or sometimes a triple monitor. The falling costs associated with webcams can justify their placement in pretty much every office of a large clinic, which effectively turns every office in the clinic into a potential telepsychiatry treatment origination endpoint.

Role of Compact Technologies

There may a significant role for more compact technologies such as tablets and smartphones in some practices. When portability is a primary objective, tablets prove their worth. A prime example is assertive community treatment (ACT) teams or other settings where case managers, or health care workers with similar functions, are going out into the field. The use of tablets provides access to psychiatric care for homebound or homeless patients who might be otherwise unlikely to attend a scheduled clinic appointment.

There may be a display size that proves to be too small for adequate use in clinical settings, although that size has yet to be empirically derived. Clearly, the market has spoken and has chosen to move in the direction of *ubiquity, simplicity,* and *affordability.* Whether the other end of this continuum—in the form of three-dimensional life-sized images projected at both ends of a link—ever becomes a reality may not depend on economics alone.

A Model for the Near Future

With the advent of cloud-based services, the lines of distinction between the different modalities are becoming blurred. In the near term, the most likely next step from a technology viewpoint is the movement away from proprietary closed systems and toward an environment where cloud-based virtual meeting space is created and secured in a way that is compliant with the Health Insurance Portability and Accountability Act (HIPAA). With this move toward virtual meeting spaces, a variety of devices can be supported, and technical solutions can be closely tailored to particular budgets and needs. Implementation of these virtual meeting spaces requires, along with assurance of HIPAA compliance, close partnering with the organizations setting up these virtual spaces.

HOW TO CHOOSE THE RIGHT TECHNOLOGY

There are several issues to consider when planning the technology scheme for a practice. Of paramount importance is how technologies will integrate with one another to achieve the goals of the practice. Acquisition of the appropriate technology allows the plan to move from concept to reality.

The steady progress of technology has allowed the practice of telemedicine to become widely available and generally affordable. Although the type of technology used has great impact on a clinical program, technology type is not always an easy choice. The latest and greatest available technology is not necessarily the most appropriate choice for every venture. In addition to other factors, the size and scope of the program will determine the type of technology that will best fit the need.

Innovations are constantly being introduced that are added to the plethora of technology options. While new technologies perpetually disrupt the status quo, there is a place for older technologies in the technology ecosystem. For example, while telegraph communications are now rare, Alexander Graham Bell's telephone (albeit in sometimes radically modified forms) is still much in use. Predictions made upon the introduction of each new technology platform often seem to suggest the inevitable disappearance of some precursor, but true "technology category killers" have proven to be rare.

Organizations interested in integrating technology into clinical settings for the purpose of improving patient care face an array of options. These include not only cutting-edge developments but also older computer systems and technologies that are established and proven. Prior to deciding on the technology, the leadership must first assess the needs of the organization. Figure 3–1 depicts a continuum of technologies available for use in clinical settings (Caudill and Shore 2015).

It is essential to choose tools that are effective, yet cost-efficient. Whereas in a perfect world, clinical interactions at a distance would take place with life-sized three-dimensional images of each participant placed in a rich and realistic virtual environment, to date such technologies remain prohibitively expensive for routine clinical encounters.

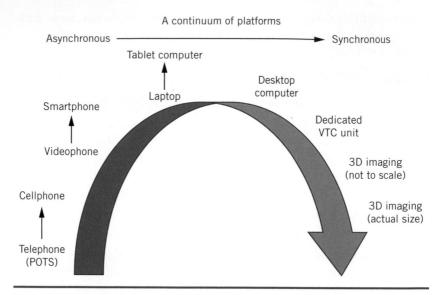

FIGURE 3–1.   A continuum of technologies.

3D=three-dimensional; POTS=plain old telephone service; VTC=video teleconferencing.

Source.   Reprinted from Caudill RL, Shore JH: "Telemedicine, Smart Devices, Social Media, and the Human/Technology Interface," in *Psychiatry,* 4th Edition. Edited by Tasman A, Kay J, Lieberman JA, et al. Chichester, United Kingdom, John Wiley & Sons, 2015, p. 2016. Copyright 2015, John Wiley & Sons Ltd. Used with permission.

CASE EXAMPLE 1: CHOOSING THE BEST AVAILABLE TECHNOLOGIES FOR TODAY AND TOMORROW[1]

Dr. Jones, a private psychiatrist with a thriving practice, knew an opportunity when he saw it. In 2005 new technologies were making it possible to deliver high-quality psychiatric care to geographically isolated communities, but the dedicated VTC units of the time were large, bulky, complicated, and expensive. Still, he had to have one—no, make it two. Dr. Jones had seen the fate of some of these units in other clinic settings, where they wound up gathering dust after the initial enthusiasm wore off, but he had a vision of practicing telemedicine for the long haul. So while the units were expensive, he was in the game, and his telepsychiatry practice launched and blossomed.

   In the meantime, personal computers were getting faster and smaller, and Dr. Jones discovered that he could have a similarly rewarding clini-

---

[1]Case provided by Robert Lee Caudill, M.D.

cal experience working from his PC as he had previously done using the larger dedicated VTC units with which he could connect using the PC-based software. He found, after he became accustomed to working from a dual monitor set up on his PC, that any trade-off in the form of a smaller image size of the patient was offset by the ability to have the patient's EMR simultaneously up and on screen. Dr. Jones knew where the field was headed, though, and by 2014, delivery of telemedicine services directly into the patient's home was where he wanted to be. He bought a cloud-based videoconferencing system that provided the necessary levels of encryptions and privacy, and for the price of a small monthly subscription these services worked well. Dr. Jones still hopes for the day when he can interact with patients in their homes as a three-dimensional holographic image, and he keeps his technological knowledge up to date so that he can be an early adopter of the next generation of such software.

▍ KEY CONCEPTS

Choosing the best available technology is always going to involve aiming at a moving target.

Change is unavoidable and is one of the exciting aspects of working in this area. Flexibility and creativity are rewarded.

RELATIONSHIP BETWEEN TECHNOLOGY AND REIMBURSEMENT

There is robust evidence supporting the clinical use of simple technologies such as the telephone, but unfortunately, payers have been reluctant to reimburse for medical services provided via the telephone. Many other service industries are unencumbered by such arbitrary policies. To illustrate the irrationality of such policies, we can explore the example of the visually impaired physician, who is overrepresented in psychiatry as compared with other medical specialties. Two factors may explain why. First, it may be easier for training programs to provide accommodations for a visually impaired trainee to obtain education in psychiatry than other medical specialties. Second, psychiatry may be a safe landing pad for other types of physicians who are compelled to change their specialties as a result of deteriorating vision (American Foundation for the Blind 2011; Walhof 1985).

Visually impaired psychiatrists have essentially audio-only interactions with patients but have historically been reimbursed for their services only when "seeing" a patient in person and not when speaking with the same patient by telephone. Regardless, it was the advent of videoconferencing that began to break down barriers to reimbursement of care at a distance, and for unclear reasons, payers decided that video was necessary for reimbursement, despite the success of visually impaired psychiatrists using only audio for in-person visits. This decision demonstrates the arbitrariness of some of the decisions payers make regarding reimbursement of medical services and suggests that payers ought to consider reimbursing for services that employ a variety of communication modalities.

Reimbursement for psychiatric consultations has been a continuing problem and is very different state by state. While with mental health parity, and multiple legislative changes in the past decade, it is true that overall reimbursement for telepsychiatry consultations has dramatically improved, it is still essential for psychiatrists who plan to develop a telepsychiatry practice to investigate the reimbursement situation in their own states. The best place to begin this task is the American Telemedicine Association (ATA) Web site, where a continuous running update on reimbursement and policy changes in all 50 states is posted (American Telemedicine Association 2016).

HIPAA AND THE BUSINESS OF TELEMEDICINE

Freely available software allowing for videoconferencing has been commonplace since 2003. The inclusion of reasonable-quality videoconferencing features in smartphones has been routine since 2010. However, for reasons discussed in the following paragraphs, these platforms may not be adequate or appropriate for clinical encounters. It is not so much an issue of technical deficiencies in the software as it is of these systems' relationship to HIPAA compliance.

For the nontechnical, think of the videoconferencing system as being a solid pipe and the clinical data as being fluid that flows through it. The pipe must be solid and unbreakable, with no fluid leaking from it, and the maker of the pipe must not be able to examine the fluid or have any idea what color, type, or viscosity it has. The fluid has to have uninterrupted passage to and from specific points in the pipe and cannot be interfered with in any way. The bottom line is that any technology provider has to be able to guarantee not only that their technology is technically secure and encrypted but also that they themselves are unable to look at any clinical data that passes through their systems, hence keeping all personal health information completely secure and private.

In a telemedicine session, patient and clinician information may be transmitted via video, voice, and text. HIPAA's definition of a business associate relationship specifies that both the clinician and the carrier are responsible for the HIPAA-compliant transmission and storage of this information. Telepsychiatry must be practiced in concert with HIPAA-compliant partners. HIPAA compliance is documented through a Business Associate Agreement (BAA) between the clinician and the technology partner. The security practices and data encryption measures of the technology partner must be contractually spelled out in any BAA. Short message service (SMS), text messaging, e-mail, and most free videoconferencing platforms lack these safeguards, and the companies that provide them have historically been unwilling to enter into BAAs with health care providers and organizations, especially if they have cloud-based systems, where security guarantees can be more difficult to make (HIPAA Journal 2016).

The most-quoted example of a non-HIPAA-compliant videoconferencing system is the free version of Skype, which many clinicians—in blissful ignorance that it is not HIPAA compliant—have used with patients. The main problem with this version of Skype is that it is possible for users to see the usernames of other users. Imagine how you would feel if all of your patients could access your clinic software to see one another's names—a serious HIPAA breach. The commercial enterprise version of Skype does not have this problem and is classified as HIPAA compliant.

Thankfully, increasing numbers of software-based videoconferencing companies are willing to enter into BAAs with clinical enterprises and have worked out technical systems that allow them to provide end-to-end encrypted technologies surrounding a clinical data stream that they cannot access and that therefore remains private and HIPAA compliant.

COMPLEMENTARY TECHNOLOGIES

Certain partnered technologies are often employed when the clinician is practicing telepsychiatry. Prior to the mandate for development of near-universal electronic health care records, electronic prescribing (e-prescribing) technology was a routine part of telepsychiatry. This pairing made sense on many levels. Given that the clinician and the patient are not in the physical presence of each other, sharing a paper prescription was always going to be problematic. Fortunately, good freestanding electronic prescribing software was readily available and was generally reliable in the years prior to widespread implementation of EMRs. One of the first things most EMR systems did (apart from building out the billing features of existing practice management software) was to integrate the prescribing aspects of these freestanding prescribing platforms into the documentation of progress notes for clinical encounters.

Another technology commonly used in association with telepsychiatry is instant messaging in some form. Instant-messaging platforms also have to be HIPAA compliant to allow for communication of protected health information, but it is still not uncommon for some physician groups to use a noncompliant instant-messaging platform, in which case additional training is necessary for all users to allow the application to be used without compromising protected information. An example of such a process would be to refer to "the patient scheduled at 3:15 P.M." rather than disclosing any sort of information that might compromise the identity of the patient. Larger, more integrated health care systems may address this problem by placing their instant-messaging software behind a firewall so that all data in the software are in a HIPAA-compliant environment. On the whole, if you are planning to use a proprietary software package, it is strongly advised that you choose one for which the manufacturer is willing to provide a BAA attesting to its security practices and HIPAA compliance.

In summary, the choice of an appropriate technology solution for a given clinical setting inevitably requires individualization. Different clinics will have different needs. Different patient populations will also vary in their needs. Fortunately, a wide range of options are currently available. The field has reached a point where relatively inexpensive hardware and software solutions are available, and there is less need for expensive consultants to help you choose your technology and train you in its use. Most current off-the-shelf videoconferencing and related technologies are quite adequate for routine telepsychiatry consultations as long as they come with BAAs and are certified as being HIPAA compliant. Looking ahead, the option of meeting in three-dimensional, virtual digital spaces may yet come to pass; for now, however, the basic needs of most clinicians can be met using off-the-shelf and readily available inexpensive technical solutions.

How Can Clinicians Ensure That Their Practices Comply With Regulations Governing Telemedicine?

A common sentiment is that the rules and regulations governing the practice of telemedicine have lagged behind telemedicine practice. Nevertheless, we are beholden to the existing rules and regulations, which are complicated by the myriad jurisdictions that may be relevant to the delivery of services and by variations between states and from federal law.

Fortunately, most of the rules and regulations affecting telemedicine are manageable. The first step in complying with the law is to review the definition of telemedicine in the jurisdiction where the patient is being examined, which is where the provider will be deemed to be practicing medicine. All states include some form of video in their definitions of telemedicine, with some only allowing video to meet the definition, while excluding interactions on the telephone or secure messaging and e-mail.

STANDARDS OF CARE

According to the ATA, telemedicine is a tool to augment, not replace, the clinical judgment and expertise of a health care provider. Unfortunately, some states institute more stringent standards for physicians when using telemedicine and may require an in-person visit in addition to any clinical examination performed via telemedicine (Thomas and Capistrant 2016). For example, as of January 2016, Arkansas requires an in-person visit before most telemedicine encounters, while Georgia and Texas require an in-person follow-up after a telemedicine encounter (Thomas and Capistrant 2016).

WHERE TO LOOK FOR RULES AND REGULATIONS

Since changes in the field of telemedicine are incremental but ever present, the best way for clinicians to ensure that they are practicing within the rules and regulations is to check with the appropriate licensing board in both their own jurisdiction and that of the patient (e.g., board of medicine, pharmacy, nursing). Licensing boards in most states have issued rules, regulations, or position statements on telemedicine. A position statement does not have the force of law but is instrumental in putting the public on notice as to what is the appropriate standard of care for that licensing board.

When you are reviewing the appropriate rules and regulations for telemedicine, keep in mind that many requirements remain the same, regardless of the modality of care delivery. For example, use of telemedicine does not remove the need for maintaining medical records and training staff. The ATA provides regularly updated information that assists individuals engaged in research on the telemedicine requirements for their particular jurisdiction and has published recommendations for practitioners on this topic, such as the various practice guidelines for mental health care services, which are described in detail in Chapter 5.

It is worthwhile to summarize the core regulatory issues that must be addressed to set up a telepsychiatry practice. More details are provided in Chapter 5.

Licensing

Licensing is currently a significant challenge for the field of telemedicine. Unlike a driver's license, a medical license in one state does not automatically grant a physician the authority to practice in another state. The lack of professional licensure portability places limits on the growth and development of telemedicine. Fortunately, the Federation of State Medical Boards has instituted a compact that includes a growing number of states that will recognize one another's licensing standards to enable physicians to gain an expedited license (although not a cheaper license) for out-of-state practice.

The U.S. Department of Veterans Affairs (VA) employs a progressive model whereby physicians need only to be licensed in one state in order to assess and treat patients in VA facilities anywhere in the country. In addition, as of July 2017, there is a legislative proposal to allow veterans to receive telehealth services in their own homes across state lines. Furthermore, state medical boards vary in their dispositions toward the practice of telemedicine, and in general, most medical boards require that physicians be fully licensed in the state in which the patient is physically located. There are, however, some exceptions. For example, Washington, D.C.; Maryland; New York; and Virginia have adopted language that would permit licensure reciprocity from bordering states (Thomas and Capistrant 2016).

State medical boards also vary in their approaches to physician-to-physician consultations. Some states allow physicians with out-of-state medical licenses to consult with in-state physicians on patient care, whereas other states require an in-state medical license to do so. Furthermore, some state medical boards grant conditional telemedicine licenses. This type of limited license typically allows physicians to practice out-of-state via telemedicine but limits or prohibits them from physically practicing within the state. A state-by-state summary of information related to physician licensure is offered in the ATA publication *State Telemedicine Gaps Analysis* (Thomas and Capistrant 2016).

Credentialing

Credentialing is a legally necessary process by which health care organizations ensure that a physician has the requisite training and qualifications to provide appropriate care to patients. Physicians practicing telemedicine, just as in conventional medical practice, must possess the requisite credentials in order to assess and treat patients.

Traditionally, physicians have had to be credentialed separately at each health facility where they wished to work. Although a thorough credentialing process can consume time and resources, it was not historically an overly burdensome process because physicians rarely worked at more than two or three health systems simultaneously. However, the advent of telemedicine gave physicians the ability to serve a multitude of sites remotely. The prospect of credentialing physicians for many different hospitals became a major administrative barrier (Yellowlees 2016).

As a result, the Centers for Medicare & Medicaid Services in 2011 issued new credentialing rules providing a much-needed precedent that benefits the telemedicine industry. The new rules mean that physicians are no longer required to undergo a full credentialing process for every site at which they provide telepsychiatry services. Instead, hospitals may now rely, when granting telemedicine credentials and privileges, on the credentialing and privileging decisions of a distant-site hospital or telemedicine entity with which they have a written agreement that meets Medicare requirements (Centers for Medicare & Medicaid Services 2011). This new method is called *credentialing by proxy*.

The rule allowing credentialing by proxy should have substantially reduced the burden and duplicative nature of the traditional privileging process for physicians intending to provide telemedicine services to multiple sites. Unfortunately, many hospitals and credentialing departments are still not aware of credentialing by proxy (Yellowlees 2016).

Informed Consent

Most states do not require formal informed consent for treatment via telemedicine, although some (e.g., California) require verbal consent. A handful of states do require a formal consent process, however, and Colorado, Delaware, and Washington, D.C., require written acknowledgment of consent from the patient before a telemedicine encounter can begin.

Prescribing

Prescribing noncontrolled substances is straightforward and is routinely done in telepsychiatry practice. Prescribing for patients seen via telepsychiatry has a number of similarities to and differences from prescribing for patients seen in person. Obviously, before prescribing any medication, the clinician must know patients' relevant vital signs, weight, and laboratory test results. These can be obtained from multiple sources, including from patients themselves and from the clinician's own or other EMR systems, depending on the setting of the consultation and the prescribing situation. It is also necessary to be licensed in the state in which the patient resides and to have a local Drug Enforcement Agency (DEA) number relevant for that state and practice if scheduled drugs are being prescribed.

The main issue in prescribing is whether a medication is defined as a controlled substance, and most medications used by psychiatrists are not so defined. For all noncontrolled substances, such as antidepressants, antipsychotics, and mood stabilizers, prescribing remotely can occur in exactly the same way as prescribing in person. Here it is allowable to use the phone, fax, or mail for prescriptions, which can be sent direct to a pharmacy—or, more frequently, to use e-prescribing, typically via an embedded EMR system. For noncontrolled medications, state laws apply and should be consulted. While many states require that a physician perform an adequate physical examination before prescribing any medication for a patient, some states explicitly exempt psychiatry from this requirement. North Carolina's position statement is similar to position statements in other states and provides that physicians must conduct "an appropriate evaluation prior to diagnosing and/or treating the patient. This evaluation need not be in-person if the licensee employs technology sufficient to accurately diagnose and treat the patient in conformity with the applicable standard of care" (North Carolina Medical Board 2014).

In essence, a physician can write a prescription for a noncontrolled substance if the standard of care is met.

Clinicians who intend to prescribe controlled substances via telemedicine must proceed cautiously, because controlled substances are a different matter. If in doubt about prescribing controlled substances via telepsychiatry, just do not do it. Prescription of controlled substances is overseen by the U.S. Food and Drug Administration (FDA) and the DEA and falls under the jurisdiction of the Comprehensive Drug Abuse Prevention and Control Act of 1970, which has since been amended several times (U.S. Department of Justice, Drug Enforcement Administration, Diversion Control Division 2017). Drugs are "scheduled" under federal law according to their effects, medical uses, and potential for abuse. Of relevance to psychiatry, stimulants (amphetamines) are categorized as Schedule II; ketamine, buprenorphine, and dronabinol as Schedule III; and benzodiazepines as Schedule IV.

Whereas the federal regulations regarding prescribing controlled substances are reasonably consistent, state regulations show a high degree of variability, with some states requiring duplicate and paper copies of prescriptions; others allowing e-prescribing, although often with extra identity checks on providers; and still others insisting on use of prescription drug monitoring programs. Prescribers must check their state regulations or the regulations of the states in which their patients reside or are being treated.

Difficulties with prescribing scheduled drugs are substantial when doing so across state lines, unfortunately, and have been made complicated by an unexpected consequence of the Ryan Haight Online Pharmacy Consumer Protection Act of 2008. This act was created following the overdose death of Ryan Haight, an 18-year-old who was obtaining narcotics from an unregulated online pharmacy. The act was created to regulate online Internet prescriptions and is enforced by the DEA. The act requires that any practitioner planning to issue a prescription for a controlled substance must conduct "at least one in-person medical evaluation of the patient" before doing so, although it does allow exceptions under special circumstances (e.g., covering prescribers working within a federal health system, such as the VA or the Indian Health Service).

In general, physicians can prescribe under the act if they conduct at least one in-person medical evaluation of the patient before remotely prescribing any controlled substances. *In-person medical evaluation* means a medical evaluation that is conducted with the patient in the physical presence of the practitioner, without regard to whether portions of the evaluation are conducted by other health professionals.

Providers who want to prescribe under the telemedicine exemption of the act must file for a special registration; however, the special registration process has not been clearly defined by the DEA. Therefore, it is prudent to consult with a telemedicine attorney prior to prescribing controlled substances via telemedicine. Recently, the DEA has been exploring implementation of a provision of the act for a special registration process for some newer appropriate clinical practices and service arrangements, such as regarding the prescription of stimulant medications for adolescents with attention-deficit/hyperactivity disorder in rural locations, but this provision is not yet finalized.

Malpractice

Nowadays, most insurers cover telemedicine, but they often ask for a description of the proposed services, so you should contact your malpractice provider and tell them in writing that you are commencing to see patients using telepsychiatry. Clinicians should also consider cyber liability insurance or check that their telemedicine policies include cyber liability coverage to ensure that they are covered in the event of a data breach, whether accidental or through malice (e.g., hacking). Some policies will explicitly require that the clinician's technology platform demonstrates compliance with HIPAA.

Safety Issues

Throughout the course of the clinician–patient relationship, mental health care providers should always be cognizant of patient safety issues. The assessment and management of risks associated with suicide, violence, and health conditions should always be at the forefront of any clinician's mind, regardless of whether the sessions are conducted via telemedicine or in person. However, telemedicine presents unique safety risks that must be carefully managed, and these are fully covered in Chapter 5. Safety plans and policies need to be in place for use wherever patients are being seen—in clinics, hospitals, or their own homes. The key to all of these plans is being able to rapidly communicate by phone, text, or video with someone who can assist patients in distress and take them to a place of safety. This means 1) having phone numbers of people (family, other providers, support people, and friends), including local police, who are physically close to the patient and can help him or her if necessary; and 2) knowing the exact location of the patient during your clinical encounter with him or her, as well as the locations of the nearest places of safety, such as local emergency departments.

Rules for Communication

It is essential that providers, patients, members of the treatment team, and hospital/clinic personnel all have a common understanding of how care using telepsychiatry will be conducted and coordinated and how and when the parties involved will communicate with each other. For example, texts and e-mails might be acceptable to coordinate schedules and arrange prescriptions, but they are not suitable for clinical discussions or urgent situations; for such communications, phone or video is best. Patients should be educated on calling 911 or going to their local emergency department in the event of a medical or psychiatric emergency, and the telepsychiatrist should have the full phone number of the patient's local police, because 911 calls always only go locally to where the 911 call has come from. In summary, the ground rules for communication should attempt to close gaps in communication, avoid loose ends, and ensure that patients receive the care they need within an appropriate time frame based on the level of urgency.

CASE EXAMPLE 2: STARTING A TELEMENTAL HEALTH CARE BUSINESS[2]

After the Iraq and Afghanistan Wars started, the country was not well prepared to treat soldiers who were returning with posttraumatic stress disorder. The problem for returning soldiers was that the perceived stigma was high, the need was great, and the access was limited. The perfect recipe for disaster—or a solution.

An entrepreneur thought she had the solution, which was to provide therapy via secure e-mail, telephone, and video. After writing a business plan, she sought funding through government channels but was not able to obtain it. Her efforts to secure funding did, however, lead her to an accrediting organization where the counselors volunteered their time to treat soldiers. On a shoestring budget, the first technology platform was developed and a pilot was launched.

---

[2]Case provided by Tania Malik, J.D.

Using the lessons learned from the pilot, the business plan was revised, and a road show began to attempt to secure outside funding from angel investors.[3] Several accredited investors form an angel group and invest as one group in the startup.) Once the funding was received, a new technology platform was built, a national network of counselors was developed, and implementation began. As important moves happened in the industry and it looked like this small company might get crushed, the entrepreneur did what any good entrepreneur would do and went to Starbucks for some caffeine-stimulated cogitation. It became clear that it was time to seek strategic partners or a buyer. Again, the road show began, but with a different set of investors and a different goal. Once that goal was reached, the company was finally able to address market needs, but this time with a seasoned board, talented management, and secure funding.

▌ KEY CONCEPT

Entrepreneurs can build sustainable companies if those companies solve real problems, have dependable funding, and are able to address market needs.

WHAT COMMERCIALIZATION AND FUNDING MODELS ARE AVAILABLE FOR LAUNCHING A TELEPSYCHIATRY PRACTICE?

REIMBURSEMENT

There are many different ways of funding a telepsychiatry practice. Reimbursement is a crucial issue, of course, because without it your telepsychiatry practice is unlikely to be successful. Most clinicians who are integrating telepsychiatry into their office practices start out by charging conventional consultation fees based on Current Procedural Terminology (CPT) codes, with an added "GT modifier" (which indicates a telemedicine visit), or based on relative value units (RVUs) paid as if the patients were being seen in an in-person clinic, as is possible in most states.

Inevitably, payments vary across states and between insurers, private and federal. It is imperative that clinicians preparing to launch a telepsychiatry practice carefully analyze the potential reimbursement options associated with the various associated payers. The ATA Business & Finance Special Interest Group (www.americantelemed.org/membership/

---

[3] "Angel investors" invest in startups to give seed funding and receive equity or convertible debt in return. Usually the amount invested is small ($50,000–$250,000).

member-groups) offers a dynamic and engaging forum for discussion of these issues.

Telepsychiatrists and commercial telepsychiatry companies have, in recent years, moved toward charging on an hourly basis for their services. These sorts of contracts are particularly suitable for telepsychiatry consultations conducted in emergency departments and inpatient units. In these settings, it is often difficult for the provider entity to bill patients directly. It is more feasible for the hospital to bill the patient and to pay the provider directly based on an established rate. This fee-for-service model can also be useful for provision of services to geographically distant places where patients may be uninsured or underinsured.

GRANTS

Traditionally, many telepsychiatry services have been set up from academic centers using grants obtained from foundations or federal or state funds. There are a number of ways to obtain grants to help fund the development of telemedicine programs or projects, and this source of funding can greatly enhance the sustainability of a telepsychiatry program. Historically, many of the grant programs have focused on promoting the development of telehealth care in rural areas, but in recent years, the scope of grant programs has expanded to include other frontier or underserved communities, including those located in urban areas.

Many grant organizations are looking for innovative ways of utilizing telepsychiatry to improve access to health care. Grant money is often used to obtain telemedicine hardware and software, to set up the telemedicine network infrastructure, and to obtain technical assistance and instruction for using telemedicine technologies.

There are multiple sources for grants that may fund your telemedicine project, ranging from public agencies to private organizations. Telemedicine grants ranging in amount from several thousand to several million dollars are available. A wise strategy is to consult with local, state, and federal government agencies in areas that are struggling to meet the health care needs of the respective population. It is prudent to be familiar with the needs of the populations the grant agency serves in order to design a relevant proposal.

The grant organization will likely have detailed information on its Web site regarding grant opportunities. In addition, agencies often have listservs that post bulletins and updates on grant opportunities. Such listings help potential applicants to identify appropriate opportunities early so that they can meet crucial grant deadlines.

The grant review process usually involves a panel of reviewers. The use of multiple reviewers helps to reduce personal biases and achieve a fairer review process. However, many of these reviewers do not have significant experience or knowledge about telemedicine. Therefore, your grant proposal must be written in a way that is easily understood by all reviewers, regardless of the degree of their exposure to telemedicine.

Reviewers often need to contend with hundreds of applications, and their time is often short. A high percentage of submissions are eliminated during the first round of reviews—mostly because they do not meet the basic parameters established by the granter. Proposals that are confusing or unclear will not survive this first round. A proposal that specifically includes the goals of the grant program has a higher rate of acceptance. It is prudent to ensure that your proposal lines up, point by point, with as many of the grant criteria as possible. Explicitly addressing each criterion makes it easy for reviewers to give an application a favorable score and improves the applicant's chances of obtaining funding.

OTHER NON-VENTURE FUNDING SOURCES

The following potential funding sources are all currently being used in differing settings, and many can be combined with conventional clinical consultation billing and successful grantsmanship.

Consulting

Many providers do some part-time consulting in telepsychiatry. Such consulting is an excellent way of being paid to help colleagues set up their practices, especially for practitioners with a broad informatics and policy background. Many start-up companies require physician or other provider consultants who are knowledgeable about clinical, technical, and administrative issues. These companies often establish advisory boards or hire consultants on a paid or unpaid (share option) basis.

Membership-Based Fees

Membership-based fees, perhaps with a "per-member per-month" recurrent fee as well as a reduced visit fee, is an approach that has become increasingly popular with "concierge" practices, where fees are charged on an annual or monthly basis and frequently include telemedicine services to the home. A number of commercial companies also charge large employers on this basis—a small monthly charge for each member can soon add up when there are many thousands of members.

Payment Based on Measured Quality Outcomes for Patient Groups

The federal government and many insurers and payers are currently and rapidly introducing reimbursement models in which payment is based on measured quality outcomes for groups of patients. It is envisioned that these payment plans will replace many CPT code–driven payment plans with capitated systems of care, wherein clinicians are hired to provide, for instance, all psychiatric services for a certain population of patients, perhaps many thousands of individuals. This Medicare payment reform typically goes by the overall acronym of MACRA (Medicare Access and CHIP [Children's Health Insurance Program] Reauthorization Act of 2015), with two other acronyms, APMs (alternative payment models) and the MIPS (Merit-based Incentive Payment System) being the actual payment systems that physicians will have to choose between. Physicians in private practice will need to understand these payment models, and it is likely that a lot of telepsychiatry practices will use them, because the practice of telepsychiatry in this new outcome- and measurement-based capitated environment is likely to expand substantially, especially in integrated and collaborative primary care environments.

Shared Savings From Avoided Costs or Reduced Utilization Rates

This model of payment has been implemented in several places already and essentially allows telemedicine providers to share in any savings that result from reductions in inpatient and emergency department visits in the patients whom they treat. Such programs are particularly attractive to hospitals that have emergency departments overcrowded by psychiatrically ill patients, as well as to employers and those running employee assistance programs.

Payments for Technology Innovations

"White-label partnerships" with telemedicine companies that have created specialist software, technical plug-ins, or components that can be added to larger software systems are always popular. These represent a financial opportunity for providers who enjoy coding and developing their own technologies. The same is true for those who are able to create tools or apps for monitoring chronic diseases, especially if the charges for these can be bundled in a capitated payment for a group of patients.

INVESTMENT OR VENTURE FUNDING

Another avenue of funding is through investors, for clinicians who are feeling entrepreneurial. Keep in mind that there are already many privately developed telepsychiatry companies in existence. Like most companies, the majority fail early or are bought out much more rapidly than their original founders had planned. At the earliest stage of an enterprise, investment sources will typically be friends, family, or angel investors. Angel investors can fund the first dollar of a venture but usually invest only small amounts (e.g., $50,000). Angel funds are available in almost every city in the country. Angel networks represent individual angel funds and should be one of the first potential sources of investment capital approached by entrepreneurs.

Entrepreneurs will need to take on debt or offer equity to investors. Offering equity is the most common practice, but the former should be considered. With debt, the entrepreneur does not give up any equity but does have to service the debt. In either situation, the value of the company will be a pivotal point. Often an owner's valuation of his or her company will be higher than the investor's assessment. Therefore, the owner and the investor will need to negotiate a mutually agreeable valuation. Most negotiations fail when entrepreneurs are not realistic about their valuations or cannot objectively justify them. After the entrepreneur raises the first dollar for the project and produces outcomes, the next round of funding will be easier to obtain. In some cases, additional rounds may not be necessary if the revenue exceeds expenses.

After angel investment or if the business is somewhat mature, the next avenue of funding is usually venture capitalists, especially if grants are not available. In comparison with angel investors, venture capitalists invest more money, take more equity, and expect greater results. The benefit of venture capitalists is that they usually also bring experience and connections that can assist the business. It is incumbent on the business owner to engage in the community and to network to determine which venture capitalist company will be the most interested, as venture capitalists specialize in specific areas of investment (e.g., financial services, health care).

For both angel investment and venture capitalist investment, a solid business plan is needed to begin the process of receiving outside funding. Most investment Web sites allow the entrepreneur to submit the executive summary online. Although that is an option, a better approach would be for the entrepreneur to find, through networking, a member of the investment firm who believes in the company and will internally champion its ideas and goals. This inside champion can more easily introduce the entrepreneur to the investment firm and assist in the process.

If, after reviewing the executive summary of the business plan, the investment firm wants to continue the process, the next step is a presentation by the entrepreneur to specific members of the investment firm (perhaps the investment committee). Anyone who has seen the television show *Shark Tank* will have an idea of what occurs in this presentation. A savvy entrepreneur will anticipate questions and will prepare his or her answers accordingly. It is mandatory that the entrepreneur be able to justify the valuation of the company, demonstrate a firm grasp of the financials, and articulate why the business is better than or different from others that currently exist.

If the investment firm decides it is interested in proceeding to the next step of the investment process, a period of due diligence begins. During this phase, the entrepreneur will provide additional information for the investment firm as it continues to deliberate on whether to invest. When the due diligence period is complete, the parties will begin to negotiate a "term sheet" that identifies the terms of the investment agreement. A term sheet is legally binding; therefore, it is prudent to consult with specialized legal counsel prior to signing the term sheet. After the term sheet is signed, additional information will be exchanged as lawyers work to close the deal. Once the term sheet is signed for venture capitalist firms, the entrepreneur will not be permitted to shop his or her idea to other organizations but is expected to keep running the business.

If the deal is closed, the entrepreneur will receive the capital investment and will solidify his or her role with the company. New members will join the board, and a new level of accountability will likely be established. With a successful round of investments, the company is expected to have an improved rate of growth and development, and the pressures on the founders will gradually increase over time as the company moves toward the planned exit and/or growth pathway.

CASE EXAMPLE 3: LESSONS LEARNED FROM THE TELEPSYCHIATRY PROGRAM IN CALIFORNIA PRISONS[4]

Regardless of the differences between telemedicine programs run by government agencies and those developed in the for-profit world, success can often be predicated on time-tested principles of business:

1. Identifying a need.
2. Developing a business plan to meet the need.
3. Making a pitch to obtain resources for the project.
4. Choosing appropriate resources and technology.
5. Structuring the program to align with the mission while satisfying rules and regulations.

An excellent example of business principles applied to public agencies is the California prison system. For decades, psychiatrists shunned the notion of spending their careers in a bleak prison environment, but in 2010, the medical director for San Quentin Prison, Edward Kaftarian, M.D., noticed that it was much easier to recruit doctors who wanted to work near metropolises like San Francisco and wondered whether telepsychiatry might provide the answer to the prison workforce problem.

Dr. Kaftarian pitched his case, including a business plan, to a variety of stakeholders, including the secretary of the prison system, and the plan was accepted. The choice of technology was important, and the decision was made to move away from large, expensive "legacy" telemedicine machines. Instead, less expensive, more readily available personal computers were chosen. Inexpensive peripheral devices such as cameras, speakers, and microphones were added as plug-ins to the USB ports. These practical technology choices removed the historic price barriers of implementing a telepsychiatry program. This, combined with the development of thorough policies and operating procedures, allowed the telepsychiatry program to meld seamlessly into the overall mental health program. Today, after only 5 years, the California Department of Corrections runs the largest and most comprehensive correctional telepsychiatry program in the world, employing approximately 60 telepsychiatrists and serving more than 20 institutions across the state.

▌ KEY CONCEPT

Government agencies can enjoy great success if they include proven business practices as part of their overall plans.

---

[4]Case provided by Edward Kaftarian, M.D.

HOW SHOULD CLINICIANS APPROACH THE TASK OF IMPLEMENTING A BUSINESS PLAN?

BASIC ELEMENTS OF A BUSINESS PLAN

Anyone proposing to develop a telepsychiatry practice should consider writing a business plan. Depending on the size of the planned venture, of course, only some of the elements discussed here may be necessary. The most important questions that anyone can ask themselves before considering starting a new business are as follows:

- What problem(s) is the business trying to solve (e.g., lack of providers in rural areas? improved convenience for existing patients?)?
- How does the business propose to solve these problems better than other businesses in the field?
- What is the competitive landscape, and what will be the business's market differentiator?
- What can be learned from the mistakes of competitors?
- What can be learned from the successes of competitors?
- What will it cost to start the business, and what are the expected revenues, expenses, and profits?

Starting a business is thrilling and worthwhile, but there will be unknown costs as the business moves to being fully independent. One thing to keep in mind about a financial model is that it is always wrong. The real question is, by how much? It is important to be realistic and to follow the financial model as closely as possible. As you learn, you can realistically adjust.

The following practical issues must be addressed:

- A plan for the overall implementation of video services and teleconsultations to provide the contemplated therapy
- The types of technology to be used—likely a cloud-based commercial videoconferencing service that is HIPAA compliant and requires a broadband Internet connection, a webcam, and an echo-canceling speaker
- A needs analysis that includes the types of contemplated services, whether existing patients would be interested, the capacity of other providers, the ability to change practice style, and workflow

- Technical and media training, the clinical policies required, knowl-edge and implementation of administrative and safety guidelines, and possible staffing and role changes
- Business aspects, including need for a business plan and understand-ing of local regulations and legal, licensing, credentialing, billing, and payment issues

Most practices also need to address the following clinical issues:

- Release of information and informed consent as required by your state
- Intake procedures, appointment scheduling, synchronization of schedules across all sites, delineation of staff roles and responsibilities
- Procedures for ensuring privacy and confidentiality in the use of EMRs, including transmission of prescriptions, lab orders, and prog-ress notes as necessary
- Licensing, liability, and malpractice insurance and safety protocols
- Integration with any other clinical or administrative software and apps

Any good business writes a business plan. If you intend to seek fund-ing for your venture as opposed to self-funding it, then any investor or granter will want to see your business plan.

WRITING A BUSINESS PLAN FOR IMPLEMENTING A HEALTH TECHNOLOGY PROGRAM

There are many ways of writing a business plan; templates and section outlines for such plans can be easily found on the Internet. Most business plans are "living documents" and are regularly updated as the environ-ment and program or business changes over time. It is generally good practice to review the business plan in a formal way at least annually.

The following section headings have been taken from a business plan-ning course for telemedicine run by Dr. Yellowlees for over a decade as part of the University of California Davis Informatics Master's program. These headings have been amended slightly to accommodate the needs of telemedicine professionals who do not work within a large institution (e.g., independent practitioners). Although these section headings are designed for a generic telemedicine business plan, they can of course be modified and customized for any individual plan.

1. Executive Summary

Think of the Executive Summary as almost the same as an academic abstract for a paper but containing what the business world calls an "elevator pitch"—literally what an entrepreneur would say if he or she met somebody in an elevator and had about 1 minute to describe the core of the business plan to that person. Focus on why your particular business is needed, who is going to run it, and what benefits—both clinical and economic—the business will provide.

2. Introduction and Rationale (What Problem Are You Trying to Solve?)

In this section, provide much more detail about the "why" of the business. This will involve conducting a background literature search for both academic papers and reports, especially ones that include solid data on clinical outcomes and costs. In this section, quote a number of studies and perform a "gap analysis" demonstrating the need for the services.

3. Proposed Services (How Will This Business Solve the Problem?)

Specify the detailed aims and specific goals of the proposed services, being extremely specific and detailing exactly the goals and over how long and in what manner they will be achieved. Goals should be measurable, time based, and clear. Additionally, provide a broader description of the actual proposed clinical services. It is often good to include a generic case study illustrating how the proposed services will work in the real world and how patients and providers will interact.

If you are an independent practitioner, state what your "secret sauce" is. Describe how the business will solve the problem better than anyone else would. If the business already has some outcomes data, here will be one of the many times that this information is repeated.

4. Personnel or Management

Introduce any key personnel who are likely to be employed to execute the plan and provide their proposed hire dates. Include short biographies of the individuals (if they are known) or a description of the skill sets needed. In telemedicine, it is common to identify "clinical champions" and telemedicine coordinators (or "patient navigators"), as well as the likely full range of administrative and clinical positions found in any new health service.

A business plan for the independent practitioner may not include patient navigators or other support personnel, so if you are an independent practitioner, highlight the extensive experience of your management team, yourself, and/or your cofounders.

5. Needs Assessment or Competitive Analysis

This section requires a much more detailed review of clinical, business, and technical needs at any sites or in any health systems or programs and partners involved. This step may involve collecting epidemiological and public health data about the region and combining it with knowledge of past referral patterns and information about the types of providers currently practicing in a geographic region.

If you are an independent practitioner, do a competitive analysis. Evaluate the competition by giving a summary of the competitor's work and comparing it to your approach, showing the features and benefits that are different and highlighting how your business is the one that can solve the problem (mentioned earlier in the plan). The competition may be a large hospital system or a group of other practitioners. The competition is specific to the proposed services and may include several different types of groups. For example, a hospital may provide only part of the bundle of proposed services, with a physician group providing another part. If you are raising money and making a pitch, the financial model in this section will be the fodder for many questions.

6. Market Analysis

Conduct a market analysis. The easiest way of evaluating the market is through a SWOT (Strengths, Weaknesses, Opportunities, and Threats) analysis. There are many good examples on the Internet, but the overall aim is to develop a good set of business reasons, whether these be clinical, financial, ethical, philosophical, or whatever, for undertaking the program. It is also helpful to be aware of both the barriers and the weaknesses that exist. The market analysis is also a good place to provide a summary review of any competitors in the space.

If you are an independent practitioner, see discussion of competitive analysis above.

7. Technology and Vendors

Describe the potential vendors and the intended technologies—cloud-based or locally run systems, types of videoconferencing, differing EMRs, scheduling systems, and the like. It is best in a business plan to be as specific as possible and to compare and contrast major options and choices to provide clarity about the final choice the business has made.

If you are an independent practitioner, and if the business is raising money based on results, these decisions may have already been made, so simply include why the business made the choice it did.

8. Telecommunications Infrastructure

Assess the telecommunications infrastructure required. This process may be very straightforward if the contemplated project is in a major health system. However, there are still many parts of the United States that do not have broadband in all rural areas, and this section is basically a check to verify that the business can undertake the contemplated services.

9. Program Operations

Describe the program operations, the nuts and bolts of the proposed program—including operation of the services, location of any clinical sites, clinicians or other staff needed, and information on how professionals will be trained and how the training will incorporate sustainability. A workflow of a patient consultation from start to finish, incorporating all administrative and financial aspects, is a useful exercise here and demonstrates that the business is thoughtful about the detail of the operational aspects.

If you are an independent practitioner, it is a good idea to also outline the workflow of a patient encounter and to incorporate into the financial model information about potential hires and when those expenses will occur.

10. Policy Issues or Legal and Regulatory Considerations

Give careful consideration to a variety of policies, requirements, and guidelines related to, among others, privacy and security, clinical quality, and safety and accreditation, as discussed earlier in this chapter. HIPAA compliance is particularly important. It may also mean becoming accredited by the Joint Commission, the ATA Accreditation Program, or both. There are other policies on licensing and credentialing, especially proxy credentialing for partner sites, that need to be reviewed and incorporated.

If you are an independent practitioner, address legal and regulatory issues. Depending on your size, accreditation may not exist. For the smaller independent practitioner, it is important to know the rules and regulations pertaining to the business's practitioners and reimbursement.

11. Costs and Financial Sustainability

Include a financial pro forma—essentially a draft budget that identifies revenue and expenses and describes how the business will be financially sustainable. For example, a business plan based on a grant model may simply specify that the business will not pursue other grants for the first 2 years. Then, after 2 years, the business will plan to pursue another grant. Even with that approach, there needs to be a plan for financial sustainability related to what happens when the grants run out, as they always do.

The costs and financial sustainability section is often the most important single portion of any business plan and is the topic that health provider entrepreneurs often find most difficult to characterize. For many, it would be prudent to seek expert financial advice and assistance to ensure that this component of the business plan makes good sense. If this part of the plan is weak, it is very unlikely that the business will be funded.

If you are an independent practitioner or are not pursuing grants, investors will review your plan and test the credibility of the numbers. It is quite rare that a business will write a pro forma, receive funding based on that pro forma, and operate the business to exactly match that pro forma. As the business operates, adjustments will be made, but at the outset, the independent practitioner must be able to justify the numbers and articulate why he or she is confident that those numbers are correct.

12. Planning Process

In this section, one that is often forgotten but is very important, describe the more mundane aspects of how the business will be started up. While writing a business plan is part of that planning process, there is more. Include details such as where the headquarters of the business will be located, what space is available, how much time is expected to be invested, and who is going to physically set up the infrastructure, negotiate early contracts, and buy furniture and equipment. What is the early governance process, and will this change? If so, when? Who will write the grant or funding proposals? Who will develop and implement training programs? For each area, specify time lines and deliverables that are transparent and clear.

13. Quality Improvement

This section is also frequently overlooked in business plans, but it is essential to continually improve the proposed project or program and to have some sort of quality improvement process in place. Start by planning to deliver certain things, measure what has been delivered, plan again to improve what is being delivered, measure again, then once more plan to improve again, and re-measure, and so on. Another way of thinking of the quality improvement process is "Plan, Deliver, Evaluate, Improve, Tweak, Measure, Continue…"

SUMMARY

Many forward-thinking entreprencurs and companies are eager to tap into the opportunity of telemedicine. However, the prospect of financial rewards must not blind clinicians to the myriad challenges and pitfalls inherent in building a quality telemedicine program. This chapter has discussed

- The barriers to implementing telepsychiatry.
- The principles that underlie success in implementing telepsychiatry.
- The change process involved in technology adoption and implementation.
- How to choose the right technology for your practice.
- How to understand the rules and regulations impacting the use of technologies—licensing, credentialing, informed consent, prescribing, malpractice, safety, and confidentiality.
- The many types of commercialization and funding models available.
- How to develop, write, and implement a business plan.

A businesslike approach to integrating technology into one's practice is strongly recommended—an approach that does not ignore safety, clinical, or regulatory issues. The right technologies need to be implemented as part of a solid business plan that is supported by an appropriate funding model. Attention to each of these issues will promote a sustainable business while allowing clinicians to advocate for the health and well-being of patients and consumers.

REFERENCES

American Foundation for the Blind: Blind Doctors in Medicine (forum), 2011. Available at: http://www.afb.org/forum/careers-in-healthcare/blind-doctors-in-medicine/12. Accessed October 12, 2016.

American Telemedicine Association: Practice Guidelines for Videoconferencing-Based Telemental Health, 2009. Available at: https://hub.american-telemed.org/viewdocument/practice-guidelines-3. Accessed November 7, 2016.

American Telemedicine Association: State Policy Resource Center, 2016. Available at: http://www.americantelemed.org/policy/state-policy-resource-center#.V50ztLgrJ4f. Accessed November 7, 2016.

Caudill RL, Shore JH: Telemedicine, smart devices, social media, and the human/technology interface, in Psychiatry, 4th Edition. Edited by Tasman A, Kay J, Lieberman JA, et al. Chichester, United Kingdom, John Wiley & Sons, 2015, pp 2011–2024

Centers for Medicare & Medicaid Services: Center for Medicaid, CHIP, and Survey and Certification/Survey and Certification Group Memorandum to State Survey Agency Directors, July 15, 2011. Available at: https://www.cms.gov/Medicare/Provider-Enrollment-and-Certification/SurveyCertificationGenInfo/downloads/SCLetter11_32.pdf. Accessed December 1, 2016.

HIPAA Journal: HIPAA Guidelines on Telemedicine, 2016. Available at: http://www.hipaajournal.com/hipaa-guidelines-on-telemedicine/. Accessed October 12, 2016.

Monegain B: Telemedicine market to soar past $30B. Healthcare IT News, August 4, 2015. Available at: http://m.healthcareitnews.com/news/telemedicine-poised-grow-big-time. Accessed October 7, 2016.

North Carolina Medical Board: Resources and Information: Position Statements: Telemedicine. Adopted July 2010, Amended November 2014. Available at: http://www.ncmedboard.org/resources-information/professional-resources/laws-rules-position-statements/position-statements/telemedicine. Accessed November 7, 2016.

Rogers EM: Elements of diffusion, in Diffusion of Innovations, 5th Edition. New York, Simon & Schuster, 2003, pp 1–38

Thomas L, Capistrant G: State Telemedicine Gaps Analysis: Physician Practice Standards & Licensure, January 2016. Washington, DC, American Telemedicine Association, 2016. Available at: https://www.americantelemed.org/policy-page/state-telemedicine-gaps-reports (Note: ATA membership is required for access). Accessed December 1, 2016.

Treister NW: Physician acceptance of new medical information systems: the field of dreams. Physician Exec 24(3):20–24, 1998 10180969

U.S. Department of Justice, Drug Enforcement Administration, Diversion Control Division: Controlled Substances—Alphabetical Order. July 17, 2017. Available at: https://www.deadiversion.usdoj.gov/schedules/orange-book/c_cs_alpha.pdf. Accessed July 25, 2017.

Walhof R: The blind in medical professions. Future Reflections, 4(3), 1985. Available at: https://nfb.org/images/nfb/publications/fr/fr04/issue3/f040303.html. Accessed October 12, 2016.

Yellowlees PM: Successfully developing a telemedicine system. J Telemed Telecare 11(7):331–335, 2005 16238833

Yellowlees PM: Who will benefit? (Chapter 2), in Your Health in the Information Age: How You and Your Doctor Can Use the Internet to Work Together. Bloomington, IN, iUniverse, 2008, pp 21–39

Yellowlees P: The Credentialing Process (video). Available at: https://psychiatry.org/psychiatrists/practice/telepsychiatry/credentialing-process. Accessed December 1, 2016.

4

Clinical Settings and Models of Care in Telepsychiatry

Implications for Work Practices and Culturally Informed Treatment

Barb Johnston, M.S.N.

Jay H. Shore, M.D., M.P.H.

Terry Rabinowitz, M.D.

There have been many different approaches to providing telepsychiatry over the years, with the majority of early projects focused on providing access to psychiatrists, mainly for patients living in rural or geographically isolated areas, and in most cases using a model in which a specialist at the hub of a health facility (e.g., hospital or clinic) was consulting on a patient located at a primary care clinic. Most of these early programs using a specialist-to-clinic model were grant funded and used a model of care that was essentially the same as that used in person, just removed at a distance. Most programs initially used a fairly typical consultation model, whereby the psychiatrist consulted on patients referred from primary care and advised on treatment, and the treatment was then carried out by the primary care provider and his or her team. In this model, the psychiatrist did not typically provide long-term therapy or take over the psychiatric component of the care; instead, he or she concentrated mainly on working with the primary care team in what would now be called a "medical home" model. This model has continued over time, but gradually an increasing number of programs started providing direct care, including not just consultations and assessments but also psychotherapy, medication management, team care, and long-term follow-up. In a number of health systems, other models gradually evolved to include patients seen via telepsychiatry in correctional facilities, emergency departments, integrated health systems inpatient units, and their own homes. Over time, telepsychiatry services have expanded and have adopted a collaborative care approach focused on improved communication between specialists and primary care in alignment with patient-centered medical home (PCMH) models.

No longer is telepsychiatry thought to be merely a replacement for in-person care for individuals who are limited by geography and unable to access mental health care locally. Telepsychiatry is frequently delivered in a hybrid environment where it is combined with in-person care and the use of multiple technologies—videoconferencing, e-mail, messaging, telephony, and electronic health records. The integration of telepsychiatry and other health technologies has led to programs that provide better care than has traditionally been possible through this improved and more flexible communication. These programs are consistent with the Triple Aim—Better Care, Better Health, Lower Costs (Institute for Healthcare Improvement; www.ihi.org/Topics/TripleAim)—to provide better individual care, to treat populations of patients, and to do so with greater efficiency and at reduced costs. In this chapter, we focus on environments in which telepsychiatry typically occurs, the various models of care used, and the changes occurring in work practices for psychiatrists, patient care sites, and members of patient care teams. New roles and team approaches are explored. Finally, we discuss the cultural components of delivering care and outline the advantages that telepsychiatry can bring to patients from differing social and ethnic backgrounds and how telepsychiatry can improve the knowledge and skills of providers involved in this practice.

WHAT SETTINGS ARE EMERGING AS TELEPSYCHIATRY BECOMES MAINSTREAM?

TRADITIONAL HUB-AND-SPOKE TELEPSYCHIATRY

The hub-and-spoke configuration has been the most common model in telepsychiatry since the first video consultations at the University of

Nebraska in 1958. In the traditional hub-and-spoke model, a patient is located in a remote clinic (originating site) and receives the video consultation from a psychiatrist who is often located at a clinic in an academic medical center (distant site). This clinic-to-clinic model can then be replicated across a network of remote spoke sites. Variations on this theme involve providers working from private practice offices or their own homes but usually consulting with a patient who is located in a remote clinic setting. The majority of grant funding for telemedicine consultations has historically been for programs working with patients who are physically located in a rural health setting such as a hospital, clinic, or other health facility.

NONCLINIC TRADITIONAL SETTINGS

Over time, the locations of patients and providers for video consultations began to expand. Psychiatrists expanded video consultations into a wide variety of locations, such as emergency departments, nursing homes, hospital inpatient settings, correctional institutions, airports, overseas embassies, ships at sea, oil platforms, and eventually patients' homes directly. As equipment gradually became less expensive and broadband became more widely available, from about the year 2000 onward, the number of potential patient sites for telepsychiatry dramatically increased, as did the use cases. Beginning in the mid- to late-1990s, a number of large hub-and-spoke telemedicine networks were set up in locations like the United States and Australia, where multiple providers could provide consultations to multiple originating/patient sites across large systems of care. In the United States, by the year 2000, the largest network that widely supported psychiatric consultations, as well as those of other disciplines, was in the State of Texas Correctional System, where the University of Texas Medical Branch at Galveston was providing psychiatric care to patients in more than 100 correctional institutions. Other large U.S. networks developed soon after to provide culturally informed care to Native American populations on reservations in Colorado and California, and networks in rural nursing homes and primary care clinics in rural communities were also established. In Australia during this same period, the Queensland Telemedicine Network expanded to more than 200 videoconferencing sites, and the South Australian Telemedicine Network to more than 80 sites. All of these large networks provided medical consultations in multiple specialties, but they also had telepsychiatry as their largest specialty service, with more than half of their total consultations being for mental health care. The majority of these programs provided video consultations that were very similar to in-person consultations, with the exception that primary care providers or other local referring "physician extenders" were often involved in part of the consultations. This approach became a model for the practice of collaborative care enabled by technology, even before the advent of the IMPACT (Improving Mood—Promoting Access to Collaborative Treatment) model of collaborative care, developed at the University of Washington, which involved an embedded in-person mental health care provider in primary care (Katon et al. 2012).

INTEGRATED MENTAL HEALTH CARE ENABLED BY TECHNOLOGY

The introduction of telepsychiatry into the PCMH model of primary care was first implemented at scale and in a commercial environment in 2012 in the United States when telepsychiatry was integrated into 82 primary care clinics across three primarily rural states by HealthLinkNow, Inc., a telepsychiatry medical service company based in California. This model of care was an extension of the original consultative models of telepsychiatry and allowed patients to receive mental health care locally in their own primary care physicians' offices, which provided a familiar and more convenient setting. This program reduced stigma and demonstrated improved health outcomes, reporting patient satisfaction levels of over 90% (Johnston 2015).

This PCMH model opened communication between psychiatrists and primary care providers (PCPs) and led to PCPs becoming more educated about mental health care management. A key component of the PCMH model is development of the role of new members of the health team, called "care navigators," who were responsible for supporting specialists, PCPs, and patients and who were effectively the equivalent of the embedded behavioral health care providers in the IMPACT model, but working fully online. Care navigators provide training, implementation assistance, and ongoing support for the health technology system, which includes a fully integrated electronic health record (EHR), e-prescribing, scheduling, billing, and videoconferencing system. Care navigators are also the primary point of contact for patients, conducting the initial semistructured patient intake interview via telephone and documenting the results directly in the EHR, thereby eliminating some of the administrative work of the psychiatrist, who is then able to spend more of his or her time on clinical interviewing. Care navigators remain available to patients and providers for follow up after the psychiatry consultations to ensure that further scheduling and prescription refills are completed or other issues are resolved, much as clinic office staff would do, just online. In Johnston's (2015) PCMH model, patients' PCPs are also encouraged to participate in part of the telepsychiatry session—usually the last 5–10 minutes—so that the PCP and the telepsychiatrist can discuss the findings and recommendations from the video consultation with the patient present.

CASE EXAMPLE 1: PRIMARY CARE DEPRESSION SCREENING LEADING TO REFERRAL FOR TELEPSYCHIATRY[1]

A 45-year-old woman scored positive for depression on a Patient Health Questionnaire (PHQ)–9 introduced by a telepsychiatry practice (HealthLinkNow) into a group of primary care practices to assist PCPs in identifying patients who needed psychiatric referral for possible depression. The woman's PCP knew her well as someone who came to see him frequently with multiple somatic complaints and who self-medicated with alcohol and marijuana, but he had been treating her primarily for substance abuse. The PCP was ambivalent about referring his patient because he did not see how the telepsychiatrist could help, but the patient agreed to a consultation and "second opinion." At the first telepsychiatry session, she was diagnosed with bipolar II disorder, after describing a long history of mood swings that she used substances to attempt to control. She was started on mood stabilizers and was able to reduce her alcohol and marijuana intake. The patient was also referred to an online therapist from the telepsychiatry practice, who provided therapy via videoconferencing for about 6 months, which she found very helpful. Much to the PCP's surprise, his patient improved dramatically, and a year later, her mood was stable, she was not abusing any substances, and she had found a new job. The PCP reported to the telepsychiatry practice that he had learned a lot from joining the psychiatrist in his consultations and had changed his approach to depression management with his other patients.

❚ KEY CONCEPT

Routine screening for depression in primary care is useful and can identify patients who would benefit from treatment, which can be provided as effectively by telepsychiatry as it can be in person.

---

[1]Case provided by Barb Johnston, M.S.N.

The IMPACT model at the University of Washington (Katon et al. 2012) has accumulated a very strong evidence base for a large number of integrated and collaborative-care telepsychiatry programs developed over the past few years. The original large-scale trial involved 1,800 patients in eight health systems (Unützer et al. 2002) in which embedded care managers were used to assist distant psychiatrists, with the result that patients in the intervention group had 3.5 times the odds of response (defined as a 50% or greater reduction in depressive symptoms from baseline) in 12 months compared with patients in the group receiving usual care. This model of care has since become one of the most heavily tested and proven clinical models in the mental health care field, especially in large clinics and large systems of care.

U.S. DEPARTMENT OF VETERANS AFFAIRS MODELS FOR POSTTRAUMATIC STRESS DISORDER TREATMENT AND TEAM CARE WITH PRIMARY CARE PHYSICIANS

The U.S. Department of Veterans Affairs (VA) has been providing tele-mental health care to veterans in clinics and directly to patients in their homes for more than 20 years. The VA is currently the largest single-system provider of telepsychiatry services in the United States, as well as the system that has undertaken the most rigorous large-scale research studies in telepsychiatry implementation models, with a number of academics, notably Fortney and Godleski, publishing important research studies in the past decade. In a VA study involving nearly 100,000 mainly male veterans conducted between 2006 and 2010, "the first large-scale assessment of telemental health care services," Godleski and colleagues found that after initiation of such services, patients' hospitalization utilization decreased by an average of 25% (Godleski et al. 2012). A major goal of the VA's approach was to improve health outcomes by providing mental health care to veterans in their own homes, or in local clinics as close to their homes as possible, where they are more comfortable and can avoid the stigma associated with visiting a mental health care clinic. The use of health technology allowed the provision of care to shift to where patients were located, similar to how people now shop, become educated, and are entertained. The first home-based telemental health care pilot program for veterans was conducted at the Portland VA Medical Center with 40 participants in 2009. This pilot program demonstrated high patient satisfaction and fewer no-show appointments in home-based telemental health care compared with clinic-based telemental health care (Shore et al. 2014) and led to the introduction of other home-based programs in other VA regions.

CASE EXAMPLE 2: HOME-BASED TELEPSYCHIATRY SESSIONS: A WINDOW INTO THE PATIENT'S REAL LIFE[2]

A Vietnam-era veteran was reluctant to obtain counseling for his depression, but his wife insisted. He appeared at the local community clinic and was seated in an examination room. The telepresenter turned on the large videoconferencing desktop unit, and the distantly based psychologist appeared "on TV." Introductions were exchanged, then the veteran said, "I drove 30 miles to see someone on TV?" For the next several weekly sessions, progress in treatment was nonexistent, with continued complaints about having to drive great distances to see someone on TV. The psychologist decided to transition the care into the veteran's home via webcam and personal computer. The first session took place with the patient seated at his desk in the corner of his bedroom. In the background were a cluttered bookshelf and the bust of an elk. "Okay, he's an avid reader and a hunter," the psychologist thought. During the subsequent few sessions, the topics of the patient's favorite books and fondest hunting memories integrated nicely into treatment, helping to develop the therapeutic alliance; however, change was still not meaningful. The psychologist and the veteran decided to move the session setting to another location in the man's house, the living room, with the caveat that no one else would be home during the session. The first session in the living room produced new information. In the background were various anthropological artifacts from Africa. The psychologist explored the veteran's interest in African culture, further developing the therapeutic alliance. A few sessions later, the veteran changed his location once again, this time to his attic, and in this session the veteran, surrounded by Chicago Cubs memorabilia, told the psychologist, "I'm a lifelong diehard Cubs fan—I listen to every game on the radio, go to spring trainings when I can." The psychologist replied, "No wonder you're so depressed." The veteran broke into hysterical laughter, and from that point on began to let his guard down and allow himself to feel vulnerable, deepening the therapeutic alliance. Over the next several weeks, positive changes occurred, including improved functioning and better communication with his wife.

---

[2]Case provided by Peter Shore, Psy.D.

❙ KEY CONCEPT
Mental health care delivered within the patient's home may provide more detailed information about the patient's background
and interests, leading to an improved therapeutic relationship.

The VA has also demonstrated that telepsychiatry sessions are as effective as in-person mental health care visits in identifying suicide risk in veterans. During a study reported in 2008, the VA developed best practices for
remote suicide risk assessment that included procedures for utilizing clinical assessment and triage decision protocols and for contingency planning
to optimize patient care and reduce liability (Godleski et al. 2008).

Fortney and his team of researchers working in the VA, first in Ala-
bama and then in Seattle, over the past decade have carried out a series of
studies focused on implementing differing versions of the Katon collaborative care model, underpinned by multiple technologies. Fortney's
studies have included services that are technology enabled and involve
team- and population-based approaches that are patient centered; evidence and measurement based, including the use of registries to track
patients and outcomes; and practice tested.

Fortney's team has evaluated three trials with veterans that have substantially enlarged the evidence base for telepsychiatry. The first trial, in
2007 (Fortney et al. 2007), compared the effectiveness of telepsychiatry
against usual care for depression (primarily pharmacotherapy). The trial
showed a higher response rate (twofold) in the intervention arm and
demonstrated that depression care with telepsychiatry was superior to
that with usual care. The second trial (Fortney et al. 2013), which replicated the findings of the first trial in 336 patients enrolled from eight federally qualified health centers, compared telemedicine-based collaborative
care for depression against practice-based care. The virtual model of collaborative care using telepsychiatry was found to be superior to usual
collaborative care. In the third trial (Fortney et al. 2015), in 265 veterans
with posttraumatic stress disorder (PTSD) from 11 VA clinics, cognitive-
behavioral therapy (CBT) plus medication management delivered by a
virtual team not only was superior to usual care but also significantly improved patients' engagement in the care process. Fortney and colleagues'
current trial, launched in 2016, is comparing the effectiveness of a hybrid
telepsychiatry collaborative care program (involving screening, monitoring, and consultations delivered both by video and in person) with

that of a conventional telepsychiatry referral and consultation program, as these are now the two main models of telepsychiatry integrated with primary care being delivered nationally.

EMERGENCY DEPARTMENTS

Many persons with some of the most troublesome mental health problems or issues, including first psychotic episodes, drug or alcohol intoxication or withdrawal, uncontainable violence, and suicidal or homicidal behaviors, are first evaluated in an emergency department (ED). However, lack of appropriate mental health care personnel in EDs significantly limits capacity to deal with these complex patients and their families. Although there have been few investigations that have specifically studied telepsychiatry's implementation and impact in the ED, interest in use of telepsychiatry in this setting continues to grow. A notable study by Narasimhan et al. (2015) reviewed more than 7,000 telepsychiatry encounters in the ED and compared them with control encounters in EDs where telepsychiatry was not available. They found that, compared with ED patients in the control condition, ED patients treated via telepsychiatry were more likely to receive 30- and 90-day outpatient follow-up, were less likely to be admitted to the hospital, had inpatient lengths of stay that were shorter by 0.86 day, and had 30-day inpatient costs that were more than $2,000 lower per patient (Narasimhan et al. 2015).

Delusional patients often present to EDs requesting care for perceived disorders, placing themselves at risk for unneeded treatments. Medical disorders can sometimes generate psychiatric symptoms and lead ED personnel to doubt the reported medical problems. In the context of this complexity, it can be tempting to automatically attribute strange stories to psychiatric issues. Careful assessment is important and can prevent unnecessary hospitalization.

CASE EXAMPLE 3: AN EMERGENCY PATIENT'S BIZARRE COMPLAINTS AND HISTORY TURN OUT TO BE TRUE[3]

A 54-year-old woman with a reported history of multiple head injuries and medical problems, including several types of cancer related to a genetic disorder, was brought to the ED by police after she claimed she had

---

[3]Case (and paragraph preceding it) provided by Mark Alter, M.D., Ph.D.

been assaulted. During her time in the ED, the patient was grandiose, agitated, demanding, and very tangential, but over the course of several telepsychiatry consultations, her story remained consistent, and she denied any dangerous intent to herself or others. The patient's caretaker reportedly had the smell of alcohol on his breath, was confused about the patient's care, and attempted to bring an unharnessed pit bull into the ED, claiming that it was the patient's service dog. However, the patient was able to supply phone numbers for her case manager at her insurance company, who was able to verify multiple medical claims consistent with the patient's reported medical diagnoses. Additionally, a Ph.D. psychologist who regularly counseled the patient verified her medical and psychiatric history and confirmed that the woman was frequently grandiose and paranoid but was never dangerous in any way, and that she actually did have a pit bull as a therapy dog. It became apparent that contrary to all appearances, the patient was in fact capable of navigating a complex set of needs for treatment. The woman was subsequently discharged with a plan for follow-up at her verified oncology appointment within a few days.

▌ KEY CONCEPT

Telepsychiatry allows EDs to access experienced emergency psychiatrists and to work as a team to make difficult clinical decisions.

A study by Seidel and Kilgus (2014) compared in-person ED evaluations of mentally ill patients with evaluations conducted via telemedicine. Over 39 months, the authors assessed 73 patients who were evaluated either in person or via telemedicine. Interrater agreement regarding evaluators' disposition recommendations, assigned diagnoses, and estimations of dangerousness was assessed with Cohen's kappa (κ). The investigators found an 84% agreement when both evaluators used the in-person approach and an 86% agreement when one evaluator used telemedicine and one used in-person. They concluded that telepsychiatry can be used reliably and safely in the ED to evaluate the need for a psychiatric inpatient admission (Seidel and Kilgus 2014).

Yellowlees et al. (2008) opine that telepsychiatry can be used for two types of emergency situations: single-episode psychiatric emergencies and mass disasters, with the potential to reduce ED overcrowding, deliver care to underserved (especially rural) populations, and improve access to care in the case of natural or human-caused disasters. Of note, there are published general telemental health care guidelines available through the

American Telemedicine Association (ATA) but no telemental health care guidelines for specific cohorts other than children and adolescents; an exception is emergency telepsychiatry, for which guidelines were published in 2007 (Shore et al. 2007). Although the *Emergency Management Guidelines for Telepsychiatry* have not been officially endorsed or adopted by the ATA, they encompass a practical and easily implemented collection of behaviors and approaches that will help ensure successful use of videoconferencing in emergency psychiatric assessment and treatment. Space does not permit inclusion of the complete guidelines for emergency telepsychiatry, but some key elements are presented in Table 4–1.

Using telepsychiatry in the ED or for other emergency situations makes good clinical sense: It has the potential to deliver quality psychiatric consultation and care to smaller, community, and rural EDs that have no or limited access to specialist psychiatric services. However, more robust studies of this approach are needed to demonstrate significant cost and time savings, to show how it might improve safety and outcomes, and to confirm its acceptance by patients, providers, and ED staff.

HYBRID MODELS OF CARE

Hybrid models, in which psychiatrists see patients both in person and online, are now common practice and can occur in any of the settings or models described in this chapter, as individual practitioners and programs expand beyond providing clinic-based telepsychiatry care. Providers now commonly use mobile devices and laptops, as cloud-based systems and more bandwidth are more widely available. Probably the best and most well-researched and validated hybrid model of care is that developed by Myers and her team in Washington State (Myers et al. 2015). Myers implemented a treatment program for 223 children with attention-deficit/hyperactivity disorder (ADHD), many of whom also had oppositional disorders, and demonstrated in a randomized controlled trial that a hybrid team–based care program—consisting of in-person PCP and therapy services and supported by a child telepsychiatrist and online educational programs for children, families, and teachers—was considerably more effective than usual care, which included telepsychiatry medication consultations. Her results were so successful that it was suggested that this form of care should become the new standard of care in child psychiatry (Hilty and Yellowlees 2015).

TABLE 4–1.   Selected key domains to consider in emergency telepsychiatry

Domain	Challenge(s)	Action
Administrative	Differences between provider and patient sites (e.g., patient and provider in two different states)	Learn local licensing and resource requirements and needs.
	Who can help?	Identify local collaborators and "champions."
	Patient safety	Develop emergency protocols and identify who will be responsible for carrying them out.
		Determine how 24/7 emergency coverage will be provided.
Legal/ethical	Patient, provider, and community safety	Learn local statutes and regulations regarding duty to warn, inform, and protect.
		Ensure that local personnel are available to help with containment and commitment activities.
		Query patients and family members about firearm ownership and ensure that all firearms are safely contained when indicated.
		Know what local resources are available for different (e.g., alcohol, drug, tobacco) substance abuse issues and how to access them.

TABLE 4–1. Selected key domains to consider in emergency telepsychiatry *(continued)*

Domain	Challenge(s)	Action
Community	Relative ease of dissemination of sensitive or confidential information in small, rural, or isolated communities	Take all necessary steps to protect sensitive information; be familiar with HIPAA and other pertinent regulations; be sufficiently familiar with data encryption and other techniques to protect information, or know whom to contact for assistance.

Note. HIPAA = Health Insurance Portability and Accountability Act.
Source. Adapted from Shore et al. 2007.

CASE EXAMPLE 4: HYBRID TREATMENT OF A CHILD BY TELEPSYCHIATRY IN A PATIENT-CENTERED MEDICAL HOME[4]

An elementary school–age child was being treated by his PCP for depression. The child's parents said that they had been unable to locate a psychiatrist anywhere close to them, that their marriage was in trouble, and that they had been neglecting their other two children. The closest psychiatrist worked more than 100 miles away, but her panel was full, and she did not normally see children. The parents stated that they were "at a complete loss," so the PCP decided to try telepsychiatry. The referral note said that the child was failing at school, was "sad and withdrawn" at home, had no friends, and refused to speak to his siblings and parents. The child telepsychiatrist consulted with the child, his parents, and his teacher and diagnosed major depressive disorder. A treatment plan was set in place in collaboration with the PCP and family. The child responded well to treatment—a combination of antidepressants, multimodal therapy delivered online and locally, and parent education—and returned to school, where he remains. At follow-up, he has new friends, and his family is doing well again.

▌ KEY CONCEPT

The lack of child psychiatrists nationally is worsening, but services provided by telepsychiatry can support local providers and yield good outcomes.

CARE IN INPATIENT UNITS

It is unfortunate in the United States that even when a bed on a psychiatric unit is available for a person in need, it may go unfilled because a nurse or physician is not available to provide necessary or mandated oversight and care for the patient. Although provider shortages may occur in both urban and rural communities, they are more likely in the latter for several reasons, including 1) financial compensation is often lower in rural hospitals; 2) even if a provider lives in a more urban location, travel to rural areas for work may be too burdensome, especially in inclement weather or when rural road conditions are unfavorable; and 3) small community or rural hospitals may be unjustifiably judged to be less intellectually stimulating compared with larger academic medical centers. Add to this

---

[4]Case provided by Barb Johnston, M.S.N.

some potential providers' reluctance to live in or practice in urban areas, where there is a real or imagined increased risk of adversity, and the result is an absolute shortage of appropriate providers. Using telepsychiatry to offset regional disparities in access to specialist care is a promising but relatively new way of dealing with this challenge.

Holden and Dew (2008) were among the first to report on this use of telepsychiatry. McCurtain Memorial Hospital in Oklahoma, a small, rural medical–surgical hospital in a medically underserved area, transitioned to coverage via psychiatric telemedicine in 2005 to staff its 14-bed unit rather than close the only geropsychiatric unit in the region. To learn how the new care model worked, McCurtain Memorial adapted the hospital's Patient/Family Satisfaction Survey, which contained six items, each rated on a Likert-type scale ranging from 1 (poor) to 5 (excellent). For example, one item asked, "How would you rate the physician's availability and attentiveness to you?" Surveys were performed 12 months before implementation ($n=211$) of telepsychiatry (i.e., "usual care") and for 12 months following implementation ($n=155$). Although no statistical analyses were performed, the authors reported postimplementation scores for every item that were better than preimplementation scores and concluded that these preliminary findings could serve as a starting point from which to build further assessment measures. This modest but important investigation supports the feasibility of using telepsychiatry to provide inpatient psychiatric care for a complex patient cohort: elders, often with cognitive disorders such as dementia or with mood disorders, as well as one or more comorbid nonpsychiatric conditions. Similar results were obtained by Grady and Singleton (2011), who investigated patient and staff responses to telepsychiatry coverage of an inpatient psychiatry unit for 1 week during a transition period (approximately 2 months) when a permanent on-site attending psychiatrist was not available. Of note, some patients with psychosis incorporated video teleconferencing into their delusional systems, and patients rated development of rapport and effectiveness of treatment higher than did staff. Because the average daily census was only seven patients, the findings are not generalizable, but they do support the feasibility and utility of this approach.

Telepsychiatry can be used to perform psychiatric consultations for medical–surgical inpatients and to the intensive care unit. DeVido et al. (2016) reported that telemedicine equipment was provided to four consultation–liaison psychiatrists and one consultation–liaison resident, and mobile telemedicine carts and equipment were made available to nurses who were trained in use of the equipment and who brought the carts to patients' rooms. In total, 30 patients (ages 19–87 years; 50% female) were seen for initial evaluation, and 17 received follow-up visits by telepsychiatry. The most common requests were for management recommendations for depression, dementia, or anxiety, and the authors found that when evaluating patients with dementia or delirium, they were able to administer tests of cognition reliably using the technology. They also noted that having remote pan, tilt, and zoom capability in the patient-side camera enhanced their ability to perform the consultations by allowing them to view personal items in the room as well as to determine whether family members or friends who might provide collateral information were present. The authors reported general satisfaction with the technology from patients, providers, and consultees. However, there were some rare and generally minor technical problems, such as signal loss requiring rebooting of the equipment. In addition, there was some skepticism on the part of some physicians and social workers who did not think psychiatric patients could be evaluated by video technology. Our (T.R.) team has performed consultation–liaison consultations to patients at an affiliated but distant rehabilitation hospital in a similar fashion and with good results.

CARE IN SCHOOLS

Although telepsychiatry has the potential to deliver care to more persons in need, a potential impediment to its use is unavailability of appropriate equipment. While smartphones and tablet and laptop computers seem to be ubiquitous, there are many persons who cannot afford the technology or who have difficulty using it due to physical or cognitive limitations. In addition, although it often seems that everyone is "connected," many cannot connect because local coverage, cellular or otherwise, is simply unavailable at a specific location, such as a home or office, especially in rural communities. Providing telemental health care services to schools may be one way to address this challenge.

Telemedicine has been used to deliver health care to schools for many years. For example, Bergman et al. (2008) conducted a prospective study in three urban schools to assess the feasibility of using telemedicine to deliver asthma care. Ninety-six children ages 5–12 years who had a diagnosis of asthma and who were not under the care of an allergist were enrolled in the study; 83 completed the study. Each child participated in four encounters: at baseline and at 8, 16, and 32 weeks after enrollment. At the end of the study, 94% of parents rated the program as excellent or good on a 5-point Likert-type scale. At the end of the intervention, children showed improvement in the physical and social domains on the Children's Health Survey for Asthma (Asmussen et al. 1999). There was also significant improvement in child and parent asthma knowledge. Similar successes were reported for school-based telemedicine diabetes and acute illness care.

Telepsychiatry can be used in school settings as well, with appropriate adaptations specific to mental health care encounters. Lending support to this approach is a presidential task force endorsement for increasing mental health care in schools (Office of the White House 2013). Stephan et al. (2016) reviewed the potential benefits and limitations of school-based telemental health care. A key point they made is that although there are often several mental health care disciplines that can be accessed through schools, including social work, psychology, nursing, and psychiatry, psychiatry is least available because of high costs and provider shortages. In addition, when a psychiatrist is available for in-person consultations at a school, there is often an inefficient use of time, because much of it is spent in travel to and from the school or in waiting for the patient and family to present for appointments.

Most school-based telepsychiatry applications, including pharmacotherapy, have "passed" the feasibility and satisfaction hurdles, but to date there are few convincing outcome studies (Cain and Sharp 2016). Nonetheless, telepsychiatry in schools is used not only for medication management but also to evaluate students for support services (e.g., individualized education programs [IEPs]), psychotherapy, and diagnostic clarification. Moreover, it can be used to deliver knowledge, by enabling the telepsychiatrist to educate teachers, other school staff, and administrators about psychiatric conditions and their management (Stephan et al. 2016).

A focus group of six child and adolescent psychiatry fellows has reported on the advantages and disadvantages of school telepsychiatry (Stephan et al. 2016). Advantages included greater efficiency (including decreased commuting times and easier scheduling), ability to serve more students and schools, and increased access to care. Disadvantages included patient privacy issues and concerns about the psychiatrist's ability to engage with families without being face to face (Stephan et al. 2016). Overall, telepsychiatry for schools has great potential and makes intuitive sense. More studies examining the efficacy of school-based telepsychiatry and greater efforts to optimize privacy for students are recommended.

CARE IN NURSING HOMES

There are 1.3 million people living in U.S. nursing homes, and a large proportion of these residents have one or more mental illnesses that often interact with preexisting nonpsychiatric conditions, to the detriment of both. Although these persons constitute one of the most vulnerable and underserved cohorts, many, especially those in rural areas, go without adequate psychiatric consultation and care despite government mandates requiring that all nursing home residents have access to competent mental health care services. This lack of access to specialist care is especially egregious given that many elderly or frail individuals have to deal with a potentially disabling mental condition, and their mental disorder(s) is often missed, misdiagnosed, or undertreated. Moreover, they are also at greater risk of developing serious side effects from psychotropic medications.

Telepsychiatry has been used to redress deficiencies in access to specialist care and has been shown to be as effective as in-person care (Hilty et al. 2013). In addition, this approach saved time and money; was well received by patients, their families, and nursing home staff; and, most important, provided a service that would not otherwise have been available.

To expedite and facilitate these telepsychiatry visits, a nurse is always present at the originating site to present patient histories or updates, to help with assessments (e.g., to present intersecting pentagons to copy as part of the Mini-Mental State Examination), and to help with positioning of the patient. A social worker is often present to provide essential family information, and family members are encouraged to attend in order to see how the telepsychiatry service is delivered and, of course, to let the telepsychiatrist know how their loved one is getting along. Minimum data set information is sent to the telepsychiatrist before the initial visit and provides a useful summary of the resident's functioning in multiple domains. Because periodic minimum data set assessments are mandated for all nursing home residents, there is no added burden to nursing home staff in performing these assessments (Rabinowitz et al. 2010). Recently, trials of asynchronous telepsychiatry consultations in nursing homes have been conducted by Xiong and his colleagues at the University of California Davis, with early results showing that these types of consultations are feasible and well accepted by patients, family members, staff, and psychiatrists (see "Pilot Study of Asynchronous and Synchronous Telepsychiatry for Skilled Nursing Facilities" [ClinicalTrials.gov Identifier: NCT02537093]; available at: https://clinicaltrials.gov/ct2/show/NCT02537093). A longer-term outcome trial is planned.

CASE EXAMPLE 5: NURSING HOME CARE FOR A CONFUSED SENIOR[5]

The patient, an 80-year-old widow residing in a skilled nursing facility, was confused and repeatedly combative to the point that some staff threatened to quit after she assaulted them. The woman had been sent via ambulance several times to the local ED for psychiatric evaluation and treatment without improvement. The patient's daughter was distraught about how her mother's mental state had deteriorated so much within a relatively short period of time. The woman's PCP requested a telepsychiatry consultation at the skilled nursing facility. The telepsychiatrist met with the patient and the staff who usually cared for her; established a diagnosis of delirium (likely caused by polypharmacy-related interactions of drugs being prescribed for the woman's multiple medical and psychiatric problems); and, in conjunction with the PCP, simplified her medication regimen. The patient improved significantly, stopped being combative, and no longer required trips to the local ED. At 6-month follow-up, the patient remained stable and was able to communicate well with her daughter, was not confused, and had a markedly improved quality of life.

❚ KEY CONCEPT

The patient-centered medical home model works well in skilled nursing facilities, where PCPs, facility staff, and telepsychiatrists are able to collaborate to provide optimal patient-focused care.

CARE IN PRISONS

Some of the largest telepsychiatry programs have been set up in correctional facilities in several states across the country. The main goals of these programs have been to improve access to mental health care for patients located in geographically isolated or difficult-to-access prisons and to lower overall costs. Provider compensation for telepsychiatry in prisons

---

[5]Case provided by Barb Johnston, M.S.N.

has been sufficient to recruit and retain telepsychiatrists. Each state has a different logistic approach. For example, 27 prisons across California have telepsychiatry programs, as described in Chapter 3 ("The Business of Telepsychiatry"), but these programs require the current workforce of about 40 full-time-equivalent psychiatrists to work from one of three Department of Corrections and Rehabilitation facilities located across the state. These specialists are not allowed to provide telepsychiatry from their own homes or offices. By contrast, the University of Texas Medical Branch does allow its telepsychiatrists to work from their own offices. Inmates who may be violent or destructive frequently require prison staff to be present during the consultations, which mirrors what happens when such consultations are performed in person in prisons. Inmate satisfaction with telepsychiatry consultations has consistently been shown to be equivalent to satisfaction with in-person consultations (Deslich et al. 2013). In addition, this approach may be much safer for providers and patients when the patient is paranoid, guarded, frightened, aggressive, impulsive, or intoxicated, and female psychiatrists in particular have reported feeling much safer working in corrections via telepsychiatry.

CARE FOR ELDERLY PATIENTS

Regular users of telemedicine are not surprised that many older persons readily accept and adapt to videoconferencing technologies for health care, because this population has been using the technology for some time, although not for medical purposes. For example, grandparents, close friends, and many others refuse to let great distances prevent them from sharing meaningful events in their loved ones' lives, such as births, graduations, religious milestones, or a first piano or ballet recital. Thus, they have become proficient in the use of various hardware and software applications that allow them to keep in touch from a distance. In another example, "snowbirds" are retirees who "fly south" for the winter, leaving their cold permanent residences for more temperate regions. They keep in touch with their families and friends using smartphones, tablets, or other technologies and rarely miss important occasions. Likewise, they communicate with physicians, psychotherapists, and other health care providers using the same equipment and software.

DISEASE-SPECIFIC PROGRAMS

Children and adolescents with cystic fibrosis lead challenging lives. They often require hospitalization for respiratory infections, they must live with the knowledge of a likely shortened life, and they frequently miss school, work, or social activities because of exacerbations in their illness. Perhaps worse than any of these complications is the fact that the disease imposes separation from other affected individuals—because of the risk of cross-infection, people with cystic fibrosis should not have in-person contact with each other, so that these young people cannot easily experience the benefits of support from peers with CF who would understand their experiences. A dedicated and creative team at the University of New Mexico met this challenge head on by developing and implementing a "Cyber CF" program—a "peer support group for teens with cystic fibrosis to share ideas, feelings, and support each other via videoconference sessions." The program is the first and thus far the only program of its kind and is almost completely adolescent run, with support provided as necessary by the professional team. Adolescents who have participated have found it to be life-enhancing and supportive, and it has enabled them to have frank discussions about their illness and what it means to them. This program represents an especially creative adaptation of videoconferencing technology and telepsychiatry.

PTSD is a serious condition, with certain occupations, including military personnel and first responders, at increased risk due to greater trauma exposure. Many individuals with PTSD do not seek care because of concerns about stigmatization or privacy, because of apprehension about being perceived as emotionally weak, or because long distances make it impossible or impractical to access care. A recent pilot study by Olden et al. (2017) examined whether exposure therapy for PTSD could be delivered via videoconferencing and whether medication (i.e., the cognitive enhancer D-cycloserine) could be administered safely with potential side effects monitored from a distance. Eleven adults with PTSD enrolled, and seven completed 12–15 sessions. There were significant decreases in PTSD and depression symptoms. Subjects reported high satisfaction with both the therapeutic alliance and their treatment, as well as with telemental health care. In addition, there were no significant technical, medication, or safety issues, leading the authors to conclude that it may be feasible to conduct clinical PTSD research and to increase access to PTSD care using a videoconferencing approach.

These findings are important, because PTSD awareness continues to increase, making it more likely that more cases will be diagnosed, with an increased need for PTSD care from mental health care providers. Using a telemedicine approach to deliver some of this care will increase the likelihood that it will be available to larger and more diverse populations, especially to trauma survivors in rural and other underserved areas.

Although palliative care does not squarely fall under the rubric of telepsychiatry, it often contains mental health care components that contribute to its quality. Menon et al. (2015) performed a review of telemedicine family conferences for critically ill patients whose providers requested transfer from their community hospital to a larger tertiary care center. This study sought to learn whether palliative care consultations for critically ill patients via telemedicine are feasible and to identify barriers to providing these consultations. The investigators performed 12 palliative care consultations via telemedicine prior to transfer. After consultation, 8 (67%) patients were transferred to the tertiary-care center, and 4 (33%) patients received care at their regional hospital. Of the patients who were transferred, 7 (88% of those transferred) returned to their community after a stay at the tertiary-care center. The investigators concluded that palliative care consultations can be provided via telemedicine with relative ease and that these consultations may be especially important for patients in smaller community hospitals, enabling their care providers to help them die in familiar surroundings rather than be transferred to a larger, less-well-known facility for their final days.

INTERNATIONAL TELEPSYCHIATRY

Telepsychiatry has been leveraged as an important tool for addressing mental health problems in the developing world. Four hundred fifty million people worldwide have mental disorders, representing 13% of the global burden of disease, with more than 75% of this cohort receiving no treatment (World Health Organization 2012). Telepsychiatry has been used to treat specific clinical populations (e.g., refugees) and respond to specific crisis situations. Care models applied in the developing world have had a population-based focus, such as supporting national health services' missions through training and increasing the ability of local health care providers to deliver evidence-based best practices to their patients.

Individual providers or organizations providing care in these settings need to be knowledgeable not only about national rules and regulations and health care systems but also about local cultural frameworks around health and illness. Strong partnership and collaboration with in-country organizations and local expertise is essential for successful international services (Augusterfer et al. 2015).

TELEPSYCHIATRY RESEARCH PROGRAMS

Although research in telepsychiatry has been conducted since the late 1950s, and many studies have found that telepsychiatry could be provided efficiently, was cost-effective, led to improvements in outcomes, and was well accepted, most of these studies were limited by small and heterogeneous samples, making findings potentially less generalizable and therefore less convincing (Rabinowitz et al. 2008). This shortage of robust telepsychiatry studies was responsible in part for the lack of telepsychiatry's acceptance as a viable alternative to face-to-face care for many decades, even though many individual telepsychiatry providers knew it "worked." More recent studies have benefited from the lessons learned from these early investigations, and the two broadest evidence-based reviews (Bashshur et al. 2016; Hilty et al. 2013) both concluded that there is robust research support for telepsychiatry's efficacy across a wide variety of clinical settings and interventions used in telepsychiatry practice. Compared with research evidence for all other areas of telemedicine, that for telepsychiatry is supported by more randomized controlled trials, with larger sample sizes, greater statistical power, and more highly focused hypotheses. In addition, telepsychiatry's instrumentation has become increasingly more reliable and user-friendly, and telepsychiatry providers and staff are generally better educated about and proficient in using the equipment currently available on the market. These advances contribute to better telepsychiatry investigations and findings that are reproducible and compelling and that can be used as the basis for more powerful and costly studies, because potential funding sources are more likely to be convinced that these investigations will be fruitful.

One important and burgeoning area of telepsychiatry/telepsychology research is assessment. Several investigations have shown that some psychiatric, neuropsychiatric, and neurocognitive assessments can be performed by videoconference with results comparable to those of assessments performed face-to-face. These findings are important because they demonstrate that both qualitative and quantitative assessments can be performed from a distance, with the potential to provide more frequent and timely evaluations in order to track patients more closely and to detect important changes earlier in their occurrence (Amarendran et al. 2011; Galusha-Glasscock et al. 2016).

TELEPSYCHIATRY EDUCATION PROGRAMS

Formal telemedicine/telepsychiatry courses or programs have been added to some medical, nursing, psychology, or other health care provider curricula. In addition, telepsychiatry is being informally offered or taught in many programs. The most common way it is taught is through a quasi-apprenticeship approach. In this method, a learner interested in telepsychiatry will first sit in on a telepsychiatry session with an experienced telepsychiatry provider, observing the provider–patient interaction and perhaps working the telepsychiatry apparatus controls and so forth. At the next session, the "apprentice" might initiate the telepsychiatry encounter and perform an assessment or provide treatment under supervision. At subsequent sessions, the learner might provide some telepsychiatry treatments, with the instructor not physically present at first but joining the encounter at the end of the visit, as is often the approach with an in-person consultation. In this way, the interested student has a chance to see how telepsychiatry is done, develop his or her own approach while receiving constructive feedback from the instructor, and eventually, after amassing a number of "solo" encounters, teach others how to be a telepsychiatrist.

Telepsychiatry education fits very nicely into the "see one, do one, teach one" approach, a common and effective methodology in medical education. An encouraging trend at some health care education programs is that telemedicine training is finding its way into the general curricula. A recent review of all psychiatry residency programs in the United States (Glover et al. 2013) indicated that about 15% of them offered some form of telepsychiatry training for residents, usually hands-on experiences as just described, but in some cases, such as at University of California Davis, month-long electives for final-year residents or specific telemedicine courses such as telepsychiatry or telehome health care for residents are available as part of a department's or division's collection of offerings. Of particular importance, telepsychiatry is slowly gaining a foothold as a component of mainstream health care education.

Training in telepsychiatry, and especially in the clinical and media skills components, is discussed in greater detail in Chapter 5 ("Media Communication Skills and the Ethical Doctor–Patient Relationship").

The American Medical Association has more recently been encouraging medical schools to include new curricula in health care technologies, including EHRs and telemedicine, to meet the needs of new-generation physicians (American Medical Association 2016).

WHAT MODELS OF CARE ARE MOST COMPATIBLE WITH TELEPSYCHIATRY?

There are several models of psychiatric care that can easily be adapted to a telepsychiatry approach (Table 4–2):

1. *Direct psychiatric consultation and treatment.* This model identifies the consulting psychiatrist as the primary psychiatric care provider. He or she examines the patient, develops the treatment plan, prescribes medications, writes orders, and when indicated provides psychotherapy. This model can be used in any setting but is often the default model in rural communities that may have a small community hospital but are generally some distance away from larger and/or teaching hospitals.
2. *Consultation–liaison model.* Here, the telepsychiatrist performs assessments for a primary care or another provider, with the referring provider implementing the recommendations. Ideally, the referring provider is present at and takes part in the consultation with the patient, and can help ensure that the joint plan created is understood and approved by the patient. However, in some consultation–liaison models, the psychiatrist performs the patient assessment and then transmits his or her recommendations (by secure note, telephone, text message, etc.) to the primary care provider. The consultation is expedited by use of a common/shared medical record—an EHR is ideal. Provision of consultation–liaison services for inpatients or ambulatory outpatients at a particular hospital may require the consulting telepsychiatrist to have privileges at that hospital and to be licensed in the state where the patient is located at the time the consultation is performed.
3. *Collaborative/integrated care model.* Here, the psychiatrist typically works as part of a team reviewing populations of patients as well as individual patients, and potentially undertaking both direct and indirect consultations either electronically or in person.

TABLE 4–2.　Telepsychiatry models

Model	Description	Comments/examples
Direct psychiatric consultation and treatment	Consulting psychiatrist is the primary psychiatric care provider.	This model is most often seen in smaller, rural communities that are some distance from larger, teaching hospitals.
Consultation–liaison (inpatient or outpatient)	Physician requests consultation, an evaluation is performed, and recommendations are made.	This model can be used when local experts are not available or when an additional expert's opinion might be helpful. Be mindful of privileging and licensure requirements.
Direct (focused) consultation	Telepsychiatrist has responsibility for specific decisions/recommendations but not for ongoing psychiatric care.	This model is used for forensic psychiatry evaluations, transplant evaluations, and addictions evaluations.
Traditional referral (outpatient)	Patient is referred to psychiatrist, who provides the care in a behavioral health clinic or private office.	Telepsychiatrist can consult with patient at clinic, private office, patient's home, or elsewhere.
Collaborative care/embedded service (outpatient)	PCP and psychiatrist provide care; psychiatrist is available at specific times, usually when consultee is also available; at times psychiatrist and referring physician (and sometimes others) meet together with patient.	Telepsychiatrist availability is enhanced, given the decreased need to travel, and there is greater flexibility in scheduling.

TABLE 4–2. Telepsychiatry models *(continued)*

Model	Description	Comments/examples
Store and forward (asynchronous telepsychiatry; inpatient or outpatient)	Patient interview/examination is performed locally and recorded; consultant reviews results at a later time and makes recommendations.	Telepsychiatry consultations can be performed across multiple time zones, with support from native/expert speakers/translators, at any time of day or night, without significant disruptions to patient or consultant schedules.

Note. Asynchronous telepsychiatry consultation is ordered as an alternative to direct consultation (see Chapter 8, "Indirect Consultation and Hybrid Care").

Source. Adapted from Rabinowitz and Hilty 2016.

3A. *Direct (i.e., focused) consultations* are used to assess or monitor patients periodically, or to assess certain patients for specific purposes (e.g., prior to transplant or bariatric surgery, prior to starting a course of interferon) or for a forensic psychiatry examination. In this model, the telepsychiatrist is responsible for specific decisions and/or recommendations but not for ongoing psychiatric care.

3B. *Indirect psychiatric consultations* are used for any of the following purposes:

- Case review of patients with positive scores on routine screening (e.g., with PHQ-9, Generalized Anxiety Disorder–7, or Alcohol Use Disorders Identification Test [AUDIT]), along with all patients referred for care coordination, conducted by multidisciplinary teams including psychiatrists. In this model, the reviewing team provides feedback and treatment planning suggestions to the patients' PCPs via EHR messaging.
- Review of registries of patients with specific disorders by psychiatrists with specific interests in those disorders.
- Phone/e-mail/EHR "curbside" consultations between PCPs and psychiatrists connected to their clinics (see Chapter 8, "Indirect Consultation and Hybrid Care").
- E-consultations between PCPs and psychiatrists conducted via EHR messaging, with psychiatrists responding to PCP questions (see Chapter 8).

HOW IS TELEPSYCHIATRY TRANSFORMING WORK PRACTICES IN PSYCHIATRY?

Telepsychiatry is undoubtedly changing the work practices of many psychiatrists quite radically. It is now possible to work full- or part-time from home or when traveling. Patient-centered care models are requiring more psychiatrists to be available 24/7. Boundaries and limits of the doctor–patient relationship are becoming more flexible and less clear, as discussed in Chapter 5. While telepsychiatry makes these changing practice styles easier to adopt, the shortage of psychiatrists nationally limits the availability of providers willing to take on "after hours" work. Psychiatrists need to change the way that they work so that they increasingly perform larger numbers of indirect consultations, manage more populations of patients, and limit the numbers of private patients they see (either in person or using telepsychiatry) by focusing on the more difficult patients and relying on their primary care and mental health care colleagues and physician extenders to manage those patients with relatively straightforward problems. Many of these issues are discussed in detail in Chapter 8 ("Indirect Consultation and Hybrid Care").

Telepsychiatry allows specialists to work from their homes, thus avoiding travel at night for the specialist covering 24/7 shifts as well as for the patient. Mid-level practitioners and physician extenders are being included on more telepsychiatry teams to preserve psychiatrist resources by shouldering certain administrative tasks such as intake and data capture for EHRs. Mid-levels, psychiatric nurse practitioners, and virtual care navigators are increasingly being included in telepsychiatry programs (Chan et al. 2015; Yellowlees and Nafiz 2010). Virtual care navigators are able to complete patient intake information and some administrative tasks in a more cost-effective way than using psychiatrist time for this (Johnston and Yellowlees 2016). The psychiatrist can view the intake patient data recorded by a nonphysician staff member prior to a video consultation and in turn utilize his or her time more judiciously.

These work practice changes are likely to be accelerated under the soon-to-be-implemented new U.S. financing models in health care (as described in Chapter 1, "Psychiatric Practice in the Information Age"), in which payment for medical services is increasingly going to be related to quality, clinical outcomes, and results over time for populations of capitated patients. This environment is likely to strongly support the expansion of telepsychiatry programs, the costs of which will be covered by the capitated block funding available, and such programs may become standard of care for certain groups of patients that are known to have better outcomes at less cost when psychiatrists are involved. The primary patients of interest here are those with chronic medical problems, such as diabetes, chronic heart failure, and chronic respiratory disease. Studies have shown that many of these patients have depression and anxiety, and that if these mental disorders are effectively treated, patients' overall utilization of medical services (e.g., admissions, ED visits, investigations) is generally halved, and their medical and psychiatric outcomes are better.

There are many different models of care and approaches to providing telepsychiatry services, but they are all implemented within an overarching environment affected by the culture of both patients and providers. Therefore, it is crucial to understand the cultural influences impacting clinical practice from the perspectives of both the individual patient and the broader population.

What Are Culture, Cultural Competence, and Cultural Humility?

The term *culture* has wide application of use and meaning. In academic circles, there is no universally accepted definition, and a large number of definitions have been offered. Adopting a functional approach, we use a definition here of culture as "learned shared behavior and knowledge." Culture is knowledge related to how one interfaces with the world that is non-innate (i.e., it has to be learned either consciously or unconsciously) and is based on shared behavior and understanding between people. Culture encompasses beliefs, values, rituals, and customs and defines frameworks and models for understanding the world. There cannot be a culture of one, although culture may exist both in small social networks (two or more) and across millions of people. There are macro-cultures, as exemplified in the traditions and rituals of major religions with millions of followers, and micro-cultures, as exemplified in work environments where shared strategies of employees aid them in successfully completing duties. Culture heavily influences personal identity and defines group membership. All individuals belong to multiple macro- and micro-cultures, including those of gender, sexuality, ethnicity, religion, employment, and recreational interests, to list a few.

Anthropology uses *-emic* to describe inside/insider perspectives on a particular culture and *-etic* to describe outside/outsider perspectives. *Ethnocentrism* is the bias toward one's own culture based on the assumption that it is superior to other cultures. The concept of *cultural competence* broadly used in health care refers to health care organizations' and individual providers' ability to work successfully with and address the health care needs of patients from other cultures. Through training and education in other cultures, providers are thought to become "competent" to interact with and render care for members of the culture engaged in treatment. A more recent construct, *cultural humility,* which contrasts with cultural competence, emphasizes that it is extremely challenging to become fully competent in a culture of which one is not a member. This construct encompasses an attitude of unassuming openness to and acknowledgment of the inherent biases and perspectives one brings from one's own culture(s) to cross-cultural interactions and striving to understand a patient's background and perspective in an ongoing manner. Cultural competence represents a destination, whereas cultural humility is a journey.

WHAT ARE PSYCHIATRIC PERSPECTIVES ON CULTURE?

There is a rich history of the interplay of culture and psychiatry, and there are many current frameworks and approaches. One of the most commonly known and official frameworks comes from the *Diagnostic and Statistical Manual of Mental Disorders* (DSM). The fifth edition (DSM-5; American Psychiatric Association 2013, pp. 749–750) proffered an Outline for Cultural Formulation (OCF) for addressing cultural issues in psychiatric treatment through a five-component model:

1. Cultural identity of the individual
2. Cultural conceptualizations of distress
3. Psychosocial stressors and clinical features of vulnerability and resilience
4. Cultural features of the relationship between the individual and the clinician
5. Overall cultural assessment

Although all of these elements are important to attend to, numbers 1 and 4 have particular relevance to the use of technology in psychiatric care. The cultural background of the patient, including his or her individual and cultural experience and knowledge of technologies, impact how the patient regards and uses technology to receive care. The specific technology, including its structure, has important impacts on and implications for the patient–provider relationship. Both of these aspects are discussed in more detail in the sections below.

DSM-5 also built on the OCF to offer the Cultural Formulation Interview (CFI; DSM-5 pp. 750–754) to support clinical understanding and decision making. This semistructured interview focuses on the following domains:

1. Cultural definition of the problem
2. Cultural perceptions of cause, context, and support
3. Cultural factors affecting self-coping and past help seeking
4. Cultural factors affecting current help seeking

While this interview provides guidance toward a more systematized approach to eliciting cultural issues in treatment, it has less focus on the impact of technology in patient–provider dynamics than does the OCF.

How Can Technology Affect Cultural Issues and Communication During Psychiatric Treatment?

Technology is becoming the medium in which provider–patient interactions occur. As providers and patients interact across cultures, they also interact through the additional lenses and filters of a specific technology (e.g., mobile, videoconferencing, e-mail, Web platforms, EMR portals). Backgrounds, past experiences, and "technological literacy" levels can play critical roles in what both patients and providers bring to the psychiatric encounter. Attitudes toward use of technology in patients' or providers' cultures will influence their individual levels of comfort and use. Generational issues also come into play, such as whether individuals are digital natives (born after the 1990s) or digital immigrants (born before this period), and, for individuals coming later to technology, to what extent they use it in their daily activities.

The specific technology itself also brings its own framework and biases into the clinical setting. The majority of technologies deployed in Western medicine not only have been developed within Western frameworks but also are often created in and driven by the English language. A false assumption, proven wrong by numerous examples, is that technology is inherently unbiased or culturally neutral.

The mix of cross-cultural interactions and technology creates risks for misunderstanding and miscommunication between mental health care providers and the patients with whom they work. A few examples are as follows:

1. Adaptation (or lack of adaptation) of clinical style and process over videoconferencing to accommodate differing cultural communication styles
2. Proper attire and room setup for direct in-home videoconferencing
3. Differing understandings around the use of voicemail and expectations about returning calls when a message is not left
4. Alternative meanings for text messaging abbreviations (e.g., LOL = laughing out loud or lots of love)

5. Differing understandings and expectations regarding immediacy of response to e-mails

WHAT ARE THE POTENTIAL DOWNSIDES OF TECHNOLOGY-ENABLED DELIVERY OF CARE AT A DISTANCE?

Modern technologies in health care allow us to instantaneously traverse immense distances to reach patients, reducing travel burden and improving and creating access to mental health care. This rapidity often can transport providers into a clinical setting where they have little or no contextual knowledge of the patient's environment, culture, and resources. For example, a psychiatrist providing remote care for patients over videoconferencing at a medical facility may make assumptions about culture and environment based on the generic nature of the medical setting. Many videoconference-based services use a hub-and-spoke model locating providers at major academic or organizational headquarters, often in urban settings, to provide treatment to patients in remote or rural areas. Urban providers may or may not have knowledge and experience about important issues of providing treatment in rural environments (e.g., gun ownership, boundaries and relationships, local health care resources). Other technologies, such as e-mail, may give even less environmental or cultural context about the patient. For example, psychiatrists providing e-mail in "doc-to-doc" consultations may miss and make assumptions about important cultural factors in cases, especially if they lack familiarity with the setting in which the colleague they are consulting with is located.

WHAT ARE THE BENEFITS OF TECHNOLOGY FOR CROSS-CULTURAL TREATMENT?

Despite the challenges and pitfalls discussed, the integration of technology into mental health care confers multiple benefits for both patients and providers.

- *Increased access to care.* Telepsychiatry, in the form of live interactive videoconferencing, has demonstrated its utility to deliver culturally appropriate care to a wide and diverse array of populations, including notable examples with Native American and Alaska Native communities, Hispanic populations, and international settings and across a range of populations, ages, settings, communities, and environments. Specific culturally adapted clinics and technologies have helped to increase both the quantity and the quality of care available, especially for many underserved and minority communities challenged by both cultural and geographic barriers.

- *Outreach, education, and community engagement.* Technology can be leveraged in creative ways to work to better engage and educate communities around mental health care services, with these efforts tailored and targeted to specific populations and subgroups through a range of platforms.
- *Translation services.* Technology is making translation services more readily available, historically via telephone but now via videoconferencing as well as text-based, mobile, and voice recognition services.

How Can Clinicians Use Technology in a Manner That Supports Culturally Informed Treatment?

Strategies for dealing with cultural issues and technology can be classified into two categories: those intended to deepen awareness and understanding of how cultural and technology interact in a clinical setting, and those intended to adapt clinical processes to increase the cultural fit of treatment. These assume that clinicians are committed to and engaged in working on developing cultural competence and/or humility with the populations they are serving and using tools such as those offered by DSM to navigate cross-cultural issues.

STRATEGIES TO DEEPEN AWARENESS AND UNDERSTANDING

- Clinicians should develop insight into their own levels of technological competence, literacy, and regard for technology and how their backgrounds, cultures, and education have influenced these levels.
- Clinicians should be aware of their own possible biases, assumptions, and expectations regarding the specific technology platform(s) they use to interact with patients.
- In the initial assessment and engagement with patients, clinicians should include a review of patients' experiences with and perspectives on various communications technologies and the potential cultural influences of these perspectives.

- Clinicians should work to become familiar with the cultures, environments, and resources in the communities in which their patients live. These efforts should include learning about local communication styles, norms, and patterns.

STRATEGIES TO ADAPT CLINICAL PROCESS TO INCREASE CULTURAL FIT IN TREATMENT

- After the initial assessment of technology, clinicians should perform ongoing assessments of patients' reactions to, comfort with, and regard for the technologies used.
- Clinicians should educate their patients about the technologies they are using; inform patients about how these could impact clinical processes, communication, and rapport; and initiate an ongoing dialogue with patients around technology's impact on the clinical relationship.
- Clinicians should consider modifying their clinical workflows, processes, and communications technologies as appropriate to accommodate the cultural norms and preferences of their patients. Such modifications may require consultation with individuals who have greater familiarity with the culture, including colleagues, staff at the patient site, and cultural facilitators. Clinicians should adapt their communication patterns to local cultural styles and seek to acquire local cultural knowledge.
- Clinicians may want to develop formal working relationships with cultural facilitators and incorporate these facilitators into their clinical processes.

How Can Mental Health Care Organizations and Systems Support the Provision of Culturally Informed Treatment?

Mental health care organizations and systems should support the development of their clinicians in striving for cultural competence/humility in the use of technology. Such support includes promotion of educational, training, and experiential activities (e.g., site visits) that help individual providers to improve their knowledge and understanding of the populations with which they are working.

Mental health care organizations and systems should recognize the interplay of culture and technology and the influence of technology on clinical processes and content. When proactively developing mental health care services that use technologies, organizations should consider obtaining the input, in iterative processes, of social science and community members. A possible stepwise process for developing a specific service could be

- Stage 1: Identify community.
- Stage 2: Build relationships.
- Stage 3: Learn the local cultural environment.
- Stage 4: Choose setting of care.
- Stage 5: Choose model of care.

SUMMARY

Telepsychiatry has shown efficacy in a wide array of populations, settings, and care models. To be successful and sustainable, a telepsychiatry practice must first select an appropriate model of care and then adapt and fit this model to the specific clinical services it will provide. Models of care include direct care, integrated care, and indirect and asynchronous telepsychiatry. Attention to both clinical and administrative aspects of technology use is critical to providing patient-centered care that is effective and culturally appropriate.

REFERENCES

Amarendran V, George A, Gersappe V, et al: The reliability of telepsychiatry for a neuropsychiatric assessment. Telemed J E Health 17(3):223–225, 2011 21443440

American Medical Association: AMA encourages telemedicine training for medical students, residents (press release), June 15, 2016. Available at: https://www.ama-assn.org/ama-encourages-telemedicine-training-medical-students-residents. Accessed April 3, 2017.

American Psychiatric Association: Diagnostic and Statistical Manual of Mental Disorders, 4th Edition. Washington, DC, American Psychiatric Association, 1994

American Psychiatric Association: Diagnostic and Statistical Manual of Mental Disorders, 5th Edition. Arlington, VA, American Psychiatric Association, 2013

Asmussen L, Olson LM, Grant EN, et al: Reliability and validity of the Children's Health Survey for Asthma. Pediatrics 104(6):e71, 1999 10586005

Augusterfer EF, Mollica RF, Lavelle J: A review of telemental health in international and post-disaster settings. Int Rev Psychiatry 27(6):540–546, 2015 26576720

Bashshur RL, Shannon GW, Bashshur N, Yellowlees PM: The empirical evidence for telemedicine interventions in mental disorders. Telemed J E Health 22(2):87–113, 2016 26624248

Bergman DA, Sharek PJ, Ekegren K, et al: The use of telemedicine access to schools to facilitate expert assessment of children with asthma. Int J Telemed Appl 159276, 2008 18369409

Cain S, Sharp S: Telepharmacotherapy for child and adolescent psychiatric patients. J Child Adolesc Psychopharmacol 26(3):221–228, 2016 26745771

Chan S, Parish M, Yellowlees P: Telepsychiatry today. Curr Psychiatry Rep 17(11):89, 2015 26384338

Deslich S, Thistlethwaite T, Coustasse A: Telepsychiatry in correctional facilities: using technology to improve access and decrease costs of mental health care in underserved populations. Marshall Digital Scholar, Management Faculty Research, Summer 2013. Available at: http://mds.marshall.edu/mgmt_faculty/85/. Accessed July 1, 2013.

DeVido J, Glezer A, Branagan L, et al: Telepsychiatry for inpatient consultations at a separate campus of an academic medical center. Telemed J E Health 22(7):572–576, 2016 26701608

Fortney JC, Pyne JM, Edlund MJ, et al: A randomized trial of telemedicine-based collaborative care for depression. J Gen Intern Med 22(8):1086–1093, 2007 17492326

Fortney JC, Pyne JM, Mouden SB, et al: Practice-based versus telemedicine-based collaborative care for depression in rural federally qualified health centers: a pragmatic randomized comparative effectiveness trial. Am J Psychiatry 170(4):414–425, 2013 23429924

Fortney JC, Pyne JM, Kimbrell TA, et al: Telemedicine-based collaborative care for posttraumatic stress disorder: a randomized clinical trial. JAMA Psychiatry 72(1):58–67, 2015 25409287

Galusha-Glasscock JM, Horton DK, Weiner MF, et al: Video teleconference administration of the Repeatable Battery for the Assessment of Neuropsychological Status. Arch Clin Neuropsychol 31(1):8–11, 2016 26446834

Glover JA, Williams E, Hazlett LJ, Campbell N: Connecting to the future: telepsychiatry in postgraduate medical education. Telemed J E Health 19(6):474–479, 2013 23570291

Godleski L, Nieves JE, Darkins A, Lehmann L: VA telemental health: suicide assessment. Behav Sci Law 26(3):271–286, 2008 18548515

Godleski L, Darkins A, Peters J: Outcomes of 98,609 U.S. Department of Veterans Affairs patients enrolled in telemental health services, 2006–2010. Psychiatr Serv 63(4):383–385, 2012 22476305

Grady B, Singleton M: Telepsychiatry "coverage" to a rural inpatient psychiatric unit. Telemed J E Health 17(8):603–608, 2011 21939381

Hilty DM, Yellowlees PM: Collaborative mental health services using multiple technologies: the new way to practice and a new standard of practice? J Am Acad Child Adolesc Psychiatry 54(4):245–246, 2015 25791139

Hilty DM, Ferrer DC, Parish MB, et al: The effectiveness of telemental health: a 2013 review. Telemed J E Health 19(6):444–454, 2013 23697504

Holden D, Dew E: Telemedicine in a rural gero-psychiatric inpatient unit: comparison of perception/satisfaction to onsite psychiatric care. Telemed J E Health 14(4):381–384, 2008 18570569

Johnston B: Integration of telepsychiatry into primary care: better care, better health, and lower cost. Presented at the 2015 American Telemedicine Association Annual Conference, Los Angeles, CA, May 5–7, 2015.

Johnston B, Yellowlees P: Telepsychiatry consultations in primary care coordinated by virtual care navigators. Psychiatr Serv 67(1):142, 2016 26725496

Katon W, Russo J, Lin EH, et al: Cost-effectiveness of a multicondition collaborative care intervention: a randomized controlled trial. Arch Gen Psychiatry 69(5):506–514, 2012 22566583

Menon PR, Stapleton RD, McVeigh U, et al: Telemedicine as a tool to provide family conferences and palliative care consultations in critically ill patients at rural health care institutions: a pilot study. Am J Hosp Palliat Care 32(4):448–453, 2015 24871344

Myers K, Vander Stoep A, Zhou C, et al: Effectiveness of a telehealth service delivery model for treating attention-deficit/hyperactivity disorder: a community-based randomized controlled trial. J Am Acad Child Adolesc Psychiatry 54(4):263–274, 2015 25791143

Narasimhan M, Druss BG, Hockenberry JM, et al: Impact of a telepsychiatry program at emergency departments statewide on the quality, utilization, and costs of mental health services. Psychiatr Serv 66(11):1167–1172, 2015 26129992

Office of the White House: Now Is the Time: The President's Plan to Protect Our Children and Our Communities by Reducing Gun Violence. Washington, DC, January 16, 2013. Available at: https://obamawhitehouse.archives.gov/sites/default/files/docs/wh_now_is_the_time_full.pdf. Accessed April 6, 2017.

Olden M, Wyka K, Cukor J, et al: Pilot study of a telehealth-delivered medication-augmented exposure therapy protocol for PTSD. J Nerv Ment Dis 205(2):154–160, 2017 27441461

Rabinowitz T, Hilty D; Academy of Psychosomatic Medicine: Telepsychiatry for vulnerable and underserved populations. Psychiatric Times 33(5):24F–24G, May 2016. Available at: http://www.psychiatrictimes.com/printpdf/217310. Accessed April 6, 2017.

Rabinowitz T, Brennan DM, Chumbler NR, et al: New directions for telemental health research. Telemed J E Health 14(9):972–976, 2008 19035810

Rabinowitz T, Murphy KM, Amour JL, et al: Benefits of a telepsychiatry consultation service for rural nursing home residents. Telemed J E Health 16(1):34–40, 2010 20070161

Seidel RW, Kilgus MD: Agreement between telepsychiatry assessment and face-to-face assessment for emergency department psychiatry patients. J Telemed Telecare 20(2):59–62, 2014 24414395

Shore JH, Hilty DM, Yellowlees P: Emergency management guidelines for telepsychiatry. Gen Hosp Psychiatry 29(3):199–206, 2007 17484936

Shore P, Goranson A, Ward MF, Lu MW: Meeting veterans where they're @: a VA home-based telemental health (HBTMH) pilot program. Int J Psychiatry Med 48(1):5–17, 2014 25354923

Stephan S, Lever N, Bernstein L, et al: Telemental health in schools. J Child Adolesc Psychopharmacol 26(3):266–272, 2016 26982886

Unützer J, Katon W, Callahan CM, et al; IMPACT Investigators (Improving Mood-Promoting Access to Collaborative Treatment): Collaborative care management of late-life depression in the primary care setting: a randomized controlled trial. JAMA 288(22):2836–2845, 2002 12472325

World Health Organization: Global burden of mental disorders and the need for a comprehensive, coordinated response from health and social sectors at the country level. 130th Session of the World Health Organization Executive Board; Agenda item 6.2, Document EB130.R8; January 20, 2012. Available at: http://apps.who.int/gb/ebwha/pdf_files/EB130/B130_R8-en.pdf. Accessed August 29, 2017.

Yellowlees P, Nafiz N: The psychiatrist-patient relationship of the future: anytime, anywhere? Harv Rev Psychiatry 18(2):96–102, 2010 20235774

Yellowlees P, Burke MM, Marks SL, et al: Emergency telepsychiatry. J Telemed Telecare 14(6):277–281, 2008 18776070

5

Media Communication Skills and the Ethical Doctor–Patient Relationship

Peter Yellowlees, MBBS, M.D.

Lisa Roberts, Ph.D.

Peter Shore, Psy.D.

In this chapter, we focus on the clinical skills and information that mental health care professionals need to practice effectively online. The emphasis in the majority of the chapter is on real-time online communication skills.

WHAT TYPES OF ONLINE CONSULTATIONS CAN BE CONDUCTED VIA TELEPSYCHIATRY?

Broadly there are two types of online consultations: *direct* (also known as "real time" or "synchronous") and *indirect* (also known as "store and forward" or "asynchronous") (Figure 5–1). Direct behavioral health consultations are what most people think of when they use the word *telepsychiatry* and are clinically similar to in-person clinic consultations but delivered at a distance using videoconferencing technology. Patients are typically seen in a distant location, such as a clinic or an emergency department; a correctional institution; or (increasingly) their own homes. These are the main settings that are the focus of this chapter.

Indirect psychiatric consultations, which are increasingly being used in the stepped-care integrated primary mental health care model (Yellowlees et al. 2011), are summarized briefly here and discussed in more detail in Chapter 8 ("Indirect Consultation and Hybrid Care"). Examples of indirect consultations include the following:

- *Evidence-based screening consultations* involve multidisciplinary (including psychiatrists) team–based reviews of panels of patients or individual cases. These team reviews often include routine screening of patients using instruments such as the Patient Health Questionnaire–9, the Generalized Anxiety Disorder–7, and the Alcohol Use Disorders Identification Test (AUDIT). Feedback and treatment planning suggestions are then returned to the patients' primary care physicians (PCPs) electronically using electronic medical record (EMR) messaging or similar electronic systems. Most of these approaches are based on the seminal studies at the University of Washington by Wayne Katon, M.D., and Jurgen Unützer, M.D., over the past several decades (Raney et al. 2014), and are backed up by more than 80 clinical trials that demonstrate the clinical and outcome effectiveness of these methods.
- *Patient registry consultations* involve reviews of registries of patients with specific disorders, such as depression or bipolar disorder, by psychiatrists with specific interests in those disorders. Such registries, which are supported by multiple data sources, can yield information about the quality of care being provided to these patients—for instance, whether all patients taking lithium are receiving annual renal and thyroid function tests, or whether all patients with depression are being offered therapeutic doses of antidepressants and appropriate psychotherapies. If certain patients are outliers or seem not to be receiving guideline-based care, the reviewer is able to contact the PCP and local treating team to reinforce whatever is missing.
- *Online provider-to-provider (in-person or telephone) consultations*— "curbside" consultations between PCPs and psychiatrists—have long been common, and most PCPs have a network of specialist providers whom they can phone or e-mail with questions about their patients when they are looking mainly for broad directions or ideas to improve the care of individual patients but where relatively little detail about the patient tends to be given.

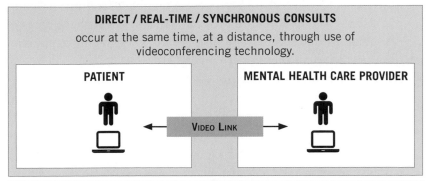

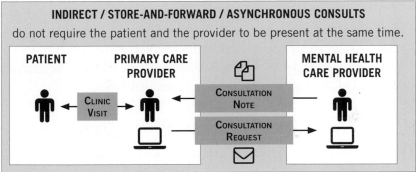

FIGURE 5–1. "Direct" versus "Indirect" consultations.

Source. Diagram and illustrations by Steven Chan, M.D., M.B.A. Used with permission. Icons are open source under SIL International's open font license (OFL) 1.1. Font Awesome, by Dave Gandy (http://fontawesome.io).

- *Online provider-to-provider (electronic) consultations*—usually consisting of psychiatrists responding to PCP questions via EMR messaging—are becoming increasingly common, as is discussed in Chapter 8. These "e-consultations" essentially are an enhanced form of curbside consultations, but in this case the psychiatrist 1) receives a formal referral or a set of questions from a PCP, perhaps with some algorithmically developed responses to questions; 2) ideally, reviews the patient notes in a shared EMR or reviews whatever detailed information is sent by the PCP; and 3) responds with an opinion and treatment suggestions for the PCP to consider. These sorts of consultations are increasingly being supported by templates that many psychiatrists and PCPs develop so that consultations can be conducted more rapidly, frequently within 10–15 minutes. A number of commercial companies have set up software programs that support these types of consultations, and some health insurers are now agreeing to pay relatively small fees for them to be conducted.

- *Asynchronous telepsychiatry consultations*—in which a patient is recorded during a semistructured interview conducted by an expert interviewer—are beginning to be used more frequently. The recording is then sent to a psychiatrist, who reviews the data from the interview as well as other relevant and available collateral information and writes an opinion and treatment plan that is sent back to the referring PCP for consideration. These types of consultations, which in some respects constitute a very much improved form of e-consultation, are discussed in greater detail later in this chapter, as well as in Chapter 8. Asynchronous telepsychiatry consultations are likely to be increasingly used as an alternative to direct consultations.

HOW DO TELEPSYCHIATRY CONSULTATIONS DIFFER FROM TRADITIONAL IN-PERSON CLINIC CONSULTATIONS?

The traditional in-person psychiatric consultation is straightforward and consists of collecting a history and other relevant information from the patient, his or her family, and potentially outside sources and then arriving at a diagnosis or differential diagnosis. Following discussion with the patient and, potentially, a review of relevant lab or imaging results, a treatment plan is created and carried out if the patient is in agreement. Much of this process occurs through the doctor–patient relationship, and the treatment plan often evolves gradually and iteratively over multiple sessions as the patient and physician get to know each other. The overall process is tried and tested and works well, and—with most patients being seen on videoconferencing in real time—is not so different from the process of seeing patients in person, as described later. At University of California Davis, we use a standard telepsychiatry consultation template similar to that shown in Figure 5–2.

Patient Name:	Consultant:
Medical Record No.:	Specialty: Psychiatry
Date of Birth:	Referring PCP:
Gender:	Referring Site:
Race:	
New/Follow-Up Patient:	Date of Telemedicine Consultation:

CHIEF COMPLAINT:
HISTORY OF PRESENT ILLNESS:
Brief Summary of Positive Aspects:
Symptom Information:
Developmental History:
Past Medical/Psychiatric History:
Family History:
Medication History/Current Medications:
Abuses/Trauma:
MENTAL STATUS EXAMINATION:
Physical appearance:
Behavior:
Speech:
Mood:
Affect:
Thoughts:
Suicidal or homicidal intent present?
Psychosis:
Cognition:
Insight:
IMPRESSION AND CODES:
1. Psychiatric Diagnosis:
2. Medical Diagnosis
SELF-HARM/VIOLENCE POTENTIAL:
TREATMENT RECOMMENDATIONS:
1. Lifestyle: *(e.g., education on illness/medications, sleep, exercise)**
2. Recommended medication changes: *(up to 3 medication and dosage alternatives)*
3. Discuss cautions/side effects for use of medication.
4. Referrals required *(e.g., labs, tests, other specialists)*
5. Psychotherapy: *(e.g., CBT/psychodynamic therapy, couples counseling, substance abuse treatment)*
6. Psychoeducation *(e.g., book/Internet resources on illness)*
QUESTIONS FOR PCP TO FOLLOW UP OR CLARIFY:
COMMENTS ON INTERVIEW:
FOLLOW-UP:
Primary care: *(e.g., PCP to see patient in ___ weeks after intervention)*
Psychiatry: *(e.g., telepsychiatry in ___ weeks prn or doc-to-doc consultation by pager or e-mail)*

FIGURE 5–2. Sample telepsychiatrist consultation note.

*Italicized entries are examples of recommendations.

CBT=cognitive-behavioral therapy; PCP=primary care physician.

Source. As used at University of California Davis.

WHAT MEDIA AND CLINICAL SKILLS DO CLINICIANS NEED TO WORK SUCCESSFULLY ONLINE WITH THEIR PATIENTS?

MEDIA SKILLS

Why do we need to have good media skills? Simply put, clinicians with good media communication skills will interact better with their patients, will find using communications technologies more interesting and fun, and will ultimately be better physicians whose patients have better outcomes. Eric Topol, M.D., recognized as a clinical innovator/entrepreneur, used the phrase "webside manner" (instead of "bedside manner") to refer to the new ways to interact with patients using technology. What are the communication and media skills we need to use when interacting online on video with our patients?

When you are seeking information on media and clinical skills, the first place to begin is the Web site for the American Telemedicine Association (ATA; www.americantelemed.org). Here there is a large amount of information, with several sets of clinical guidelines (for both adult and pediatric patients) available for downloading, as well as numerous streamed lectures and PowerPoint-driven courses available in the learning center, once you have joined as a member. The quickest way of learning about how to practically deliver mental health care services via video is to attend the ATA annual meeting. This meeting is attended by mental health care professionals from a wide range of disciplines (e.g., nurses, social workers, psychologists, psychiatrists) who work in clinics, private practice, institutions, and businesses. There are specific workshops, presentations, and networking events to provide access to individuals who want to further the adoption of online telemental health care and increase their networks of colleagues globally. There are also discipline-specific resources. The American Psychiatric Association also has a formal committee on telepsychiatry (www.psychiatry.org/psychiatrists/practice/telepsychiatry) that has developed an excellent toolkit of more than 30 short videos (presented by many of the authors of chapters in this book) on most aspects of telepsychiatry, including a short video on media communication skills presented by Peter Yellowlees, M.D. The American Psychological Association has developed guidelines for psychologists (Joint Task Force for the Development of Telepsychology Guidelines for Psychologists 2013).

CASE EXAMPLE 1: TELEPSYCHIATRY WITH ALASKA NATIVES: LEVERAGING TECHNOLOGY IN PROVIDING CULTURALLY RELEVANT AND PATIENT-CENTERED CARE[1]

A 43-year-old Alaska Native woman is referred to see a male telepsychiatrist for treatment of chronic problems with sleep and anxiety. These symptoms are complicated by a childhood and adult history of sexual trauma perpetrated by several significant male relations. The patient is hesitant to meet with an outsider who is male over a videoconferencing system but has enough trust in her local PCP to attend the initial visit. The psychiatrist greets her with a traditional greeting from her tribal language. He then takes time to explain the videoconferencing system, the telepsychiatry service, and his relationship with the local tribal health care system. After discussing the patient's previous experiences and exposure to video conferencing, he reviews the purpose and process of the initial session. The psychiatrist then talks briefly about his recent visit to the community, mentioning several local staff members and community leaders he had the pleasure of visiting with. He asks the patient if the weather has been affecting the fishing season. After checking in with the patient to see whether she has additional questions, the psychiatrist proceeds with an initial assessment, making sure to take a detailed cultural history. At the conclusion of the session, he shares his impressions, recommendations, and next steps, including coordination with on-site providers. He finishes by asking the patient how she feels about the session. She replies that after she got used to the format, she felt fairly comfortable, and meeting a male psychiatrist by video gave her a sense of control and safety in the session, allowing her to share her difficult history of trauma. The psychiatrist refers the patient to a local therapist for trauma-focused anxiety management and continues to work with the patient on an ongoing basis, prescribing medications and providing overall case consultation to the therapist.

▎ KEY CONCEPTS

Telepsychiatry can be a powerful tool to improve cross-cultural care when integrated into the patient's environment.

For patients with a history of trauma, telepsychiatry may offer empowerment by giving patients a sense of safety and control via the clinical distance and virtual space created.

---

[1]Case provided by Jay H. Shore, M.D., M.P.H.

Video media skills are similar to those used by TV anchors and need to be practiced and learned. We have all seen flat and relatively unemotional interviewees on television who are talking in their natural voices and not trying to emphasize their words or beliefs with changes in tone, manner, or movement. Contrast this with the experienced TV anchor, who is interesting, credible, and alert. As clinicians, our goal should be to learn specific media communication skills so that we come across to our patients like an experienced TV anchor.

Exercise

Turn off the sound on your TV and study a number of anchors. Observe their nonverbal behaviors. Notice how they use facial expressions and movements much more than they would in an in-person conversation. Now turn on the sound and listen to how they accentuate their language with extra emphasis and tone to make their points. None of this comes naturally. It all has to be learned. See whether you can do this.

There are many courses in media training available, often run by experienced TV journalists. Most of them involve the students being asked to take part in a number of recorded exercises in which they are observed by the rest of the group. They are then asked to criticize themselves after they review their recordings, before the group does the same. During the course of a few hours, with a group of three or four students, each student can generally take part in three or four interviews—as both an interviewer and interviewee and in a number of different situations. The topics chosen can be either benign ("Let's talk about what you did last weekend") or difficult ("How do you feel about our national immigration policy?"), and the interviewer can be friendly or aggressive. It is amazing how quickly you get over the initial embarrassment and performance anxiety that most of us have when seeing ourselves on video and how quickly you learn to forget about the camera and present yourself well. We strongly advise all clinicians to undergo formal media training or a similar course or, as some of us have done, do several of them with different tutors. At the end of the day you need to be able to present yourself with 120% of the energy and style that you use in your daily conversations. You must use extra gestures and vocal intonation and know how you will come across on TV so that you will not be afraid of "performing" when you see your patients. It is crucial that you learn to watch yourself and critically evaluate and improve your online presence. One way of doing this continuously when you are seeing patients is to routinely use the "picture in picture" function on your screen, if you have one, or record yourself, so that you can see yourself, and how you look (Figures 5–3 and 5–4). You will be making sure not just that you are well centered (eyes typically two-thirds of the way up the screen) and taking up about half of the total screen space, but also that you come across as warm and engaging rather than flat and defensive.

Let us first look at all the general online organizational and communication skills a clinician needs (Figure 5–5).

Dress Professionally

Lots of jokes are made about how it is possible to be wearing a smart shirt and tie and pajama bottoms and bunny slippers while consulting on video. There are at least two reasons that it is important to dress as you would for an in-person visit. First, you will behave in a more professional manner. Second, appearance models both self-care and respect for yourself and others, which can be very important for the therapeutic relationship. You will find, for instance, that a number of patients, especially elderly women, who have not been "on television" before, will actually dress up for the occasion, with more makeup than usual, well-coiffed hair, and their best clothes. We have seen this numerous times when conducting consultations in nursing homes, where the actual appearance on TV, and the extra beauty preparation involved, have been extremely therapeutic for patients. As a rule of thumb, it is best to always be smart and well presented. Color choice is important for TV and video. Dark colors such as blue or black are generally most forgiving, and white and green least forgiving. Patterns on ties, blazers, blouses, and scarves should be small. Jewelry is acceptable but should be smaller scale; if you look like you are wearing a sculpture around your neck, the person on the other side will be distracted. Remember that patients are there to see you, not your flashing gold bangles.

Be Punctual for Your Consultations

A great saying from the military is "If you are on time, you are late." Because you may need to make adjustments to the room or equipment, you will need to build in a time buffer for such fine-tuning, just as you would for a clinic session, to ensure that your audio and visual devices are work-

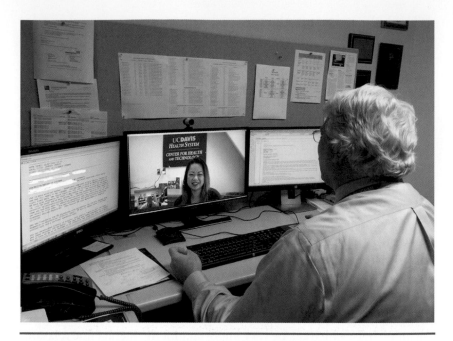

FIGURE 5–3.   Three-screen telemedicine desk setup.

Source.   Photograph courtesy of Peter Yellowlees, MBBS, M.D. Used with permission.

ing properly. Remember that audio is actually more important than video—you can do a consultation with poor video as long as you and your patient can hear each other adequately, but nothing will work, however well you can see each other, if you cannot hear. So very occasionally you may be asked, if bandwidth is low, which modality you wish to maintain quality on. Always choose audio, which anyway requires less bandwidth by itself.

Maximize Lighting and Décor

Check that the lighting in your room is sufficient and is not causing glare on the camera. The trick here is to make sure that there is no bright light behind your head causing your face to be dark and in shadow. If you are able to close all the curtains and doors and turn on the main room lights as brightly as possible, you will generally look the best. Keep in mind your background. Many health care providers use desktop systems in their usual clinic rooms or offices and sit at their desks, so frequently bookshelves or paintings behind them are an excellent backdrop as long

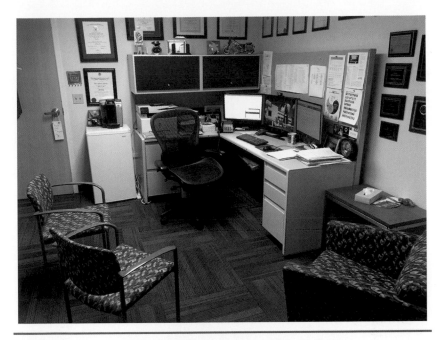

FIGURE 5–4. Clinician's office set up for both telemedicine and in-person consultations.

Source. Photograph courtesy of Peter Yellowlees, MBBS, M.D. Used with permission.

as they are not too busy and distracting. Avoid potentially divisive (e.g., political, religious) background décor.

Be Technologically Competent

Know how to operate your technology and be specifically aware of limitations such as nonmuting, poor visual definition, impaired audio, and speech delay. Despite significant improvements in hardware, software, and connectivity, there are common issues. Without a doubt, the greatest potential source of trouble is the mute button. Be extremely careful to stay aware of whether you are on mute. Imagine a scenario in which you have a student or colleague with you and you start to explain some stigmatized issue about the patient, or make some rather off-the-cuff comment about, for instance, your patient's personality style, meant only for the ears of your student or colleague, and the patient hears what you say. Whether it is a clinical consultation or an online meeting, there are numerous examples of people mistakenly thinking that they were muted

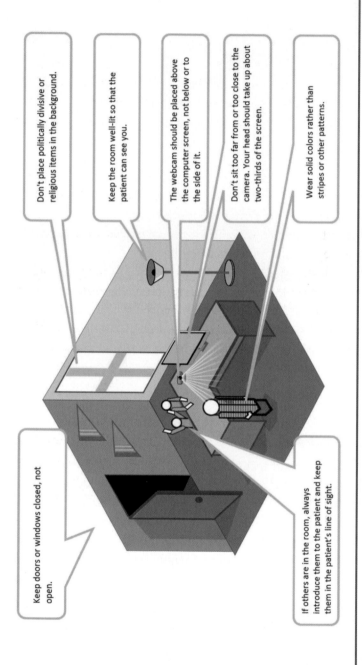

Don't place politically divisive or religious items in the background.

Keep the room well-lit so that the patient can see you.

The webcam should be placed above the computer screen, not below or to the side of it.

Don't sit too far from or too close to the camera. Your head should take up about two-thirds of the screen.

Wear solid colors rather than stripes or other patterns.

Keep doors or windows closed, not open.

If others are in the room, always introduce them to the patient and keep them in the patient's line of sight.

FIGURE 5–5. Creating a safe and professional physical environment for telepsychiatry.

Source. Diagram and illustrations by Steven Chan, M.D., M.B.A. Used with permission.

when they were not. To stay on the safe side, it is best to assume that all parties are able to hear all comments.

Maintain Good Visual Positioning

Sit comfortably in your chair and adjust the height so that you maintain good visual positioning (eyes two-thirds up) on your screen for yourself and for all participants. Do not make the mistake of sitting too close to the screen, with your head taking up more than half of the image space, or sitting over a laptop, so that observers at the far end can see the ceiling of your room behind you. This positioning is very off-putting and does not allow you to make good natural eye contact with your patients. It is usually best to be at least 3 feet away from your screen if you are using a plain camera attached to, or part of, a computer. This extra distance gives you a fairly small angle of difference between your camera height and your eye level on the screen, to make it appear that you are able to have reasonably good eye contact during the sessions.

Some systems have a pan/tilt/zoom camera that you can use to adjust your position and, often, that of others taking part in the conference at the far end, although these are increasingly less necessary if you use the very-good-quality cloud-based integrated computer systems now available.

There are many ways to set up the video/computer screens. Look at how the telepsychiatrist is sitting in Figure 5–3. He is at a height similar to the patient and is far enough away that a good angle of eye contact is achieved, but he looks closer to the patient through the use of the zoom setting (as seen in the picture-in-picture). In this setting, the telepsychiatrist has additional screens for the EMR and any other function (e.g., finding information) he needs to access during the consultation placed beside the patient's screen and out of the patient's sight. This setup allows him to touch-type his notes while he is talking to the patient, without the patient being aware that this is happening, and thus solves the problem of disrupting the patient interaction that occurs when typing notes in front of a patient during in-person consultations.

Ensure Privacy and Security

Ensure that the equipment and environment support patient privacy and confidentiality. You should know whether your video system is compliant with the Health Insurance Portability and Accountability Act (HIPAA)—all manufacturers will provide this information on their Web sites or (if you are not able to find a specific compliance statement) a contact number for more details. If you are using a laptop, you might want to check whether it is encrypted, and certainly if you are recording any of the interview—with the patient's written consent—you will need to be sure that this process is done to a secure drive or to an encrypted machine, or both. In addition to ensuring technical security and privacy, it is important to protect environmental security. The biggest potential hazards for environmental privacy breaches are open windows or doors or thin walls. Finally, make sure that you and your patient know exactly who is involved in the conference. It is vital to always introduce everyone participating in the video visits and to try to have everyone on screen at all times. There have been numerous occasions in our experience where, if this had not been asked about specifically, extra members of a patient's family would have been able to sit through a session without the clinician knowing that they were present, a situation that could be clinically embarrassing or therapeutically destructive. If students are present with the psychiatrist, they need to be introduced, the reason for their presence explained, and the patient's verbal or written consent obtained for them to observe, or be a part of, the interview.

Now let's review the clinical skills needed during the session.

CLINICAL SKILLS

Determine What Your Role Is (Direct Care Versus Consultation)

The skills required for patient consultations vary with the model of care being practiced and the environment involved. A number of differing models of care are described throughout this book. From the clinical skills perspective, the two major ones most commonly used by psychiatrists are *direct consultations,* where the patient is seen either alone or with other family members, just as though he or she were being seen in a typical outpatient clinic, and the *consulting consultation-liaison model,* where the psychiatrist works with a referring outpatient, inpatient, emergency department, or correctional provider to assess the patient and advise on management. Usually in the first model the psychiatrist is delivering treatment, including prescribing and ordering, whereas in the second model the patient's treatment is being provided by the local provider. In both models, the referring provider may be sitting in with the patient for all or just a few minutes of the session, typically the beginning to introduce the patient or the end to help with treatment planning.

Maintain Good Eye Contact

You need all the usual individual clinical skills that you need in any clinical interview, especially the skills of active listening and the capacity to effectively interpret the patient's meaning and needs and be empathic toward the patient and his or her situation, and the ability to make decisions with and for the patient during the interview. Good eye contact is especially important, and this is why your position in relation to the angle of the camera is vital, because patients find it very hard to interact well with someone who looks like they are looking away from them. One of the major advantages of seeing patients on video, and one of the reasons that patients routinely report very high satisfaction results with this form of assessment, is that good direct eye contact probably occurs for a greater proportion of the average video interview than it does for the in-person situation. While there are many factors that contribute to patient satisfaction, one that is repeatedly mentioned in the literature is the empathic connection that patients feel they can make with their telemedicine providers. In reality, for the provider, it is simply harder to look away from a screen that has a person talking to you on it than it is in a conventional clinic room, where it is all too easy for a provider's eyes to stray to the window, the desk, the pictures on the wall, or elsewhere. There is something about this eye contact online that can be intense, more substantial, and emotionally closer than is often the case in the in-person consultation, as will be discussed later. If you are also using an EMR, it is important to set up your video and computer screens in a way that maximizes your body position and eye contact with the patient yet still allows you to type during the consultation if you wish.

Practice Effective Time Management

Interviewing on video takes longer than in-person interviewing and requires more concentration, and the power relationship that you have with your patient is somewhat different from that in a conventional clinic setting. So, while you gesticulate and intonate more than usual during the interview, this is also more tiring, and you will find that you only have, effectively, about 80%–90% of the useful clinical time that you might have in an equivalent in-person interview because the interactions are just a bit slower than in person. Also, it is fairly common for a local provider to join the interview toward the end. While almost universally helpful, it does take a few extra minutes out of the planned interview time. A more subtle issue concerns the power relationship between doctor and patient, where, in the in-person relationship, the doctor typically has more authority and the psychological advantage of being in his or her own clinic or environment. With telemedicine, patients tend to feel more "in control" during video consultations and can, if they wish, literally "switch off" the doctor at their end and leave the consultation without any physical embarrassment or loss of face. Fortunately, this has not yet happened to us, although occasional patients have walked out of interviews, just as can happen in a clinic. Much has been written about power issues between doctors and patients (Hilty et al. 2013; Shore 2013), but it seems clear that the online relationship, in most situations, tends to be more egalitarian than that which occurs in person. This more balanced dynamic is something that today's patients, with their expectations of more patient-focused care approaches, greatly value, but can take time for some practitioners to get used to.

Practice Effective Task Management

What is really different about seeing patients on video versus in person is the management of the video session itself. It is a good idea at the beginning of the session to spend a little more time on introductions than is usually the case, and engaging in some small talk is often helpful to put patients at their ease if they have not used video before. Such preliminaries are of course less frequently necessary today, as so many people use video in their personal relationships and lives. Because the session allows you slightly less clinical time, you have to be even more organized than usual and should get into the habit of always planning your patient sessions. It is sensible, if you have time, to pre-read the medical notes or referral notes and, whenever possible, summarize these notes for the patient at the beginning of the session. This not only shows patients that you are interested in them and understand them but also gives them the opportunity to correct any misunderstandings that you might have, and it is a much more time-efficient way of handling the session than asking patients to repeat a lot of information that you have already read. During the session we suggest that you regularly summarize your knowledge of sections of the patient's history to ensure that you have got them right and to give the patient an opportunity to add other relevant information. It is often also helpful to mark certain times to ensure that you can finish on time by reminding the patient, for instance, that you are halfway through or that there is only 5 minutes to go. At the end of the session, we typically spend more time on summing up and working out a treatment plan—ideally in association with a local provider who has joined the patient toward the end of the session—than occurs in an in-person consultation.

Ensure Safety, Security, and Privacy of Patients, Providers, and the Community

Safety and privacy issues are of great importance in telemedicine and have been very carefully thought through for patients being seen at a distance in primary care clinics and other health facilities, as well as in the home (Figure 5–6). The guidelines from the ATA can be downloaded free from the ATA Web site (www.americantelemed.org), with the 2009 telemental health care guidelines focusing on care in health facilities (American Telemedicine Association 2009b) and the 2013 guidelines on the home (American Telemedicine Association 2013b). There are a number of basic principles that need to be followed to ensure the safety and privacy of patients, providers, and the community.

1. Be certain that you are using an encrypted videoconferencing system that meets HIPAA requirements.
2. Confirm the physical address at which the patient is being seen for the consultation to ensure that you, as the provider, are professionally licensed in the state where the patient is to receive care.
3. Make sure that you know exactly who is on the call at both (or all) ends of the videoconference, that their role and the importance of confidentiality is understood (family, spouse, children, student, guardian, health provider, support person), and that the patient agrees to their presence.
4. Check that doors and windows are shut at both ends and that physical privacy is possible.
5. Ensure that there is always an alternative way of contacting the patient or others close by (usually a phone number) in the event of a technical breakdown or clinical emergency.
6. If the patient is being seen at home, obtain the contact information (phone number) of the designated patient support person for use in an emergency.

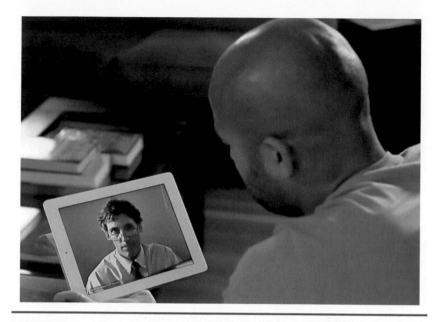

FIGURE 5–6.   Example of home telepsychiatry on an iPad.

Source.   Photograph courtesy of Peter Yellowlees, MBBS, M.D. Used with permission.

7. Ensure that you are familiar with the requirements of and documentation governing mental health "holds" in the state in which the patient resides and that you have the correct phone numbers for local police or health services so that you can arrange a hold if you need to. You cannot call 911 in this instance, as 911 calls only go to the locality that the caller is in, so you actually need to know the local number of the police in the state/city/region of the patient.

Coordinate Care With the Patient's Local Provider

How do you best integrate a patient's local PCP into the interview? First, it is very useful to have the local provider physically with the patient, and they frequently can add helpful information about the patient or have very specific questions to ask. Sometimes local providers want to sit in for the whole session, but in our experience this is relatively rare, as they do not have the time. If they do wish to do this, though, it can be an excellent teaching opportunity for both of you—we have certainly learned a lot about local culture from such interactions, and the literature contains a number of studies demonstrating how effective video consultations can be for improving the psychiatric skills of PCPs as they watch psychiatrists work with their patients. Certainly, we always encourage local providers to take part, and when they come to the interview, it is polite to ask them to summarize what their concerns about their patient are. Most of the time the patients really appreciate seeing their PCP talking to a specialist about them, and we are always extremely careful to be highly respectful of the PCP and never be critical in any way. Sometimes the PCP wishes to consult with you without the patient present, and that is fine—just ask the patient to wait in the waiting room for a few minutes using some pretext. We frequently finish the interview by asking the patient to tell the PCP about the discussion the patient has had with us—what their likely diagnosis is and what treatment plan has been decided on. We find that approach very helpful with most patients. It not only keeps the patient as the center of the interview but also allows us to check the patient's understanding of the diagnosis and treatment plan, and it cements the patient's dyad with his or her PCP, who is likely going to carry out much of the treatment plan anyway, with you, as the specialist, acting as a consultant.

Practice Effective Group Skills to Accommodate Multiple Participants

Group skills are a core required skill for any clinician using video consults if he or she is working as a consultant, in a consultation-liaison manner, to a PCP, as often happens when providing care in collaborative or integrated care environments. They are of course also vital if seeing children or families or when teaching with colleagues or students at either or both ends of the consultation. Video consults can be done in exactly the same way as in-person group consults, in that everyone involved must be introduced and given the chance to speak and say hello, and people can be moved in and out of the overall group for periods of time at either end or at any of several ends in some situations. Just as in any group, it is necessary for someone to be the group chair or coordinator at any one time, but that role can be shifted to several other people in the group during the consultation process. It is common, for instance, for us to give that role over to the patient or to his or her PCP at the end of a session when feedback and follow-up planning are occurring. During the sessions, it is important to involve the other clinicians or family members at the patient's end and to avoid side conversations that would exclude them; if you wish to have such conversations with a colleague, tell the patient and mute the system. It is a good idea to move the camera away from you or to move out of the camera angle in this situation.

How Can the "Virtual Space" of the Online Doctor–Patient Relationship Be Used to Improve Care?

Skills for understanding and using the virtual space in which the video relationship evolves are essential and take many clinicians a while to learn. As discussed earlier, the video relationship addresses the two major weaknesses of the in-person relationship—lack of physical access and the power differential between patient and provider—and adds a third component that is clinically useful: the existence and use of a "virtual space" between the patient and doctor. The physical separation of patient and provider that occurs in telemedicine has, in the past, typically been assumed to be a disadvantage of telepsychiatry, but it is now clear that sensitive use of the virtual space within which video consultations take place can improve the overall standard of care delivered by psychiatrists and other therapists to their online patients (Figure 5–7).

There seem to be two components of the virtual space that affect both providers and patients: physical and psychological (Chan et al. 2015; Yellowlees et al. 2015). At the most basic level, the *physical space,* along with the separation for providers, allows providers to give much more direct feedback to patients than might happen in consultations where the patient is physically present in the room, especially if this is difficult feedback that the patient may not wish to hear about or may disagree with. This experience—when the psychiatrist consults in a primary care environment—is clinically useful and may allow the psychiatrist to play the role of the "bad cop" to ensure (for example) that a patient with poor insight receives treatment, while preserving the patient's good relationship with his or her PCP, who is the "good cop" and is not blamed for the patient requiring such treatment (see Case Example 3, later in this chapter). From the patient perspective, the physical distance is helpful for individuals living in small communities (where specialist care is increasingly delivered via telemedicine), who for privacy reasons often prefer to see a physician who does not live in their community and who they are not likely to meet at the local store. From the provider perspective, the physical space has been shown to enhance a feeling of safety, particularly

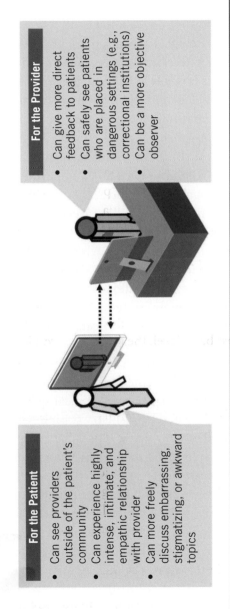

For the Provider

- Can give more direct feedback to patients
- Can safely see patients who are placed in dangerous settings (e.g., correctional institutions)
- Can be a more objective observer

For the Patient

- Can see providers outside of the patient's community
- Can experience highly intense, intimate, and empathic relationship with provider
- Can more freely discuss embarrassing, stigmatizing, or awkward topics

FIGURE 5–7. Advantages of the virtual space in telepsychiatry.

Source. Diagram and illustrations by Steven Chan, M.D., M.B.A. Used with permission.

when patients who are physically dangerous or who inhabit potentially dangerous environments, such as correctional institutions, are being seen (Deslich et al. 2013). This feature of telepsychiatry has been noted to be particularly important for female psychiatrists and has made it more comfortable for them to work in such environments.

The *psychological space,* and distancing, is perhaps more important than the physical space, although its effects are different for providers than for patients. We all know that it is possible to have intense, intimate, and empathic relationships through videoconferencing. Many long-distance relationships are started and maintained on Skype, FaceTime, Google Hangouts, and similar easily available videoconferencing software platforms all around the world, in all cultures, and, in recent years, on smartphones. Fifteen percent of U.S. adults report that they have used online dating sites or mobile dating apps (Smith and Anderson 2016), and today's high-quality, high-definition systems allow users to clearly show and detect emotions, connect with each other, and interact empathically, as seen daily on television news programs where emotion-filled long-distance interviews are routinely presented. The psychological extra distance that both partners in the consultation frequently notice initially tends to dissipate markedly after a few minutes, and anyway this feeling of psychological distancing is much less significant than in the past, when poor audio and visualization made the separation of the parties in the interview more obvious. For providers, the psychological space enables them to be simultaneously part of the consultation but also an objective observer. This dual potential of the psychological space is most commonly used to good advantage in telepsychiatry sessions with children who have behavioral disorders, in which it is possible for psychiatrists to engage initially with the child's parents to take a history from them while at the same time being able to observe, through the video, the child's behavior; the interactions between the child and the parents; and the parents' parenting and disciplinary skills. It has been argued that for some children, this use of the psychological space online can lead to better-quality assessments than are possible in the traditional office setting and that online assessment should in these cases be the new standard of care (Hilty and Yellowlees 2015; Pakyurek et al. 2010).

The psychological space is even more important for patients and frequently allows them to have more intimate conversations with their providers than they would have in a physical consultation. When the topic of discussion is potentially embarrassing, stigmatizing, or awkward, people find it easier to converse on video or online, and the computer science literature is full of human–computer interaction studies demonstrating that individuals being interviewed in a "virtual space" environment tend to respond more honestly than do those being interviewed in person (Rogers 2003). For instance, a man with depression and sexual dysfunction may feel uncomfortable speaking to a young, attractive female, or an adolescent female who has been abused may feel uncomfortable talking to someone she might meet locally. There are many instances where it is easier to talk about experiences with someone who is physically more distant on video rather than in person, just as it is more embarrassing to reveal something problematic about ourselves to a friend or family member than to a relative stranger. Some have suggested that video communication in some instances may actually encourage intimacy and emotional intensity in a relationship, more so than in person (Yellowlees 2008). Religions around the world have understood the importance of this virtual space for centuries, because the same dynamic occurs in the confessional box, where parishioners are able to tell intimate stories about themselves to a priest close by whom they know well but who is not physically seen and thereby more distant.

CASE EXAMPLE 2: VIRTUAL ASSESSMENT OF A CHILD WITH OPPOSITIONAL BEHAVIOR[2]

An 8-year-old boy, Nathan, is referred for assessment and evaluation of symptoms of possible attention-deficit/hyperactivity disorder (ADHD), oppositional disorder, or both. Nathan moves weekly between his divorced parents, who share custody, and only his single mother attends the session. As usual, the telepsychiatrist explains to her that he will take a history from her initially, while asking Nathan to sit and listen, and indicating that he was welcome to interrupt and add comments to his mother's answers if he wanted. The mother is told to manage Nathan's behavior in whatever way she usually does. The session rapidly deteriorates as Nathan continually interrupts his mother; sits calmly with his feet up on a chair, ignoring the telepsychiatrist; and in general behaves in a highly disrespectful, rude, and entitled manner. It is clear to the telepsychiatrist that Nathan is in charge and that his mother has minimal parenting skills and no way of managing her child. The mother responds

---

[2]Case provided by Peter Yellowlees, MBBS, M.D.

to Nathan's unruliness by telling the telepsychiatrist that this behavior shows why her son needs to be medicated for "ADHD." After about 15 minutes, by which time it is clear to the telepsychiatrist that Nathan does not have ADHD, the telepsychiatrist decides to see how Nathan responds to some clear control and direction. He, for the first time, addresses Nathan directly, insisting that he sit up straight, take his feet off the chair, and pay attention. Nathan, in shocked surprise, responds surprisingly appropriately, at which stage the mother is asked to wait outside and the telepsychiatrist is able to start exploring Nathan's anger and the discordant messages he is receiving from his separated parents' very different parenting styles—harsh punishment or being ignored at his dad's home and total lack of authority and boundaries at his mom's.

▌ KEY CONCEPT

Telepsychiatry offers the opportunity of observing patients when they do not realize they are being observed and frequently allows the psychiatrist to more easily assess children in particular than if they were in an in-person office, where the psychiatrist would inevitably be more part of the group dynamics.

WHAT STRATEGIES CAN HELP CLINICIANS MANAGE UNUSUAL PATIENTS OR SITUATIONS?

There are no absolute clinical contraindications to use of telepsychiatry, unless the patient refuses treatment or actively demonstrates violence toward the self or others at the time of the interview. Difficult patients can often be seen by engaging an assistant at the patient's end of the interview, either to calm the patient and act as a "supporter" or to help with administration of questionnaires or neuropsychological tests, or even to explain the process and assist the patient while a specific physical examination, such as the Abnormal Involuntary Movement Scale (Shore et al. 2015), is being conducted

There are some predictable symptoms and situations that one might think would be challenging for patients and providers to manage:

1. *Patients with psychotic symptoms such as hallucinations and paranoia, or with delusions incorporating technologies.* We have seen a number of such patients, and they can usually be managed with sensitivity and care. Patients who have active psychotic symptoms incorporating the monitor on which you are appearing can still usually under-

stand the difference between you and any other hallucinations they might have that are appearing from the screen or that relate specifically to them. Certainly, in our experience, it is possible for patients to separate out the practitioner's voice, for instance, from the psychotic voices, but this may need to be specifically explained. Somewhat more difficult are those patients who are very paranoid about the monitor and believe that they will be harmed by it. When this has occurred, it was helpful to suggest that patients sit out of the angle of the camera at their end (they can see that they are not being filmed in the "picture in picture" on their screen if that is available). Once such patients are out of the picture, it is possible to continue talking to them and therefore to continue the assessment until they feel comfortable coming back on screen. For many patients, both psychotic and anxious, we have found that asking them to move away from the camera and get off screen has been therapeutic and has allowed them to calm down and eventually resume the consultation more normally. On some occasions, it has been possible to interview paranoid patients on video using this technique, where it is highly unlikely that they would have continued the interview in the in-person world.

2. *Patients who are malingering or have factitious disorders.* These patients may be difficult to interview at the best of times, and frequently their histories need to be checked with third parties and others with knowledge of their daily functioning and physical and mental states, as these occur outside of the psychiatric consultation. Malingering is a particularly significant issue when seeing patients within the correctional system, and for those patients, validated screening questionnaires designed to identify malingering, such as the Miller Forensic Assessment of Symptoms (M-FAST; Miller 2001), are essential and can certainly be conducted via videoconferencing.

3. *Elderly patients with sensory deficits or cognitive impairment.* Sensory deficits, especially auditory and visual, may impair patients' ability to interact over videoconferencing. Recommendations for assessing these patients are included in the 2009 ATA guidelines, where it is suggested that physicians use interviewing techniques and any available assistive technologies that can help patients with visual or auditory impairment, as well as cognitive impairment, and particularly involve family members or carers. Patients may well need more explanation and a slower interview approach, and carers or assistants at

the patient's end may need to help with giving a brief cognitive screening test such as the Montreal Cognitive Assessment.

4. *Very young or nonverbal children.* Children usually respond very positively to videoconferencing, and in general their assessment can be carried out as it would be in an in-person consultation. It is very important that families and/or legal guardians provide consent and be involved, as clinically appropriate, and ideally the room at the patient's end should be large enough for the children's motor skills to be assessed as they move around the room and play, separately from the parents. Children can be asked to wait outside the room with a carer for parts of the interview, as can parents or other family members, just as occurs in the clinic, so that issues can be discussed privately with individuals as necessary rather than with a whole family group. A separate table, paper, and age-appropriate toys need to be available for children to use, and the assessments should follow the guidelines of the American Academy of Child and Adolescent Psychiatry (Myers et al. 2008) and the American Telemedicine Association (2017).

5. *Patients with limited English proficiency.* It is common to see patients on telepsychiatry whose first language is not English and who speak little or very limited English. Ideally a professional interpreter should be used in this situation, and a number of commercial companies are available who can provide such access, with the consultation becoming a three-way video link between the patient, psychiatrist, and interpreter, or even linking in by telephone ideally at the psychiatrist's end. Unfortunately, interpreters are not always available or may be costly, and the next-best option, although not ideally recommended, is to work with a staff member at either end of the consultation who speaks the patient's language. It is strongly recommended not to use a family member for interpretation unless there are no other options and the family is prepared to fully consent to this and understands that this is not the preferred solution. It is not uncommon for the best English language speaker in the family to be a child who has learned English at school, and for that child to be used to translate for his or her parents, but to have such a child translating a psychiatric consultation, with the many potential family issues and traumas, is not appropriate in terms of the protection of the child and the need for privacy for the parents. On the occasions when we have had no alternative but to work with children as interpreters for their parents, it

has been possible to modify history taking and have a more limited conversation covering primarily urgent issues and then attempt to have a second, more detailed follow-up consultation at a later time with an interpreter. As discussed in Chapter 8, early studies of automated interpretation systems are already happening, and it is likely that within a few years it will be possible to use such systems to translate patients' languages in real time during consultations, hence resolving this difficult communication issue.

CASE EXAMPLE 3: GOOD COP, BAD COP[3]

Neville, a 25-year-old single man on a disability pension who has a long-standing diagnosis of schizophrenia and lives in a very isolated rural environment, is referred for an urgent telepsychiatry assessment because he has stopped taking his oral antipsychotic medications and has become acutely paranoid and threatening. Neville's PCP is confident that his patient's situation meets criteria for a psychiatric hold and involuntary admission, which would involve a 2-hour ambulance drive to the nearest psychiatric unit. The telepsychiatrist had previously seen Neville twice for annual reviews of his treatment, which was always prescribed by the PCP, and thought that he had a reasonable relationship with the patient. Unfortunately, Neville's psychosis is now severe, and he immediately starts yelling and shouting at the telepsychiatrist, so the PCP is called in to assist, because the clinic is in an uproar. Neville has a close and excellent relationship with his PCP and does not want to be admitted to the hospital. In the end, the telepsychiatrist is able to convince Neville to receive a stat injection of a long-acting depot antipsychotic medication given personally by his PCP, which he has not been on before. Neville also agrees to receive regular visits from the clinic nurse and to see his PCP at least weekly, as well as to take some oral medication at night to help him sleep better, with the understanding that he will not be certified and sent out of town to the hospital, which was the original plan. This community-based plan works very well, and over the next few weeks Neville's psychosis remits, and he remains on depot medications long-term, finally agreeing to see the "bad cop" telepsychiatrist intermittently while continuing to see the "good cop" PCP regularly.

▌ KEY CONCEPT

The capacity for two physicians to see a patient at the same time, and for the telepsychiatrist to play the role of "bad cop" who in-

---

[3]Case provided by Peter Yellowlees, MBBS, M.D.

sists on needed treatment for a patient, in contradistinction to the "good cop" PCP, is a rarely needed but potentially very helpful telepsychiatry intervention that in this instance prevented a several-weeks-long hospital admission, thereby more than paying for the telepsychiatry service.

WHICH GROUPS OF PATIENTS PREFER TO RECEIVE MENTAL HEALTH CARE ONLINE RATHER THAN IN PERSON?

Most patients having telepsychiatry consultations are from rural or psychiatrically underserved areas and are still consulting online primarily because of poor access to care in their communities. Many of them prefer to see psychiatrists at a distance because they live in small communities and are likely to be seen going into a local psychiatrist's or therapist's office, if such an office exists, or might know those individuals socially and be reticent to see them as patients. For these patients, the capacity to see an individual from outside of their community is important, and the avoidance of the need to travel, a related motivating factor.

However, patients are increasingly asking to be seen online, rather than in-person, for a range of reasons related to stigma avoidance, personal preference, the nature of their psychiatric disorders, and convenience and cost.

The largest group of these patients who are seeing telepsychiatrists in preference to having in-person consultations are unfortunately from that group of many patients who are afraid of seeing psychiatrists, and with whom PCPs often still have to work hard to get them to agree to accept a psychiatric referral. They are the individuals who see this referral as an indication that they are "crazy" or "mad." They are worried by the stigma of visiting a psychiatrist's office and potentially being seen by someone they know either in the waiting room or entering the offices. This is a particularly important issue for celebrities or people who are well known in their communities, as there have unfortunately been a number of examples of Hollywood actors being "outed" by the media while visiting a psychiatrist. So, a consultation by video is much more private and potentially less stigmatizing, and it is evident that some people feel calmer about the process if they can have the consultation on video, either from their primary care clinic or, increasingly, from home, while at the same time saving them travel time and being more convenient.

There are now numerous telepsychiatry companies providing video consultation services to the home, sometimes as part of concierge practices marketed as a more convenient time-saving service that improves access to physicians and psychiatrists. The companies are targeting individuals who are "VIPs" or celebrities or who are professionals with public reputations to maintain (e.g., lawyers, doctors, business executives) who have psychiatric or substance-related disorders or other stigmatized medical conditions, or who simply prefer enhanced privacy. These patients often prefer to pay cash for all of their consultations so that their insurance carriers do not find out that they have been seeing psychiatrists. Employee health plans are also increasingly adopting virtual care as a benefit for their employees. This reduces time away from work due to travel and the time for in-person visits.

Generational issues are important here as well. Young males are notorious for their avoidance of physicians for both physical and psychiatric reasons, but they—along with their female counterparts from today's younger generations—are likely to see video interactions as being not only normal but preferred. For these young people, convenience and time saving are the most important drivers, and seeing a psychiatrist online from their own home meets their needs much better than visiting a clinic. This group in the future is especially likely to accept hybrid forms of care, where they attend in person on occasion and online at other times.

Other individuals who do not want to see psychiatrists in person may be anxious, avoidant, shy, or paranoid and are not keen to leave their home or surroundings that they know well. This is particularly the case for patients with agoraphobia, who may be stuck in their homes, afraid to leave for months on end, or for veterans with posttraumatic stress disorder (PTSD), where the nature of the illness, like agoraphobia, makes them more avoidant and less prepared to attend a clinic. Some recent fascinating research with veterans (Fortney et al. 2015) has shown that veterans attending video groups for therapy for PTSD while visiting their psychiatrists in person were actually more engaged in treatment than a control group of veterans receiving all of their treatment in person, and that the video was actually a positively engaging force for them.

Some patients prefer telepsychiatry simply because no local psychiatrists speak their preferred native language, or they may be deaf or very hard of hearing and wish to connect with a psychiatrist who can sign. Increasing numbers of patients are also seeking video opinions from psychiatrists who are known to be national or international experts in a particular area but who live in other states or countries. This option is especially important for patients with genetic or other rare diseases, such as Huntington's disorder.

In What Situations Might Telepsychiatry Represent Better Clinical Practice Than In-Person Care?

Over many years of practice, it has become evident that in certain situations the practice of telepsychiatry is actually better than the use of traditional in-person consultations. No longer is it appropriate to try to prove that telepsychiatry is "no worse than" or "as good as" in-person consultations. A large amount of data from randomized controlled trials is available to support that thesis and has been reviewed in detail by Bashshur et al. (2016), who concluded that there is more evidence supporting the practice of telemedicine for psychiatry than for any other medical specialty. So in what ways might telepsychiatry be better than traditional care models?

COLLABORATIVE AND TEAM-BASED CARE

Telepsychiatry gives us the ability to work more effectively in teams, across disciplines, and with patients, their families, and local providers (Fortney et al. 2015; Hilty et al. 2013; Shore 2013) in a collaborative care model, especially in integrated primary care systems, working within the concept of the primary care medical home. Here patients are treated within a primary care environment with their PCPs as the primary point of medical contact. Psychiatrists using telemedicine can collaborate more effectively with their colleagues who refer patients to them and who can join the psychiatrist and their patients during psychiatric consultations. Patients value seeing their PCPs talking and interacting with specialists to work out the best care plan for them and enjoy being part of a team decision-making process. This capacity to collaborate can be especially strong and useful in nursing homes and emergency departments, where several others involved with the care of the patient may need to be consulted.

HYBRID CARE

Hybrid care is discussed in detail in Chapter 8. In an extension of the collaboration model, Fortney et al. (2015), working with veterans with PTSD, have demonstrated that telepsychiatry, if added to usual care in a hybrid model that involves both in-person and online care components, may lead to enhanced patient engagement as well as improved clinical outcomes. The same has been found to be true for children with ADHD; Hilty and Yellowlees (2015) suggested that telemedicine-enabled care, when delivered in a hybrid in-person and online format with multiple technologies as demonstrated by Myers et al. (2015), is better than conventional in-person care and should be the new standard of care in child psychiatry.

RECORDING OF PATIENT CONSULTATIONS

Routine recording of telepsychiatry consultations is unusual, but with patient consent, recording can be easily done and is especially helpful for teaching purposes. Asynchronous telepsychiatry consultations are always recorded, and if patients consent to having these recordings become part of their medical records, such recordings can provide a valuable extra piece of clinical material, giving psychiatrists the capacity to easily and objectively compare changes in patients' mental states over time. Video documentation is something we have never been able to do in the past, but as we move to a world where "video is data," there will be many situations in which recorded examples of patients' behavior will be available in their electronic records.

SPECIFIC PATIENT GROUPS

As discussed earlier, the intimacy of the online space means that all forms of psychotherapy can be delivered effectively and often better over telepsychiatry, with support from a strong evidence base (Totten et al. 2016). Patients who are in correctional environments are another group who are often able to access better care, and care given by providers who feel less threatened, than is traditionally available. Finally, patients who have disorders that tend to make them feel threatened or anxious, as discussed earlier, or who would simply not see a psychiatrist because of perceived stigma, can now receive care of high quality.

What Skills Practiced in Telepsychiatry Can Help Clinicians Deliver a Higher Standard of Care in Their In-Person Psychiatric Consultations?

Having been practicing telepsychiatry for many years, we have found that the skills learned during these consultations, and discussed above, can be transferred to in-person consultations to improve them. What specific skills are these?

TIME MANAGEMENT AND ORGANIZATION OF SESSIONS

When you are doing telepsychiatry sessions, where several clinics may be visited in the course of a single afternoon, it is essential to learn and practice good time management. Think about the number of people involved in an afternoon of such practice. At each site, there is likely to be at least one patient, and perhaps family members, as well as a PCP and likely a telemedicine coordinator or medical assistant. There may well be extra students or observers at one or more sites as well, so that a typical afternoon of consultations may involve anywhere from 10 to 20 people in three distant sites plus your own site, all of whom have their own schedules and other work to complete. It is crucial not to get significantly behind in your clinical schedule, and this has led to an interviewing process in telepsychiatry that involves more summations of information, and regular reminders to the patient that there is a certain amount of time left.

One technique that is often employed is to briefly summarize at the beginning of a session all of the information you have about a patient (either from notes provided beforehand or from an EMR). This tells patients that you have done your homework, and it also gives them the chance to correct you if you have misunderstood something. Either way, beginning with a brief summary is an efficient way to deal with initial concerns in the interview and allows you and the patient to rapidly get on the same page. Later in the session you can summarize all of the new information for the patient and then move smoothly on to explaining your diagnosis and treatment plan, once the core data that your clinical judgment is based on are agreed upon.

All of these approaches are directly transferable to the in-person consultation and can greatly assist the organization and time management of these sessions.

PATIENT AND PRIMARY CARE PROVIDER EDUCATION

Patient and PCP education is an area that tends to be emphasized more in telepsychiatry consultations than is often the case in in-person consultations mainly because it is so common to finish a consultation by talking to the patient with his or her PCP present. In the online consultation, this is an excellent opportunity to do some education with the patient about the diagnosis and treatment. An excellent technique to demonstrate that the patient does have a good understanding of his or her situation is to ask the patient to give some feedback about the session to his or her PCP. This is something that we do almost routinely, having previously warned the patient that we are going to ask him or her to discuss the outcomes with the local provider, which as a by-product can immensely strengthen the relationship between the patient and the local physician, if he or she is to continue to be the PCP, and maintains you, as the consulting psychiatrist, in that consulting role. It is good practice to ask PCPs to summarize their concerns about their patients and to ask any specific questions that they may have, and this is often an excellent time to give some tactful education to them, which in our experience is greatly valued. It is vital to never be critical of PCPs, whatever they have been doing, because part of the role of the telepsychiatrist is to support and strengthen the doctor–patient relationship of primary physicians and their patients. While it is very uncommon to have PCPs take part in an in-person consultation, it is sometimes possible to bring them in on the phone, or to phone them later, and the practice of telepsychiatry generally significantly increases the focus on the primary care dyad and leads to an increased level of respect for how PCPs manage their patients.

WHAT ETHICAL PRINCIPLES AND GUIDELINES IN TELEPSYCHIATRY ALLOW CLINICIANS TO ESTABLISH AND MAINTAIN CORE STANDARDS?

Ethical principles for psychiatry have been developed as a result of years of discussion and clinical observation in a variety of clinical settings (Sabin and Skimming 2015). The standard of care in telepsychiatry is a work in progress and rapidly changing before our very eyes.

Let's start with a critical point: psychiatrists must uphold ethics and their professional conduct to the standards set forth by the American Medical Association (AMA) irrespective of whether they provide those services in person or via videoconferencing technology. Ethical principles do not change when the modality in which the service changes.

However, the delivery of services via the Internet and videoconferencing poses a new set of ethical challenges. Following policy is quite different from upholding ethical principles, and policy is changing at an alarming rate, whether it is *ethically sound* or not. Many practitioners face a difficult question: telemedicine technologies allow psychiatrists to help people in ways that laws and policy may not yet support for a variety of reasons, some of which are political. So then, *what is ethical?* Do you do the right thing for the patient, or adhere to the guidance that was established well before the technology existed to enable a needed service to occur? Psychiatrists should never be in this situation, yet they are now.

Ethics in the context of telepsychiatry have been discussed within the American Psychiatric Association since 1995. According to a position statement by the Board of Trustees, updated since the 1995 version, "The American Psychiatric Association supports the use of telemedicine as a legitimate component of a mental health care delivery system to the extent that its use is in the best interest of the patient and is in compliance with the APA policies on medical ethics and confidentiality" (American Psychiatric Association 2015).

In June 2016, the AMA announced that it had adopted new ethical guidance on telehealth care (American Medical Association 2016a, 2016b). The new guidance, which was developed through the AMA Council on Ethics and Judicial Affairs, is designed to help physicians better understand their responsibilities when conducting appointments via telemedicine. The guidelines are also designed to inform physicians that coordination between physicians is important to avoid potential problems with delivering services via telemedicine.

Given that numerous practice guidelines for telemedicine predate the adoption of the AMA's document on the ethical practice in telemedicine (American Medical Association 2016b), this now presents an interesting challenge to all physicians and leads to an inherent question we must confront: what if the ethics do not coincide with or complement an aspect of the practice guidelines or policies of the agency in which we are working?

Irrespective of what medical specialty one practices, the professional code of ethics should not differ significantly whether you see patients in person or via videoconferencing technology. It is the function of the technology, physical distance between the practitioner and patient, and the settings on both sides that provide additional complexity to the encounter that warrant additional considerations and planning. So, the first step, inherent in the ethical guidance issued by the AMA, is to become familiar with available practice guidelines relevant to your practice, as discussed throughout this chapter and in other chapters of the book.

There are a number of available practice guidelines and a strong literature base pertaining to telepsychiatry, as discussed in Chapter 2 ("Evidence Base for Use of Videoconferencing and Other Technologies in Mental Health Care"). The following telemedicine guidelines are recommended:

The ATA Web site provides access to several well-established guidelines, including the following:

- *Core Operational Guidelines for Telehealth Services Involving Provider–Patient Interactions* (American Telemedicine Association 2014).
- *A Lexicon Assessment and Outcome Measurements for Telemental Health* (American Telemedicine Association 2013a).
- *Practice Guidelines for Video-Based Online Mental Health Services* (American Telemedicine Association 2013b).
- *Practice Guidelines for Videoconferencing-Based Telemental Health* (American Telemedicine Association 2009b).
- *Evidence-Based Practice for Telemental Health* (American Telemedicine Association 2009a).

Other guidelines of importance include the 2008 practice parameter for pediatric telepsychiatry by the American Academy of Child and Adolescent Psychiatry (Myers et al. 2008), which was recently updated (American Telemedicine Association 2017); and a guideline document from the Royal Australian and New Zealand College of Psychiatrists (2013). This document, *Professional Practice Standards and Guides for Telepsychiatry,* also includes practice standards, one of which (Standard 4.1, Ethical Considerations) states that "The practice should incorporate organizational values and ethics statements into Telepsychiatry administrative policies and procedures, inform the patient of their rights and responsibilities and declare any conflict of interest to influence decision making" (p. 7).

In addition to seeking guidance from practice guidelines, it is important to understand your state licensing board's regulations on telemedicine, given that states vary in their regulations. If you are working within a system of care, it is important to follow the telemedicine policies set forth by both the system from which you are delivering services and the system in which the patient is located.

From the AMA's existing practice guidelines and Code of Medical Ethics, we can begin to identify and outline core ethical standards.

WHAT ARE THE CORE ETHICAL STANDARDS FOR TELEPSYCHIATRY?

It is important to understand and establish core standards that may serve as the benchmark for your standards of care. Standards of care inform ethics, and ethics influence decisions. Upon reviewing the AMA's Code of Medical Ethics, a number of well-established telemedicine practice guidelines, and a thorough review of the literature, one can extrapolate common standards that are further accentuated in the AMA's document on the ethical practice in telemedicine (American Medical Association 2016b). Through this process, we have identified eight core ethical standards worthy of further discussion. Several of these standards have been mentioned earlier in this chapter, but here we take a deliberately ethically oriented slant to their discussion.

I. EDUCATION, TRAINING, AND QUALITY (AND A STANDARD OPERATING PROCEDURE)

First, psychiatrists and any other clinicians involved should have the requisite training and competency to deliver services via any form of technology that they are personally required to use. Additionally, education and training should be an ongoing endeavor to ensure that current standards are being met.

A standard operating procedure (SOP) should be established and vetted if necessary by appropriate administrative executives and/or legal counsel well in advance of conducting the first telepsychiatry appointment. An SOP should outline protocols related to administrative, clinical, and technical requirements. Any local, state, and/or federal relevant policy and authorized regulations impacting the telepsychiatry clinic shall also be included in the SOP. A high-quality SOP is an ongoing working document that should be reviewed on an annual basis to ensure that all standards are current. It is recommended that an individual and/ or entity with expertise in quality management and improvement participate in the ongoing development of any SOP.

II. LICENSURE AND CREDENTIALING

As noted in Chapter 3 ("The Business of Telepsychiatry"), states require physicians to be licensed in the state where they practice and, in the case of telepsychiatry, where the patient is physically located during the appointment. Furthermore, physicians must be credentialed at the facility or system from which the physician delivers services as well as at the site where the patient is receiving those services. Physicians also must hold Drug Enforcement Agency accreditation at the site where the patient is seen in order to be able to prescribe controlled substances. Credentialing by proxy has been available since 2011, and this allows an individual who is fully credentialed in one health system to work at any site in another system, as long as he or she is credentialed at one of the receiving system's sites and there is a business agreement in place between the systems. Ambiguity may arise when it comes to some consultations, especially when the psychiatrist is consulting to a PCP in a shared care environment, where consultations occur only on an occasional basis, or when the patient is well known but is in another state for a short term. It is imperative to acquire the appropriate legal information related to the system of care's policy on providing consultation via telemedicine. In the context of private practice, licensure and credentialing issues would fall under the rubric of professional liability (Hyler and Gangure 2004).

III. PRIVACY, SECURITY, AND CONFIDENTIALITY

The use of telepsychiatry decreases a physician's control over transmitted information, and there is an inherent increase in potential infringement of privacy and confidentiality, although in reality this occurs seldom, and many telepsychiatry systems are much more private than the average inpatient unit, where two patients may be separated by only a curtain.

Privacy and Security

If the patient is physically located in his or her home or other location where family and/or friends may be near, there is an increased risk of interrupting the session or of deliberate or accidental eavesdropping. Whenever possible, it is recommended that practitioners use the most secure type of technology, and it is equally important to be familiar with the industry security and encryption standards. Many federal health care systems use the Federal Information Processing Standards Publication (FIPS) 140-2 (http://csrc.nist.gov/groups/STM/cmvp/standards.html) as the gold standard. The National Institute of Standards and Technology maintains a list of vendors whose products have met this standard (located under "Validation List"; http://csrc.nist.gov/groups/STM/cmvp/validation.html).

Confidentiality

Given the increased risk for a breach in confidentiality due to vulnerable technology and personal locations where appointments may occur, it is recommended that stringent measures be taken to ensure confidentiality. A process should be established that outlines the storage and retrieval of health records. The process should also specify who may access those records and what are the legal regulations related to protecting patient health information. It is highly recommended that all documentation be stored in a secure location, which must be HIPAA compliant. This is particularly important if the psychiatrist is working from a home or in another non-clinic-based setting. All precautions should be made with respect to sharing the patient's information in accord with the AMA standards.

IV. INFORMED CONSENT

Some states require written informed consent for every consultation, others require verbal documented consent, and still others do not require formal consent. It is essential to know which type of consent process applies to the state in which the patient is being seen and to meet those requirements.

Psychiatrists should include additional information in their informed consent process, and we would caution practitioners against rushing through this important part of the engagement process. Sabin and Skimming (2015) and Shore (2013) suggest providing an increased level of detail pertaining to the unique elements of the informed consent in telepsychiatry. These elements include

- Panning the camera around both offices to verify that no one else is present;
- Asking the patient about his or her working knowledge of videoconferencing and discussing the technical aspects of the video display; and
- Addressing questions regarding security of the transmission.

Other items noted by Shore (2013) include evaluating the patient's level of comfort during the informed consent process (via videoconferencing) and asking the patient at the end of the session what his or her experience was like to determine if the patient is comfortable enough to continue treatment via telepsychiatry.

It is recommended that both treating practitioner and patient mutually agree that the benefits of conducting the appointment by telepsychiatry are sufficient to work in this manner if an in-person visit is a viable alternative possibility. Furthermore, both parties to the consultation should know what will happen if video and/or audio connections are lost and reconnection is not possible. Usually, if this situation arises, the session will be completed via telephone.

V. MALPRACTICE AND PROFESSIONAL LIABILITY

There are theoretically increased risks of malpractice in telepsychiatry consultations, but very few practitioners have ever been sued, and medical defense companies do not charge increased rates to telepsychiatry providers. We strongly suggest, however, that any clinician who is about to practice telepsychiatry should inform their medical defense provider in writing of this change to their practice. As long as practitioners use the appropriate guidelines and adhere to safety practices for telepsychiatry, they are unlikely to run into trouble. Some emergency situations can be difficult to handle and require very careful documentation of what happened, and it is essential that psychiatrists be familiar with the laws governing "holds" in the state in which the patient is being seen and be able to use these correctly if necessary. Sometimes technical glitches—related to either video or audio—occur. If this happens, we recommend that practitioners make a clear note about what occurred and also document whether they felt that, as a result of the lost or impaired audio or video, they were or were not able to make an accurate clinical assessment of the patient.

VI. PROFESSIONALISM AND BOUNDARIES

In general, a telepsychiatry visit is intended to be no different than an in-person visit and, with the physical separation between patient and provider, should at a very practical level make boundary violations less likely than in an in-person consultation. Noting that while there is a "shield" or "protective glass" separating the treating practitioner and the patient, all professional conduct consistent with an in-person consultation should be the same. If the patient is in his or her home, the practitioner will be able to see their personal effects, which may in some instances provide additional clinically relevant information but may also lead to a loosening of boundaries; similarly, the patient may be less guarded when he or she is in the home environment and therefore may have increased vulnerability (Rambo 2016). Irrespective of the location, it is critical for the practitioner delivering services via telepsychiatry to maintain professionalism and to manage the therapeutic alliance in light of what is still a relatively nontraditional setting compared with the office environment.

The use of social media is another important area where ethical concerns can arise; this topic is discussed in detail in Chapter 6 ("Data Collection From Novel Sources"). The AMA stipulated, in its policy statement *Professionalism in the Use of Social Media* (American Medical Association 2011), the following: "If they interact with patients on the Internet, physicians must maintain appropriate boundaries of the patient–physician relationship in accordance with professional ethical guidelines, just as they would in any other context," and "to maintain appropriate professional boundaries physicians should consider separating personal and professional content online."

Utilizing technology to deliver services may cause lapses in ethical judgment, whether by using social media inappropriately, texting, exchanging e-mails, or agreeing to see a patient late in the evening or on the weekend because of the conveniences afforded by technology. Additional issues with boundaries may include developing a more social relationship or one that is leaning toward intimacy because of the more personal level of service being provided.

VII. CONTINUITY OF CARE

Sabin and Skimming (2015) identify *encouraging continuity of care* as one of the key ethical areas of importance. In most clinical settings, numerous physicians are involved in a patient's care. When care is delivered at a distance, it may prove challenging to share the patient with other members of the treatment team. Not being part of a local care community adds complexity to the care of the patient. When psychiatrists treat patients via videoconferencing, they are engaged in a full patient relationship with an obligation to maintain medical records, provide continuity of care, and pursue avenues to integrate all relevant medical information into the patient's overall medical and mental health history and record. The reality of telepsychiatry practice is that this can sometimes be difficult, and Tapper (1994) went so far as to suggest that "failing to address continuity of care for the patient could constitute patient abandonment just as if the patient had been seen for an initial consultation in the psychiatrist's office" (p. 3). With the increasing numbers of psychiatrists practicing integrated and collaborative care through the use of technology, the other side of this coin is that the use of such technologies can actually dramatically increase the opportunities to provide high-quality continuity of care compared with traditional office practice, and this is an area where practice standards could be significantly elevated through the use of telepsychiatry.

VIII. PATIENT SAFETY PLANNING AND EMERGENCY MANAGEMENT

Patient safety is particularly challenging in telepsychiatry and is discussed at length earlier in this chapter and in Chapter 3. There are real practical challenges (how to manage a real emergency) and more nuanced challenges (loss of perceived control). It is critical to establish a protocol that operationalizes the safety plan. For a comprehensive review of patient safety planning measures, see Shore and Lu (2014).

A well-developed safety plan should include, at a minimum, the following:

- The patient's physical address and current working telephone number.
- A working telephone number for emergency personnel/services in the patient's location.
- A contingency plan for reconnecting with the patient if a technical disruption occurs.

When patients are being seen in their homes, we strongly recommend that all providers utilize a patient support person as a backup as recommended in the American Telemedicine Association (2013b) guidelines. In the event of an emergency, the practitioner can contact this support person and ask him or her to physically go to the patient's residence. Shore and Lu (2014) also recommend developing contingency plans for other issues (e.g., medical emergencies, loss of access to transportation, natural or human-caused disasters, weather alerts, fire alarms, bomb threats, acts of violence) and establishing a referral source for additional services in the community as needed.

SUMMARY

The practice of telepsychiatry is a burgeoning industry in which access to emerging technologies has outdistanced the availability of widely accepted ethical principles to guide the provisioning of services, whether in a clinic- or a non-clinic-based setting. In this chapter, our goal has been both to provide an overview of clinical individual and group skills needed for synchronous care and to review ethical considerations. Topics addressed included the following:

- What types of online consultations can be conducted via telepsychiatry.
- How telepsychiatry consultations differ from traditional in-person consultations.
- What individual and group clinical and media skills are needed for psychiatrists and other therapists to work successfully online with their patients.
- How the virtual space in telepsychiatry consultations can be used to improve care.
- How clinicians can best manage unusual patients or situations.
- Which groups of patients prefer to be seen online rather than in person.
- In what situations telepsychiatry may be better clinical practice than in-person care.
- What skills learned from the practice of telepsychiatry can help clinicians deliver a higher standard of care in their in-person psychiatric consultations.
- What ethical principles and guidelines in telepsychiatry allow clinicians to establish and maintain core standards.

Before embarking on a career in telepsychiatry, clinicians should become familiar with the practice guidelines of the ATA. Additionally, they should know their state's jurisdictional legislation pertaining to telemedicine, involuntary commitment, suicide holds, and welfare checks conducted via technology. States vary, and laws in some states are quite nuanced. Under no circumstances should practitioners deliver services via technology across state lines unless they are licensed in the state in which the patient is physically located.

It is critically important that telepsychiatry practitioners adhere to all medical ethical standards expected for in-person appointments. While the field continues to play catch-up, clinicians must develop and maintain core ethical standards of practice guided by the available literature base. Formulating standard operating procedures to articulate those standards and becoming familiar with the policies and regulations regarding telepsychiatry set forth by their system of care are highly recommended.

REFERENCES

American Medical Association: AMA Policy: Professionalism in the Use of Social Media, 2011. Available at: https://www.adventisthealth.org/nw/Documents/AMA-Professionalism-in-use-of-Social-Media-7-25-11.pdf. Accessed August 3, 2016.

American Medical Association: AMA adopts new guidance for ethical practice in telemedicine. American Medical Association website, June 13, 2016a. Available at: https://www.ama-assn.org/ama-adopts-new-guidance-ethical-practice-telemedicine. Accessed June 22, 2017.

American Medical Association: Ethical practice in telemedicine: executive summary and recommendations, 2016b. Available at: https://www.ama-assn.org/ethical-practice-telemedicine. Accessed March 17, 2017.

American Psychiatric Association: Position Statement on Telemedicine in Psychiatry, November 2015. Available at: https://www.psychiatry.org/File%20Library/About-APA/Organization-Documents-Policies/Policies/Position-Telemedicine-in-Psychiatry.pdf. Accessed August 17, 2017.

American Telemedicine Association: Evidence-Based Practice for Telemental Health, 2009a. Available at: http://www.americantelemed.org/resources/telemedicine-practice-guidelines/telemedicine-practice-guidelines/evidence-based-practice-for-telemental-health#.V6DiAle1eoI. Accessed July 31, 2016.

American Telemedicine Association: Practice Guidelines for Videoconferencing-Based Telemental Health, 2009b. Available at: http://www.americantelemed.org/resources/telemedicine-practice-guidelines/telemedicine-practice-guidelines/videoconferencing-based-telemental-health#.V6DhaFe1eoI. Accessed July 31, 2016.

American Telemedicine Association: A Lexicon Assessment and Outcome Measurements for Telemental Health, 2013a. Available at: http://www.american-telemed.org/resources/telemedicine-practice-guidelines/telemedicine-practice-guidelines/a-lexicon-of-assessment-and-outcome-measurements-for-telemental-health#.V6Ddg1e1eoI. Accessed July 31, 2016.

American Telemedicine Association: Practice Guidelines for Video-Based Online Mental Health, 2013b. Available at: http://www.americantelemed.org/resources/telemedicine-practice-guidelines/telemedicine-practice-guidelines/practice-guidelines-for-video-based-online-mental-health-services#.V6DgyVe1eoI. Accessed July 31, 2016.

American Telemedicine Association: Core Operational Guidelines for Telehealth Services Involving Provider–Patient Interactions, 2014. Available at: http://www.americantelemed.org/docs/default-source/standards/core-operational-guidelines-for-telehealth-services.pdf?sfvrsn=6. Accessed July 31, 2016.

American Telemedicine Association: Practice Guidelines for Telemental Health With Children and Adolescents, March 2017. Available at: https://higherlogicdownload.s3.amazonaws.com/AMERICANTELEMED/618da447-dee1-4ee1-b941-c5bf3db5669a/UploadedImages/Practice%20Guideline%20Covers/NEW_ATA%20Children%20&%20Adolescents%20Guidelines.pdf. Accessed August 17, 2017.

Bashshur RL, Shannon GW, Bashshur N, Yellowlees PM: The empirical evidence for telemedicine interventions in mental disorders. Telemed J E Health 22(2):87–113, 2016 26624248

Chan S, Parish M, Yellowlees P: Telepsychiatry Today. Curr Psychiatry Rep 17(11):89, 2015 26384338

Deslich S, Stec B, Tomblin S, et al: Telepsychiatry in the 21(st) century: transforming healthcare with technology. Perspect Health Inf Manag 10(Summer), 2013 23861676

Fortney JC, Pyne JM, Kimbrell TA, et al: Telemedicine-based collaborative care for posttraumatic stress disorder: a randomized clinical trial. JAMA Psychiatry 72(1):58–67, 2015 25409287

Hilty DM, Ferrer DC, Parish MB, et al: The effectiveness of telemental health: a 2013 review. Telemed J E Health 19(6):444–454, 2013 23697504

Hilty DM, Yellowlees PM: Collaborative mental health services using multiple technologies: the new way to practice and a new standard of practice? J Am Acad Child Adolesc Psychiatry 54(4):245–246, 2015 25791139

Hyler SE, Gangure DP: Legal and ethical challenges in telepsychiatry. J Psychiatr Pract 10(4):272–276, 2004 15552552

Joint Task Force for the Development of Telepsychology Guidelines for Psychologists: Guidelines for the practice of telepsychology. Am Psychol 68(9):791–800, 2013 24341643

Miller HA: Miller Forensic Assessment of Symptoms Test (M-FAST): Professional Manual. Odessa, FL, Psychological Assessment Resources, 2001

Myers K, Cain S; The Work Group on Quality Issues: Practice parameter for telepsychiatry with children and adolescents. J Am Acad Child Adolesc Psychiatry 47(12):1468–1483, 2008 19034191

Myers K, Vander Stoep A, Zhou C, et al: Effectiveness of a telehealth service delivery model for treating attention-deficit/hyperactivity disorder: a community-based randomized controlled trial. J Am Acad Child Adolesc Psychiatry 54(4):263–274, 2015 25791143

Pakyurek M, Yellowlees P, Hilty D: The child and adolescent telepsychiatry consultation: can it be a more effective clinical process for certain patients than conventional practice? Telemed J E Health 16(3):289–292, 2010 20406115

Rambo EM: Ethical Considerations in the Practice of Telepsychiatry. Luminello Mental Health Practice Blog, March 9, 2016. Available at: https://luminello.com/ethical-considerations-in-the-practice-of-telepsychiatry-2/. Accessed July 30, 2016.

Raney L, Pollack D, Parks J, Katon W: The American Psychiatric Association response to the "joint principles: integrating behavioral health care into the patient-centered medical home." Fam Syst Health 32(2):147–148, 2014 24955687

Rogers E: Diffusion of Innovations, 5th Edition. New York, Simon & Schuster, 2003

Royal Australian and New Zealand College of Psychiatrists: Professional Practice Standards and Guides for Telepsychiatry. Melbourne, Victoria, Australia, Royal Australian and New Zealand College of Psychiatrists, 2013. Available at: https://www.ranzcp.org/Files/Resources/RANZCP-Professional-Practice-Standards-and-Guides.aspx. Accessed March 17, 2017.

Sabin JE, Skimming K: A framework of ethics for telepsychiatry practice. Int Rev Psychiatry 27(6):490–495, 2015 26493214

Shore JH: Telepsychiatry: videoconferencing in the delivery of psychiatric care. Am J Psychiatry 170(3):256–262, 2013 23450286

Shore J, Vo A, Yellowlees P, et al: Antipsychotic-induced movement disorder: screening via telemental health. Telemed J E Health 21(12):1027–1029, 2015 26125084

Shore P, Lu M: Patient safety planning and emergency management, in Behavioral Telehealth Series, Vol 1. Clinical Video Conferencing: Program Development and Practice. Edited by Tuerk P, Shore P. New York, Springer International, 2014, pp 167–201

Smith A, Anderson M: Five facts about online dating. Fact Tank, Pew Research Center, February 29, 2016. Available at: http://www.pewresearch.org/fact-tank/2016/02/29/5-facts-about-online-dating/. Accessed August 17, 2017.

Tapper CM: Unilateral termination of treatment by a psychiatrist. Guidelines of the Canadian Psychiatric Association. Can J Psychiatry 39(1):2–7, 1994 8193994

Totten AM, Womack DM, Eden KB, et al: Telehealth: Mapping the Evidence for Patient Outcomes From Systematic Reviews [Internet]. Agency for Healthcare Research and Quality Report No. 16-EHC034-EF. Rockville, MD, AHRQ Comparative Effectiveness Technical Briefs, June 2016. 27536752

Yellowlees P: Your Health in the Information Age: How You and Your Doctor Can Use the Internet to Work Together. Bloomington, IN, iUniverse, 2008

Yellowlees P, Odor A, Patrice K, et al: Disruptive innovation: the future of healthcare? Telemed J E Health 17(3):231–234, 2011 21361819

Yellowlees P, Richard Chan S, Burke Parish M: The hybrid doctor–patient relationship in the age of technology—telepsychiatry consultations and the use of virtual space. Int Rev Psychiatry 27(6):476–489, 2015 26493089

6

Data Collection From Novel Sources

Steven R. Chan, M.D., M.B.A.

Michelle Burke Parish, M.A., Ph.D.(c)

Sarina Fazio, Ph.D.(c), M.S., R.N.

John Torous, M.D.

Patient-clinician encounters—whether by in-person visits or telephone calls—have traditionally been the most important source of data used to assess and treat patients with mental disorders. There is, however, an enormous demand for mental health care services with limited supply of health care practitioners. In resource-poor countries and counties, there is a dearth of mental health care practitioners. Rural counties and Native American reservations, for example, have the lowest psychiatrist-to-patient ratios versus urban areas. On a macroscopic scale, it is projected that mental disorders will have a global economic impact of about $16 trillion in lost labor and manufacturing productivity by 2030 (Jones et al. 2014). The trend within the United States toward pay-for-performance and capitated models—and away

We gratefully acknowledge the illustration support of creative designer Jennifer Favela, using icon libraries of Font Awesome, by Dave Gandy (http://fontawesome.io), under SIL International's open font license (OFL) 1.1.

from fee-for-service models—will place increased pressure on mental health care practitioners.

Technology has the potential to alleviate a proportion of these issues. Mental health care informatics and incorporation of information technologies can boost accessibility, reduce costs, and provide a more tailored, personalized experience for patients (Lal and Adair 2014). Having usable electronic health record (EHR) systems can decrease communication delays, and data from patient prescription drug monitoring programs can help reduce the impact of substance use disorders, overprescribing, and polypharmacy.

There are some other financial factors that stimulate the use of information technologies. Although the Health Information Technology for Economic and Clinical Health (HITECH) Act of 2009 incentivized the use of electronic medical records (EMRs), these incentives did not apply to behavioral health care. As of 2017, the Centers for Medicare & Medicaid Services (CMS) provide matching funds for development of connectivity between long-term care facilities, public health, and mental and behavioral health care providers, but still no financial incentives to support core clinical information technology (IT) systems by these providers (Adler-Milstein 2016).

The technology sector sees an enormous amount of opportunity in these developments, as evidenced by a shift from traditional medical startups toward funding for mental health care and behavioral health care startups. There has been increased interest among both academic and commercial researchers in technology-assisted delivery of mental health care, as demonstrated by increases in research projects, research funding, and venture capital funding.

In this chapter, we discuss

- Information that can be gathered for clinical purposes.
- The difference between *passive data* (information gathered through sensors, messages, and databases without the patient's active involvement, and with or without the patient's knowledge or awareness) and *active data* (information that the patient submits).
- How information is gathered from the Internet, remote monitoring sensors, and health care networks.
- How to choose from available consumer apps, devices, and technologies for patient care.

- The challenges and ethical dilemmas surrounding use of these new data sources.

CASE EXAMPLE 1: INCORPORATING NONHEALTH APPS INTO A TREATMENT PLAN[1]

Ash, a 20-year-old male, presented to Dr. Oak with complaints of anxiety, because next week Ash faced final exams in animal studies and zoology. Ash had not been able to focus on his training because he said his mind kept thinking about so many different things, leading to distractibility. Ash has had struggles in the education environment since middle school, which he attributed to being very forgetful with homework and waiting until the last minute to complete projects. He even at times forgets to submit assignments and cannot complete exams on time. Concentration has even been an issue in his relationships, as Ash's ex-girlfriends have accused him of not paying attention to them during conversations.

Ash has not had disciplinary issues, has a negative legal history, and has not been tested for learning disabilities. Ash has been very successful in his extracurricular activities and gym tournaments. When given a trial of an attention medication (of unknown name), which worked, his mother had stopped it within a month and decided to give him dietary supplements instead.

Dr. Oak determined that Ash has generalized anxiety secondary to untreated attention-deficit/hyperactivity disorder (ADHD). Dr. Oak wanted to prescribe Ash an extended-release stimulant as well as psychotherapy. Unfortunately, ADHD services in the local area were only available for children and adolescents younger than 18 years, and the nearest ADHD therapist had no openings.

Given these constraints, Dr. Oak discussed using productivity software, which included a task management app and a task timer app, plus a Web site–blocking app to help Ash minimize distractions. Ash signed an informed consent form stating that he understood the privacy, security, and legal implications of using unencrypted consumer software for his condition.

I KEY CONCEPT

Habits and behaviors can be shaped by effective use of technology. Clinicians must learn how to use consumer devices and apps, which can be as important as identifying community resources, recommending self-help books, and referring to other

---

[1]Case provided by Steven R. Chan, M.D., M.B.A.

specialists. Patients must be educated about the privacy, security, and legal issues associated with use of consumer tools.

WHY DO CLINICIANS NEED TO COLLECT DATA?

Clinical data help clinicians build a differential diagnosis, propose treatments, and perform psychotherapy. These data can come from patients themselves, from patients' families and caregivers, and from other providers and organizational entities. The clinical interview and examination with the patient is often the most important source of data. Patient questionnaires, therapy homework, journal entries, and even art can help provide information outside of the patient–clinician interview.

The *patient's family and caregivers* can provide historical data, which is invaluable in establishing a baseline and longitudinal time line of the patient's functioning. School reports, family photographs, and school-grade report cards can provide childhood educational history. Family movies on videocassettes, digital video disks (DVDs), and digital video files can allow clinicians to observe patients' behavior and movements, essentially allowing clinicians to perform historical mental status examinations. Handwritten notes and drawn art can provide some insight into the patient's social history and educational level. In this digital age, photos can easily be scanned and videos digitized, making the sharing of this information simpler.

Other providers can provide progress notes, medical records, laboratory testing, neuroimaging, and psychological testing results. Integrated medical record systems and notes can give clinicians the history they need to refine a patient's diagnosis. Pharmacies can provide medications prescribed, and government databases—such as Controlled Substance Utilization Review and Evaluation System (CURES) and prescription drug monitoring programs—can give insight into a patient's medication history and potential prescription drug abuse patterns.

TRADITIONAL METHODS OF DATA COLLECTION

Traditional means of collecting clinical data have included mail, fax, telephone, the Internet, and long-distance telemedicine video systems.

- Data can be acquired by *mail*—which currently occurs in older offices not equipped with EMRs and for large datasets such as radiological imaging series.

- *Fax machines* are still in wide use for transmitting paper records quickly, but they are slowly being supplanted with PDF files as the primary, lowest-common-denominator option from EHRs.
- *Voice calls* over telephones are still used. They are a very limited method, as they do not provide high audio fidelity, much less a visual picture of the patient.
- Record systems connected to the *Internet*—such as patient portals—are also used. The U.S. federal government incentivized the use of patient portals (for Meaningful Use stage 2 requirements), which allow patients to read, download, and transmit their own health information.
- Finally, *telemedicine video systems* (described elsewhere in this book) are in wide use within large health systems, such as government (e.g., U.S. Department of Veterans Affairs [VA]), commercial (e.g., Kaiser Permanente) and academic health systems (e.g., University of California).

NEW METHODS OF DATA COLLECTION ENABLED BY NEW TECHNOLOGY

The clinical interview remains a primary source of information despite the plethora of information available to clinicians. However, clinical interviews offer only a single snapshot in time, a single view into a longitudinal and dynamic presentation of a mental illness. The skilled clinician can glean much information from this single view, but this view may be limited by a patient's memory and retrospective recollection bias.

As a thought exercise, try to recall how well you slept for the past 2 weeks. Many mental illnesses impact cognition, which can make retrospective recollection even less reliable. Compounding the problem: many patients may be ashamed of their symptoms and minimize them on examination, and co-occurring substance use disorders may affect the patient's memory, further clouding the psychiatric diagnosis.

The problem is that these are retrospective questions that—using our traditional methods of collecting data just described—rely on a person's memory if no other historical collateral information is available. Furthermore, the person's memory may be unreliable, thus giving a distorted history.

New sources of data—from social media networks, the patient's own personal mobile computers, and sensors—can help provide high-quality collateral information to help the clinician. For organizations concerned with population health (e.g., accountable care organizations, physicians operating under a capitated financial model, vertically integrated health systems), the ability to continuously assess a patient's symptoms, provide more resources, and intervene "just in time" could more quickly and reliably prevent relapses of symptoms, emergency department use, and unnecessary hospitalizations.

WHAT NEW SOURCES OF DATA ARE AVAILABLE?

New sources of data—data that are currently not typically incorporated in the traditional clinical workflow—come from information and consumer health technologies. These new sources can potentially help clinicians make more accurate diagnoses, fill in gaps in patient histories, and can potentially change the way diagnoses are made. To distinguish how data are obtained, think of these as two separate categories:

- *Active data* refers to data collected from patient surveys or other assessments that require patient participation. A mood survey that a patient takes every week at noon is an example of active data. Here, if the patient does not fill in the survey, no data are collected. A major advantage of active data is that they minimize retrospective recollection by asking patients to report what they are feeling exactly at the moment the survey is offered instead of what they think they felt in the past. Several studies (Bush et al. 2013; Moore et al. 2016; Moran et al. 2017; Torous and Powell 2015) have demonstrated the utility of active data in helping to achieve more sensitive and specific diagnostic assessments.
- *Passive data* refers to information obtained without patients' active involvement and communication. This type of data is obtained from business databases, patients' electronic devices, and indirect technology interactions. For example, users' phones automatically detect their location through their proximity to cellular towers, their available WiFi networks, and their GPS coordinates. These location data could potentially be useful in monitoring whether a patient with depression is active or sedentary or whether a patient at risk for a manic episode is suddenly moving rapidly around the neighborhood and making erratic stops at seemingly random locations.

As these two brief examples underscore, passive data involve two core challenges: First, the ethics of passive data use in mental health care is unexplored territory (Roberts and Torous 2016), and second, the collection of passive data is still new and not yet fully developed.

Finally, like many other data sources, passive data often represent only a small part of the complete dataset and may require integration with other data. For example, using machine learning, computers could determine whether a person was more or less active based on the person's historical daily step count, and even though this information cannot by itself lead to a diagnosis, numerous studies have shown the usefulness of passive data when integrated into a bigger diagnostic picture (Rabbi et al. 2011; Torous et al. 2015).

PASSIVE DATA FROM SMARTPHONES AND SMARTWATCHES

The digital divide preventing access to computing devices and the Internet is narrowing as a result of increased access to *smartphones*—integrated, pocket-sized computers containing ample memory, a large touchscreen, Internet and wireless connectivity, and the ability to run software. As of 2017, 77% of adults in the United States own a smartphone, a drastic increase from 35% in 2011 (Pew Research Center 2017). Smartphone owners tend to be younger, with higher levels of education and higher levels of income. Many are "smartphone-only" Internet users: 12% of U.S. adults access the Internet primarily using their smartphones and do not have home broadband service. And reliance on smartphones for Internet access is particularly common among younger, nonwhite, and lower-income Americans.

Smartwatches are smaller, wrist-sized computers that incorporate features of both wearable devices and smartphones. Although they are often marketed as an accessory to a larger computer (often a smartphone), smartwatches have enough computing power, memory storage, and network connectivity to operate as independent devices.

Besides serving as a means of communication, smartphones and smartwatches contain a variety of sensors that detect environmental changes (Ben-Zeev et al. 2014, 2015; McClernon and Choudhury 2013; Puiatti et al. 2011; Torous et al. 2016), and many of these sensors are built into standard smartphones that cost less than $500 per unit. Smartphones and smartwatches account for nearly all of the sensors used in mainstream consumer applications (Table 6–1). Sensor data can inform medical and psychiatric clinicians about a patient's well-being, comfort,

TABLE 6–1. Types of data captured by smartphone and smartwatch sensors

Sensor-captured data	Mainstream application examples	Potential clinical uses
Accelerometers can detect a person's movement, number of steps	Fitness tracking	Exercise, weight loss, activity level, movement and gait detection
Location triangulated through global positioning satellite (GPS), cellular towers, and WiFi networks	Maps, driving directions, location-specific photography, social media, augmented-reality games	Activity level, movement, wandering behaviors, peer support, addiction trigger avoidance
Cameras can detect light, a person's face, and a person's movements	Security, social media and chat, exercise, nutrition tracking, augmented reality	Light exposure, photographic self-reflection and photo journaling, peer support
Cameras can have depth perception and perform 3D mapping	Augmented-reality games, indoor mapping, 3D object scanning	Exposure to stressful environments or objects with response prevention
Compass	Maps, driving directions	Movement, wandering behaviors
Humidity level	Weather	Environmental comfort indicator
Temperature of environment	Weather	Environmental comfort indicator

TABLE 6–1. Types of data captured by smartphone and smartwatch sensors *(continued)*

Sensor-captured data	Mainstream application examples	Potential clinical uses
Microphone	Telephone calls, audio recording, social media and chat, voice dictation	Activity level, speech assessment, assessment of ambient noise as environmental comfort indicator, voice dictation for physical impairments
Screen taps with touch pressure intensity	Games, secondary controls	Activity level, cognitive exercises
Heart rate	Fitness tracking	Exercise, weight loss, activity level, biofeedback
Electrodermal activity (skin conductance)	Stress testing	Biofeedback

activity level, and mood. Activity-level data, in particular, could indicate either *hyperactivity*—as in anxiety or mania—or *hypoactivity*—as in depression or cognitive impairment (Vahia and Sewell 2016). Sensor data can be combined to form a rich new source of clinical information (Chan et al. 2014).

PASSIVE DATA FROM WEARABLE DEVICES

Seven in 10 adults track a health indicator, such as weight, diet, sleep patterns, or health symptoms. Rather than keeping track of this information in their heads or using paper, adults more often use some form of technology to track their health data (Fox and Duggan 2013).

Much of this technology tracking comes in the form of wearable devices that are more affordable than traditional commercial medical-grade technology. These devices can be worn as accessories—watches, patches, clothing, and even fashionable jewelry—to track different data elements about the wearer's physical activity, sleep, and vital signs (Table 6–2). Smartwatches can measure heart rate and elements of fitness, such as calories burned, steps taken, and distance traveled.

Compared with wearable devices, fitness trackers that are not attached to the body are less sophisticated, with less focused tracking abilities. Many wearable devices are also water resistant and embedded with GPS tracking. Patches can detect skin conductance and medication ingestion. The information collected from these devices can connect back to a smartphone app or Web app using Bluetooth or near-field communication (NFC). These apps—because of their larger displays—can visualize their data in graphs and charts. The health data collected can be aggregated over time, making it possible to make sense of behavioral trends. Although these consumer devices are not medical-grade devices, they still provide an important source of collateral data. Both patients and physicians can view these graphs in making clinical decisions.

Many applications use machine learning technology to analyze information collected and to provide personalized feedback on an individual's performance. Some applications also allow manual data input or integration from other health apps, such as where users can actively track their nutrition and mood.

The Health app on Apple iOS, Google Fit on Android, and Microsoft Health on Windows are examples of platform-specific apps that digest data streams from multiple wearable devices and smartphone apps.

TABLE 6–2. Consumer wearable devices and tracking applications as of August 2017, based on features listed on product Web pages, in reviews, and in press releases

		Features				
Accessory type	Device name	Step count	Heart rate	Calories burned	Sleep	Other
Watches	Android Wear–powered smartwatches	X	X	X		Global positioning satellite (GPS) location in some models
	WatchOS-powered Apple watch	X	X	X	X	GPS and GLONASS (globalnaya navigatsionnaya sputnikovaya sistema ["global navigation satellite system"]) location in some models
	Garmin Vivoactive HR GPS fitness tracker	X	X	X	X	Galvanic skin resistance; activity and exercise detection
	Fitbit Alta HR, Charge 2, Blaze fitness trackers	X	X	X	X	Automatic activity recognition and logging
	Tizen OS-powered Samsung Gear S3 smartwatch	X	X	X	X	Altitude, air pressure, GPS location
	Nokia Steel smartwatch	X		X	X	Running/swimming detection

TABLE 6–2. Consumer wearable devices and tracking applications as of August 2017, based on features listed on product Web pages, in reviews, and in press releases *(continued)*

Accessory type	Device name	Features					
		Step count	Heart rate	Calories burned	Sleep	Other	
Clothing	Sensoria Fitness Smart socks with anklet	X		X		Step cadence, foot landing technique, altitude	
	Hexoskin Smart Shirt	X	X	X	X	Breathing rate, minute ventilation, heart rate variability and recovery	
	Neopenda baby hat		X			Respiratory rate, blood oxygen saturation, temperature	
	Glasses: JINS MEME	X				Gaze and eye movements, activity detection	
	OMSignal OMBra smart bra	X	X	X		Step cadence, respiratory rate	
Posture	Lumo Lift	X		X		Posture	
Jewelry	Bellaband Leaf	X		X	X	Regularity of menstrual cycle via calendaring app	

These streams can be displayed on a comprehensive dashboard. This dashboard, if configured, can in theory be connected with an EHR. However, as of August 2017, interoperability functions and wearable data dashboards such as that shown in Figure 6–1 are not offered as part of most EHR systems' core functionality.

CASE EXAMPLE 2: USE OF WEARABLE DEVICES AND SMARTPHONE APPS FOR SYMPTOM TRACKING AND DIAGNOSTIC ASSESSMENT[2]

Mrs. Green, a 55-year-old married woman with a bipolar I disorder diagnosis and a history of 12 past hospitalizations, consults Dr. Willow because of worsening depression. Although she has been stable on valproic acid and risperidone for years, she tells Dr. Willow that she has recently become aware that she does not have as much energy as she used to, and she finds it difficult to control her worrying. On questioning, she cannot say how many hours of sleep she currently gets, but she knows that her sleep has changed and is not restful. In the course of the conversation about sleep, Mrs. Green mentions that her husband of 12 years recently purchased a fitness-tracking wristband that tracks the wearer's hours of sleep per night, steps per day, and heart rate.

Dr. Willow requests that Mrs. Green activate the wristband and start charting her sleep. He mentions that even though the accuracy is not fully guaranteed and is not the same as a medical-grade sleep study, a wrist-worn activity-tracking device could provide a rough indicator of her sleep habits that could potentially help predict a relapse of depression and give her an opportunity to seek intervention before her mood worsens. Mrs. Green agrees, saying that she typically finds she gets less sleep for about 4 days prior to her mood changing.

Dr. Willow warns that even though the fitness tracker comes with an online dashboard, he has no access to it, and there should be no expectation that a professional is monitoring the results. He stresses that in the case of an emergency, Mrs. Green should contact the on-call physician or call 911, but should not send messages through the Coach feature of the fitness tracker.

Mrs. Green begins using the fitness tracker, and when Dr. Willow sees her 2 weeks later, she shows him her smartphone app, which summarizes the sleep data captured from her wristband in the form of charts and graphics. Dr. Willow quickly discovers that on most nights, Mrs. Green apparently gets out of bed and walks around the house for about 30 minutes. Both the patient and her husband are extremely surprised to

---

[2]Case provided by John Torous, M.D.

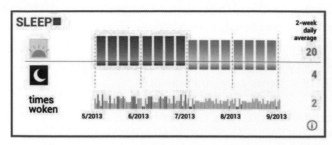

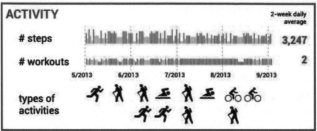

FIGURE 6–1.   Sample wearable device data visualization, from Mind Mentor, a prototype app for monitoring both physical and emotional health.

Source.   Illustration by Steven Chan, M.D., M.B.A. (see http://www.steven-chanmd.com/project/mind-mentor/). Used with permission.

learn about these sleepwalking episodes, which neither of them had been aware of. Dr. Willow, suspecting that these episodes represent a disorder of arousal from non–rapid eye movement (NREM) sleep, refers Mrs. Green to a sleep medicine specialist for further evaluation.

▌ KEY CONCEPT

Much like recommending a gym membership, clinicians can discuss and even recommend the use of fitness-promoting devices. Clinicians should set expectations and create the therapeutic frame around the interaction between clinician, patient, and device. These devices are another tool to help clinicians assess symptom patterns—like mood-tracking and sleep-tracking paper charts—and the data can be summarized for the clinician to review at each visit.

PASSIVE DATA FROM AUGMENTED REALITY AND VIRTUAL REALITY DEVICES

Virtual reality (VR) devices—in which a person wears a headset that places an up-close display to their eyes and headphones to their ears— have been researched for decades for stress relief, anesthesia, intraoperative anxiety, concussion detection, and exposure therapy for specific phobia. In fact, some therapists and psychologists in private practice use these regularly. The VA Health System has researched VR extensively for posttraumatic stress disorder (PTSD) and uses VR clinically at multiple sites around the United States.

VR technology is becoming more affordable, particularly with the increased availability and reduced price of immersive VR goggles that integrate with smartphones. Passive data collected from VR can include the quality of patients' interactions in their immersive environments and the amount of time spent in VR, as well as physiological data during use of VR devices.

Augmented reality (AR) technology has also gained interest with the popularity of AR-based smartphone games. AR overlays information in the environment, encouraging users to interact and become active with the environment. This encouragement can increase directed activity and energy levels for a patient. For example, AR glasses—which overlay a display on a device shaped like eyeglasses—have been used to assist youth with autism in making eye contact and identifying other people's moods. These AR glasses collect data on the amount of eye contact made with other persons. AR can be used for animal phobia exposure therapy by showing visual simulations of the feared stimulus in the person's environment: imagine spiders crawling around the room through a smartphone window. AR can also provide schizophrenia education by simulating visual and auditory hallucinations in the current environment.

PASSIVE DATA FROM HEALTH RECORDS

EMRs act as a hub for information—such as hospital episodes, outpatient clinic encounter summaries, medication refills, medication reconciliation, number of phone calls and e-mail messages—accumulated from the clinic, hospital, pharmacy, insurance companies, and even the patients themselves. Traditionally, the EMR consists of information documented by the clinician or provider when the patient is being seen in the context of clinical care. With the advent of wearable and smarthome technologies, more granular information can be captured in the EMR that reflects the patient's health information on a daily basis.

Analytics and clinical decision support systems can also be applied to data in the health record. These systems can quantify patients' health care and medication use by deriving counts of visits, prescriptions, and contacts with the health care system. This type of data can be used to better understand trends of health care service use for research and practice. These trends may be inferred from "big data," which may involve the health records of millions of patients and require very sophisticated informatics-driven analysis to create useful clinical results at the individual or population level.

In general, this type of technology is offered by commercial, enterprise vendors, with IBM Watson being one of the more highly advertised recent entrants to this market. It is most likely that, for you as the individual clinician, health record information will be offered by your IT team or vendor or your organization and may even be available just for patients that you have personally seen. Individual clinicians will find that their capacity to access this type of data will vary enormously and that the implementation of EMR-related data apps requires rigorous privacy and security standards and business contracts beyond the scope of this book. These standards and contracting information can be found in clinical informatics and business IT texts.

CASE EXAMPLE 3: ADDRESSING ELECTRONIC MESSAGING RISKS WITH PATIENTS[3]

Alex, a 19-year-old male, is being seen by Dr. Sycamore for depression and anxiety at Kalos Clinic, a mental health care center for at-risk and homeless adolescents. He asks Dr. Sycamore whether he can contact her on Facebook about his appointments, because he no longer has access to a phone and has no home address, so the only way he can receive messages is by checking his Facebook page from the library computer.

Dr. Sycamore is concerned about losing her contact with Alex, but she is also not sure about her agency's policy regarding the use of social media with patients. She consults with Kalos Clinic's risk management and IT experts. The experts tell Dr. Sycamore that using Facebook

---

[3]Case provided by Sarina Fazio, Ph.D.(c), M.S., R.N., and Steven R. Chan, M.D., M.B.A.

would pose a liability. Dr. Sycamore's peers also say that using Facebook with Dr. Sycamore's personal account could result in a therapeutic boundary crossing.

Instead, Dr. Sycamore arranges to set up a secure messaging account for Alex through Kalos Clinic's patient portal to communicate with him through a separate electronic messaging app.

▍ KEY CONCEPT

Using consumer social media networks exposes both clinician and patient to security and privacy risks as well as therapeutic boundary crossings and should be avoided. Clinicians should consult their organization's legal and risk management teams to determine which electronic tools are appropriate for use with patients. Clinicians who are operating independently in private practice should contact their malpractice insurance carrier for guidelines and review the recommendations in Chapter 8 ("Indirect Consultation and Hybrid Care").

ACTIVE DATA FROM SOCIAL MEDIA

Social media sites have become ubiquitous across the globe, with more than 2 billion active social media users worldwide as of August 2017 ("Most Famous Social Network Sites Worldwide" 2017). Social networking data has attracted interest from researchers and clinicians alike as a potential source of clinically useful information about patients.

Studies examining speech and language pattern recognition have evaluated publicly available social networking information and have found that, using data mining techniques, mental illnesses such as depression and posttraumatic stress disorder can be associated with particular users. These data mining studies have included publicly available social media posts and information collected for research purposes, although such information has not been used to track or evaluate individuals' symptoms or illnesses in a clinical setting. While it may be in theory clinically useful to employ such algorithms for clinician decision support through public social media tools, questions remain about *if, how,* and *when* social media should be used within the clinical setting. It is clear, however, that some popular social media applications may be particularly useful tools for accessing and engaging some patient populations online, and extensive work has occurred in this area in the political domain where differing groups of potential voters are identified and contacted through sophisticated data mining of social networking environments.

Secure, private, or closed social networking sites are, however, already a very useful tool in patient care. Private social networks allow patients to communicate not only among themselves but also with human or computer-driven artificial intelligence coaches as well as with anyone who is invited into the group, such as doctors with a specific expertise. The concept is similar to that used in group psychotherapy, group classes, and group activities to encourage intragroup communications, interactions, learning, and behavioral activation. The difference is that the closed online group operates asynchronously, over a social network that provides messaging, events, and online activities. Some commercial social networks, such as PatientsLikeMe, use similar concepts. These sites connect patients with common illnesses and encourage sharing of information about medications, side effects, and experiences related to their illnesses. Private social networks may also offer the ability to anonymize user names, but it is up to each user to decide whether to divulge personally identifiable information. Data are currently being aggregated within some of these networks, and PatientsLikeMe, for instance, runs a number of clinical trials of medications and therapies through regular contact and follow-up with members of the group, which it has then started to publish both online and in academic journals. The most dramatic example so far of this approach to data collection via social networks appeared on the PatientsLikeMe Web site in April 2011:

> PatientsLikeMe reveals the results of a patient-initiated observational study refuting a 2008 published study that claimed lithium carbonate could slow the progression of the neurodegenerative disease amyotrophic lateral sclerosis (ALS). PatientsLikeMe, a health data-sharing website with more than 100,000 patients and 500+ conditions, announces its study results in the journal *Nature Biotechnology* (www.patientslikeme.com).

ACTIVE DATA FROM MOBILE APPS

Mobile apps can collect data that users input themselves. There are health-specific and general consumer apps, and the use of such apps, just like the use of social networks and social media, comes with the benefit of interactivity and the risks of privacy, security, and discoverability.

The most prevalent of mental health–specific apps, *mood trackers,* allow patients to rank symptoms on various scales, such as irritability versus calm and depression versus happiness. Apps vary in the use of assessing these: numerical scales, iconographic scales, and continuous scales can be used in varying, subjective degrees. Look at specific apps before recommending them to patients, and make sure that the scales are useful for your needs. A variant of these are medication tracking apps, in which patients enter in whether they have taken a medication or not.

The second most common are *diary apps.* Patients can enter their thoughts and feelings in these apps much like they would in a journal. Some diary apps may allow users to post anonymously to the public or craft an online, alternate persona. Similarly, though not specific to mental health, fitness apps can allow patients to manually enter in their workouts, exercises, and goals. These apps can often incorporate passive data gathered from wearables and sensors.

These apps can help patients who have conditions that can be improved with lifestyle changes and better self-management. Many smartphone apps are associated with specific goals, such as diabetes management or smoking cessation. Some apps, in the form of video games, can even use the camera to detect whether a patient is doing physical exercises like sit-ups and push-ups, use accelerometers to detect whether a patient is dancing while the game plays pop music, and use the GPS to track a runner's location. In this respect, patients can still directly enter data, but it need not be typical mundane data entry.

Wellness apps generally aim to promote improved monitoring of health behaviors related to nutrition, physical activity, stress, sleep, and goal setting. The act of actively monitoring and receiving feedback from devices can help create self-awareness and accountability for patients who are managing complex chronic conditions. Clinicians have an opportunity to help patients derive meaning from their results and make sense of these data.

Finally, active data can be obtained from other non-health-specific apps. Patients can elect to show clinicians their social network postings and accounts on their smartphones, perhaps in lieu of traditional journaling and diary entries. The user search history within search engine apps, video apps, and music apps can show patients' interests. The built-in phone call history and contacts apps can be an indicator of their communication patterns. Patients can also use calendar apps to list their activities and even adopt such apps as a cognitive tool to gauge, journal, and assess their emotions. Task, reminder, and productivity apps could additionally help with behavioral activation, goal setting, and attention focusing. Camera, video recording, and photo gallery apps can show off items that catch patients' attention and visually record moments in their lives. Maps apps may have "timeline" functionality that shows where patients have traveled. Combinations of these apps may ultimately lead to the capacity to have an even more intimate, personal look into patients' lives, more so than has ever been previously possible.

All of the aforementioned data can be derived from devices shown in Figure 6–2.

WHAT NEW TECHNOLOGIES ARE STILL IN DEVELOPMENT?

While the technologies, software, and devices discussed already are certainly new, they have all been implemented in some form in actual clinical practice outside of the realm of research. In this section, we discuss even newer technologies that are not yet used clinically but that could potentially aid in psychiatric diagnosis and treatment in the future.

PASSIVE DATA FROM PERVASIVE COMPUTERS AND VOICE-RECOGNITION DEVICES

Pervasive computing, or ubiquitous computing, is the use of common objects for microprocessing with Internet capabilities, voice recognition, or wireless computing (Satyanarayanan 2001). Commercial devices—such as Amazon Echo, Amazon Dot, and Google Home—recognize voice commands to enable smarthome features in which items, such as lighting and air conditioning, are controlled by computers instead of the traditional on/off switch.

While pervasive computers have predominantly been used for geographical and transport-tracking systems, they are increasingly being used for home health care. Devices such as Microsoft Kinect, a webcam-style motion-sensing add-on to Xbox video game consoles, can experimentally detect movement disorders, making movement assessments, such as those using the Abnormal Involuntary Movement Scale (AIMS) or gait exams, more accurate.

PASSIVE DATA FROM MOTION-DETECTION AND EYE-TRACKING DEVICES

Eye-tracking devices are often used in business marketing for consumer advertisement testing but may also have applications in health care for

Smartphone app data

Mental health data

- Mood logs
- Medication reminders & logs
- Diary & journal
- Activity & exercise log
- Nutrition log
- Sleep log
- Stress & mindfulness log

Non-health-specific data

- Social network posts
- Search history
- Phone call history
- Contacts
- Calendar
- Productivity
  - Goal setting
  - Task management
  - Alarm clock

Smart watch & wearables data

Activity data

- Activity & exercise types
- Distance traveled
- Movement while sleeping
- Light exposure

Physiological data

- Calories burned
- Step count
- Heart rate
- Galvanic skin response

FIGURE 6–2. Types of data measured and logged in mobile devices.

Source. Illustration by Jennifer Favela. Icons are open source under SIL International's open font license (OFL) 1.1. Font Awesome, by Dave Gandy (http://fontawesome.io).

stroke and head injury detection. The University of California at Los Angeles Center for SMART—Systematic, Measurable, Actionable, Resilient and Technology-driven—Health is testing a variety of fixed sensors that can detect patient activity and can monitor individuals at home to detect indications that their conditions are deteriorating (http://risksciences.ucla.edu/smart-health/). The commercially available JINS MEME eyewear combines electrooculography sensors to detect eye movements (including accelerometers) with a gyroscopic sensor to detect motion and rotation speed to monitor drowsiness while driving, concentration during work, and even walking movements. These devices offer novel opportunities to "listen in on" patients' behavioral patterns and may enable mental health diagnoses and aid in understanding individual illness trajectories outside of the traditional clinic setting.

What Types of Challenges Are Associated With Use of Data From These New Sources?

CASE EXAMPLE 4: DOING THE RESEARCH: SELECTING
PATIENT APPS WITH DATA INTEROPERABILITY IN MIND[4]

Dr. Rowan is the psychiatric medical director of an assertive community treatment clinic that recently transitioned to a new EHR system that is hosted by an external cloud vendor. Dr. Rowan finds that several new vendors are offering new patient apps to the clinic, claiming that their apps will provide therapy and psychoeducation to the clinic's patients remotely, will boost patient satisfaction, and will extend the reach of the clinic's overworked therapists and case managers.

Dr. Rowan is most interested in Sandgem, a vendor whose app also features an attractive dashboard that shows, in graphs and visuals, the most high-risk patients within the clinic as well as statistics on the number of cases and patients seen. The vendor claims that the app is interoperable with the clinic's EHR system. Dr. Rowan quickly finds, however, that Sandgem's app can only export text files and PDF files and that other clinics have had difficulties with the vendor's unresponsiveness and poor customer service.

Dr. Rowan ultimately decides to contract with a different vendor, Jubilife, that offers this interoperability but does not have an attractive dashboard. The clinic team finds that this new app cuts down on administrative and referral tasks by 20% because patients are actively engaging with the app's content, and the app platform sends data to and from the clinic's EHR system, reducing the number of phone calls.

❚ KEY CONCEPT

Software and hardware vendors may claim particular functionalities in their marketing and sales collateral materials. Before committing to a vendor, do the research. Ask peers about their experiences with the vendor and its products and, if possible, obtain references from the vendor and follow up on them. Discuss the acquisition thoroughly with your organization's administrative, legal, and business operations teams and, most importantly, make sure that the vendor and product are approved by your IT group, as they are the experts who can vet the product's security, usability, and interoperability functions.

---

[4]Case provided by Steven R. Chan, M.D., M.B.A.

EFFECT OF WORKFLOW ISSUES AND TECHNOLOGICAL LITERACY ON USE OF APPS

Generally, individuals with lower socioeconomic status, lower levels of literacy, and less education are less comfortable with using technology to manage their own health. They may not be accustomed to charging devices daily, or may have accommodation needs, such as requiring a larger typeface for low vision. The affordability of devices, apps, and other technologies also can be a barrier, as they are not covered, in most cases, by insurance and may incur higher costs.

These barriers to the use of technology affect staff and patients alike. Staff who must take readings from wearable devices or operate apps must be trained to use them. Incorporating these technologies into the clinical workflow is not as simple as "dropping an app in." Careful thought must be given to mapping workflows and identifying opportunities for integrating technologies. Individual clinics, hospitals, and care facilities all have their own unique workflows.

An example of a mental health care outpatient clinic workflow (Figure 6–3) shows areas where apps can be used. This model is worth thinking about not only to decide which apps to introduce into a clinical situation but also to determine which ones to move with first. Customize the apps based on your available human resources (e.g., medical assistants, social workers, other case managers) and available patient resources such as in-clinic classes, group therapies, local resources, and local support groups. Your clinic's other resources such as equipment and physical space may also play a role.

Although discussing best practices in clinic workflows and process mapping is beyond the scope of this book, use of best practices is essential to successful technology adoption. Details on such practices can be found in the literature on business change management, health care operations, and clinical informatics.

TECHNICAL CHALLENGES ASSOCIATED WITH USE OF APPS

Clinicians, developers, and patients must consider a variety of factors that may decrease the efficacy and increase the danger of using mobile mental health apps. App and device security, network service reliability, and the capacity to transfer data may mean that the app will be unable to

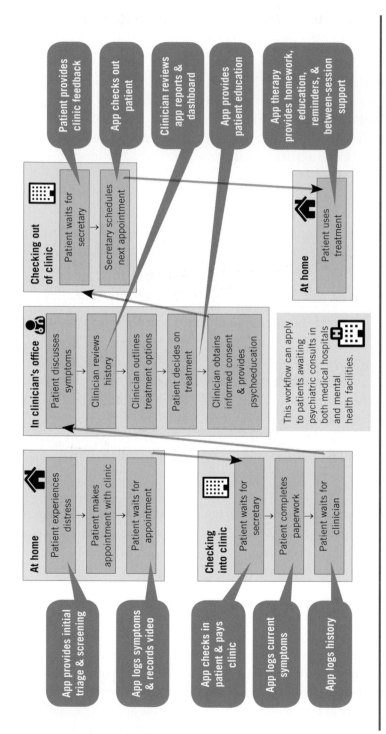

FIGURE 6–3. Typical mental health care outpatient workflow, with opportunities for nontraditional data sources.

Source. Illustration by Jennifer Favela. Icons are open source under SIL International's open font license (OFL) 1.1. Font Awesome, by Dave Gandy (http://fontawesome.io).

perform as marketed. In many respects, having such an app would be similar to having incomplete medical records or unreliable collateral data. Furthermore, the usability and appeal (or lack thereof) of some apps may have an impact on patient use of, adherence to, and engagement with them, leading to inadequate active or passive data entry.

Interoperability, data accuracy, and device constraints are just some of the challenges inherent in the use of apps on any devices. The devices themselves often require software updates or have technical glitches that can be difficult to navigate for those not accustomed to using technology. Concerns related to data accuracy are common for apps built by companies that may have little understanding of the health care environment, especially when developers are rushed to market for commercial reasons and have limited real-life reliability and validity testing for use in non-healthy populations. Individuals with cognitive and attention issues may forget to charge their devices or to connect their devices at regular intervals for accurate data collection and clinical interpretation. Sharing of a patient's device among family members, such as children or partners, may lead to accidental or intentional pollution of the patient's data. Finally, for the most part, most consumer technologies have few or no capabilities for interacting with clinicians and EHRs, so they tend to collect data in a vacuum that is much less helpful for a clinician than if it could be downloaded.

Another problem is that smartphones and wearable technologies must be charged frequently in order to capture data, and continuous connections between a smartphone, its app, and Bluetooth devices can decrease battery life. These challenges may lead to significant missing data collected from these new devices, which consequently makes them less helpful for clinical assessments.

Device loss and technical catastrophes also affect devices. While less common in smartwatches, device loss is common for wearable clips and clothing, which not infrequently end up in the washing machine by mistake. Phones are frequently stolen, or patients may inadvertently download malware and corrupt apps while using such devices, making them unreliable or unusable (Ben-Zeev et al. 2016).

All of these issues can transform a device's seemingly objective, quantifiable data into data that are unreliable and unusable.

PRIVACY CHALLENGES AND SECURITY BREACHES

Technology is continually developing at a rapid rate, faster than the rate of development of laws and regulations. The Health Insurance Portability and Accountability Act (HIPAA) in the United States covers the privacy and security of patients' protected health information and defines covered entities as organizations that transmit protected information electronically. Protected health information is individually identifiable information that is created, received, maintained, or transmitted by a covered entity (or a business associate on the covered entity's behalf) in its role as a covered entity (Touchet et al. 2004).

HIPAA is an overarching law protecting patient data and requires covered entities, such as health care facilities, to adopt policies to ensure the safety of electronically transmitted patient data. If covered entities do not ensure this safety, they may face fines and other major consequences. While HIPAA has very clear rules about protecting the electronic transmission of patient data, each organization must define policies and procedures for their employees to ensure that HIPAA standards are not violated.

All clinicians need to know and understand the limits of electronic communication with the patients they serve at their organization, and how those policies might differ from those of other organizations. Technology has become such an essential part of our day-to-day lives, it can be very difficult to parse out whether a technology or an app is compliant or not.

Take, for example, standard text messaging. Can you, as a provider, send text messages to your patients or respond to texts from your patients? The answer is not clear-cut. For several years, there has been debate and lack of clarity about whether providers can communicate with patients via unencrypted SMS (short message service) text messaging. Some entities may allow such communication with patient consent and as long as sensitive information is not communicated. Generally, covered entities do not allow for communication over unencrypted channels, however (U.S. Department of Health and Human Services Office of Civil Rights 2016).

Text messaging has clearly identifiable security risks (Cepelewicz 2014) that include, but are not limited to, devices being stolen, lost, or discarded, especially if not password protected. These unprotected missing device messages could be easily accessed by anyone. When a standard text is sent, the sender cannot be certain that it reaches the intended recipient or that the patient's privacy was not compromised.

Furthermore, electronic communications must meet HIPAA standards for retaining and storing health information. Physicians who communicate in this way without regard for these standards may open themselves and their organization up to liability. Thus, specific policies around SMS messaging must be adopted and agreed to by provider and patient (Cepelewicz 2014).

HIPAA requires covered entities to encrypt electronic transmissions to a patient over an electronic communications network. The law also states that the covered entity has a duty to warn the patient that there may be some level of risk that the information could be read by a third party.

How does HIPAA apply when considering the use of patient-generated information through apps for health care and behavior tracking sent from the provider to the patient? Under the law, if the patient consents to the data communication after being notified of the risks, the physician or entity has met the duty to warn. They will not be held responsible for unauthorized access of protected health information while in transmission or for safeguarding information once delivered to the patient.

HIPAA standards are, however, based on the assumption of a unidirectional flow of information, from the provider to the patient. It is not clear what the entities' responsibility is to protect and store data that flow in the opposite direction, from the patient to the provider, especially if that information is part of the patient's care. However, once a physician or organization begins to use patient-generated information as part of patient care, whether by uploading it to the record or writing a note about it, it becomes part of the patient treatment record and must be treated in accordance with HIPAA rules.

It is important for clinicians to understand the threats to their patients' privacy associated with use of non-HIPAA-compliant apps and electronic resources. It is difficult, if not impossible, to track where, how, and what information from these apps is shared. The extent of providers' responsibility is unclear in the event that information is leaked about their patients through apps that providers use with their patients in practice.

So what should clinicians do? Should they allow patients to use unsecured apps as part of their treatment? How should the clinician respond if a patient finds a particular app useful (e.g., guided meditation app, mood-tracking app, other health apps)? Clinicians should evaluate the pros and cons of using apps or collecting additional patient data in practice with their patients and consider the following guidelines:

1. Can patient data be collected, transferred, and stored in a way that is HIPAA compliant?
2. Will use of the app significantly improve the information-gathering process with the patient and inform care?
3. Is use of the app/data collection critical to the treatment of the patient?
4. Is use of the app within the therapeutic frame?
5. Will the additional data collected from the app be easily synthesized and evaluated by the clinician, or will it lead to information overload for the clinician, possibly to the point of diminishing returns?

A privacy breach in the area of mental health care received national attention in 2016. Following Facebook's acquisition of WhatsApp, a psychiatrist's patients were contacted by Facebook with the recommendation that they "friend" each other. Each of these patients had the psychiatrist's number stored in the contact lists on their private phone. The breach most likely occurred when Facebook's data mining and algorithmic processing of the contact information stored on the patients' phones detected a common name, that of their psychiatrist, which triggered the automatic "People You May Know" recommendations (Hill 2016).

This example underscores an important issue for providers: the existence of an entirely new world of patient privacy concerns largely beyond the provider's control, where simply storing a provider's phone number in a patient's private phone could unwittingly lead to release of sensitive information publicly online. Such data sharing and privacy breach concerns between mental health care providers and patients should be addressed through the consent process and through regular discussions about technology and privacy. These concerns are particularly salient if electronic information is to be used during the process of care, a virtually ubiquitous practice in the ever-growing digital health care world.

CASE EXAMPLE 5: ADDRESSING SOCIAL NETWORKING BOUNDARIES WITH PATIENTS[5]

Dr. Bell is an early career psychiatrist who has long enjoyed social networking with friends, family, and colleagues on a social network site—"Face Page"—that allows picture, video, and text posts through mutually selected "Face Page buddies." Dr. Bell recently completed a workplace dis-

---

[5]Case provided by Jay H. Shore, M.D., M.P.H.

ability evaluation on a patient who was unhappy with her findings. She subsequently receives a "buddy request" on this social network from the patient, with a comment suggesting that by accepting it, Dr. Bell could gain a better understanding of the patient's daily life that might change her clinical opinion. Dr. Bell declines the request but does call the patient. She explains that her own policy is not to be Face Page buddies with patients and discusses the importance of professional boundaries as a way to protect the integrity of the provider–patient relationship. She also explains her rationale for her impression and then identifies other ways for the patient to share more details about her daily life, including providing collateral contacts. She tells the patient that she will use this information to formulate the best assessment she can with the information available to her. Dr. Bell later carefully reviews her settings on Face Page, with attention to what type of information and posts can be publicly seen, and modifies her settings to better limit her information and posts to within her strict family and friends network.

❚ KEY CONCEPT

Providers as a general practice should not include patients as part of their network on open social networking sites and should be aware of what can and cannot be seen publicly in their posts and messaging. Regardless of the setting, providers should assume that whatever they post to a social network has the potential to become public and may have an impact on both their professional reputation and their boundaries with patients.

ETHICAL DILEMMAS SURROUNDING USE OF INFORMATION FROM ONLINE SOURCES

Most clinicians have information posted about themselves, either voluntarily through a practice Web site or involuntarily via the many "doctor scoring" or service-provider-scoring Web sites that allow patients to post both positive and negative evaluations of clinicians. Patients frequently Google clinicians before coming to a first consultation, but what about clinicians Googling their patients?

It depends on whether gathering information about patients from public or private sites is of value to clinical practice. This practice—referred to in academic literature as "patient-targeted Googling"—involves different levels of searching. Simply Googling a patient's name may lead to information of varying quality and reliability. A patient may be represented by a detailed social network page, by a false online persona, or by publicly available legal and court records.

Guidelines for social media policies in clinical practice are available from the American Medical Association (AMA), the American Psychological Association, and the American Association of Directors of Psychiatric Residency Training. In essence, these guidelines recommend that before using online information about patients, clinicians should ask themselves the following questions (Clinton et al. 2010):

- *Why do I want to conduct this search?* Clinicians may feel that they have a very good reason to access a patient's social networking page, such as general concern for a patient's well-being or to look specifically for signs of distress, suicidal ideation, or bullying. The clinician may simply want to review the patient's page to see if he or she has been posting any irregular or troubling information, or to get more insight into the patient's social functioning. Such access may seem to be in the patient's best interests, but it may cause clinicians to break the therapeutic frame. In general, clinicians must determine whether the Googling of a patient is for satisfying their own voyeuristic desires or is truly clinically useful to the patient's assessment and treatment.

- *Would my search advance or compromise the treatment?* Think of Internet data as a type of collateral information. Don't consider them as self-report data. Weigh them with respect to their level of utility. Also consider the data's source, context, and convergence or divergence with other data. Weigh the potential utility versus the prejudicial effects of data, if searching for and using Internet-based data. Consider the credibility of the data and whether you are qualified to understand and interpret such information. Online personas can be different from real-world behavior (Pirelli et al. 2016).

- *Should I obtain informed consent from the patient prior to online searching?* Without the patient's consent, snooping for information can be considered a violation of patient privacy, a therapeutic boundary crossing, and can therefore compromise the trust between you and your patient. However, information from the Internet may sometimes provide more benefits than risks. Circumstances in which such information might be helpful in patient care include emergencies, patients who lack decision-making capacity, and compliance with government requirements for prescription-monitoring diversion programs for controlled substances (Genes and Appel 2015). A 2012 study revealed that many physicians use public social media sites in a way that crosses the boundaries of care (Ginory et al. 2012). Nearly 20% of American Psychiatric Association respondents surveyed reported viewing patient profiles or patients' family members' profiles on Facebook without permission. Trainees were far more likely to engage in this behavior than were attending physicians.

- *Should I share the results of my online search with the patient?* Data you find online should, except in rare circumstances, be discussed with the patient. Forensic psychologists, for instance, not only discuss the possibility of search results with patients but also let them respond to it—similar to other types of collateral data—should the patient be challenged on cross-examination (Pirelli et al. 2016). One way to inadvertently "share" that you are searching is by adding patients as a connection, "Friend," or "Contact" on your own personal networking site, professional networking site, or photo- and media-sharing sites. Adding such connections should not be done at all, not just for ethical reasons but also for practical and technical reasons. Engineers and administrators of social networks continuously change the way they connect their users. These changes can inadvertently—on their part—lead to a HIPAA violation if a physicians' patients are grouped together by the social networks' automated contact suggestions.

- *Should I document the findings of the online search in the medical record?* Clinton et al. (2010) recommends documenting all relevant data, but doing so in a sensitive manner. Expect that the patient and other treatment providers may read the medical record.

- *How do I monitor my motivations and the ongoing risk–benefit profile of online searching?* Learning more about searching and patient-targeted Googling is important with new technologies. The AMA provides general guidelines for physicians to follow regarding their own use of social media and states that "physicians should be cognizant of standards of patient privacy and confidentiality that must be maintained in all environments, including online" (American Medical Association 2015). Furthermore, the AMA declares that "if [physicians] interact with patients on the Internet, physicians must maintain appropriate boundaries of the patient–physician relationship in accordance with professional ethical guidelines, just as they would in any other context" (American Medical Association 2015).

Another useful framework for evaluating clinical situations involving electronic communications and social networking was proposed by Koh et al. (2013). This heuristic model focuses on four key areas:

1. *Treatment frame:* Establish expectations with patients, avoid friending them, and consider how to respond to patients' requests to view social media posts, images, or other online information about themselves, their families, or their friends.
2. *Medico-legal concerns:* Understand your institution's guidelines and policies or create your own. Discuss informed consent, risks, and benefits with patients.
3. *Patient privacy:* How secure are the communications and devices? What online information enters the patient's chart?
4. *Professionalism:* What are the privacy settings of the online sites you use? What information is available online about you?

In summary, it is up to clinicians to understand the privacy and confidentiality limitations of social media sites. Be aware of policies governing social media interactions with patients within your organization. Include a social media and electronic contact policy in your informed consent documentation. Discuss these policies with patients early in the initial consultation and treatment planning (Sabin and Skimming 2015; Snowdy et al. 2016).

HOW CAN CLINICIANS ASSESS THE USABILITY OF APPS?

There are many ways to design or craft an app, but the aim of most programmers is to make apps easily usable by the consumer. Much like the diversity and variety of psychotherapeutic approaches, the design of apps and technologies can evoke emotional reactions from users. These designs draw from the fields of human–computer interaction, user experience design, psychology, product design, and marketing. Even the name of an app or Web site is important: such names can appear on a patient's smartphone home screen, smartwatch home screen, computer desktop, or Web browser bookmarks.

The reverse of usability—in which an app is unusable—means that something about the app discourages and prevents consumers from using it. The bitter taste of cough syrup can break young patients' medication adherence; so, too, can poorly designed software frustrate, demotivate, and eventually lead patients to quit altogether.

In general, clinicians can evaluate apps on the basis of the following criteria, as proposed in a published framework by Chan et al. (2015):

- *Satisfaction and reward*—Is the app pleasurable and enjoyable to use, or does it discourage repeat use?
- *Usability*—Can the user easily, or with minimal training, use and understand the app?
- *Disability accessibility*—Is the app usable by those with disabilities (e.g., does it incorporate screen readers for blind users or closed captions for the hard-of-hearing and deaf communities)?
- *Cultural accessibility*—Does the app work effectively with the user's culture (as defined by factors such as ethnicity and language)?
- *Socioeconomic and generational accessibility*—Does the app take into account the user's socioeconomic status and age (which have potential implications for the user's digital health literacy)?

Usability standards also extend to immersive environments provided by VR and AR apps. A common side effect of VR and AR apps is vertigo, caused by a mismatch between users' vestibular senses and what they see. VR and AR apps also, because of their novelty and difference from other technology user interfaces, require more education and up-front training for users.

Numerous standards have been proposed by professional organizations regarding usability. The simplest advice: use the software yourself. Would you want to use this software yourself a second time? A third time? Do you think others would understand how to use the app? If the software is not free, does the app developer provide sample copies, review demonstrations, and visual walkthroughs of how the app works? Is the app being fairly widely used, with user comments, or has it been sitting undownloaded from the shelves of the app store?

EVIDENCE SUPPORTING SAFETY AND EFFICACY OF APPS AND MOBILE DEVICE–DRIVEN CARE

Although the number of apps, technologies, and startups surrounding the mental health care space has increased faster than the traditional pace of research, much of the technology is not yet vetted or validated, and there is still insufficient evidence to prescribe an app. Unfortunately, numerous attempts to publicly "certify" these apps as safe and efficacious have failed due to cost and time constraints.

There are many reasons why there is no certification: the continuous new development and updating of apps plus the overwhelming costs of externally testing and validating each version tend to preclude such vetting. Sluggishly long traditional research methods (4–8 years) do not align with the rapid pace of development (a few weeks or months). Reviews available on consumer-accessible app stores are almost always written by the general public, not by expert clinicians, and Web sites that feature physician-written reviews not only review apps for a particular version and single point of time, but they likely do not adequately test apps. Guidance from the U.S. Food and Drug Administration indicates that wellness and low-risk apps will not be regulated by the federal government as "medical devices."

On the other hand, mental health care clinicians who work for larger health systems have access to IT teams that vet apps for recommendation and prescription by their clinicians. For instance, Kaiser Permanente operates its own formulary of vetted apps and has developed its own Kaiser Permanente–branded apps for internal use by its customers. The VA Health System has a similar model, available through the VA App Store, where a group of excellent apps are available for the general public to use. In the future, pharmaceutical companies may offer "digital prescription," with apps, sensors, and devices paired with medication to facilitate adherence and monitoring. In these cases, larger entities take on the risk for the apps.

Clinicians can advise patients to use publicly available apps as they would when discussing self-help books. Such books do not have to be prescribed, which would imply a mandate by the clinician and thus would incur liability, but could be part of a suggested list of resources. Common-sense guidelines for recommending publicly available apps include the following:

- Choose reputable publishers, developers, and institutions. In general, nonprofit, academic, and governmental institutions are less likely to sell or distribute user information. However, privacy is still not guaranteed, and personal information breaches happen very frequently even with such institutions. Examples of such apps are listed in Table 6–3.

TABLE 6–3. Examples of publicly available mental health apps for patients, backed by academic, nonprofit, or governmental institutions

App names (URL)	Author	Use
Intellicare, Thought Challenger, Daily Feats, Aspire, Purple Chill, Worry Knott, Slumber Time, iCope, My Mantra, Day to Day, Boost Me, MoveMe, Social Force (https://intellicare.cbits.northwestern.edu)	Northwestern University	Monitoring of depression, anxiety
SAM (http://sam-app.org.uk)	University of the West of England, Bristol	Management and monitoring of depression, anxiety
MindShift (https://www.anxietybc.com/resources/mindshift-app)	Anxiety Disorders Association of British Columbia and BC Children's Hospital	Monitoring of anxiety
ACT Coach, Breathe2Relax, CBT-I Coach, Concussion Coach, CPT Coach, Dream EZ, LifeArmor, Mindfulness Coach, Moving Forward, PE Coach, Positive Activity Jackpot, PTSD Coach, Stay Quit, T2 Mood Tracker, Tactical Breather, Virtual Hope Box (http://t2health.dcoe.mil/products/mobile-apps and https://mobile.va.gov/appstore)	U.S. Department of Defense National Center for Telehealth and Technology (T2) and U.S. Department of Veterans Affairs	Monitoring of insomnia, PTSD, TBI, nicotine addiction, depression, anxiety

TABLE 6–3. Examples of publicly available mental health apps for patients, backed by academic, nonprofit, or governmental institutions *(continued)*

App names (URL)	Author	Use
NAMI AIR ("Anonymous Inspiring Relatable") (http://www.nami.org/Find-Support/Air-App)	National Alliance on Mental Illness	Social network for individuals and caregivers
AlcoholFX (http://toosmarttostart.samhsa.gov/educators/alcoholfx.aspx)	U.S. Substance Abuse and Mental Health Services Administration (SAMHSA)	Alcohol use education
Suicide Safer Home, ASK and Prevent Suicide, Hope Box (http://www.mhatexas.org/find-help/)	Mental Health America of Texas	Suicide safety, prevention and education
My3 (http://www.my3app.org)	California Mental Health Services Authority and Mental Health Association of New York City	Suicide safety planning
The Grouchies (http://www.apa.org/about/social-media.aspx?tab=9)	American Psychological Association	Child anger education
WellMind (http://www.dwmh.nhs.uk/wellmind/)	Dudley and Walsall Mental Health Partnership NHS Trust (National Health Service)	Monitoring of stress, anxiety, depression

TABLE 6–3. Examples of publicly available mental health apps for patients, backed by academic, nonprofit, or governmental institutions *(continued)*

App names (URL)	Author	Use
The Language of Letting Go, Free Inspirations from Hazelden, Twenty-Four Hours a Day, Each Day a New Beginning, Food for Thought, A Day at a Time, Field Guide to Life, My Sober Life, Touchstones (https://www.hazelden.org/web/public/mobileapps.page)	Hazelden Betty Ford Foundation and Bookmobile	Codependency, addiction (with specific apps for adolescents, men, and women)

Note. As of September 2016. This list does not include clinical references, which typically are not for patient use.
PTSD=posttraumatic stress disorder; TBI=traumatic brain injury; URL=uniform resource locator.

- Thoroughly use and evaluate apps yourself. See if their content is sound. Being familiar with an app additionally helps you engage and teach the patient about the app.
- Do not trust online store reviews of apps. These reviews are primarily from consumers, not health care professionals.

The American Psychiatric Association's App Evaluation Work Group has put together guidance on the association's Web site (www.psychiatry.org) on how to evaluate an app. Table 6–4 shows five distinct stages of evaluation: 1) garnering basic, ground-level information about an app; 2) evaluating whether the app has adequate privacy and safety features; 3) determining whether the app is evidence-based and has demonstrated efficacy; 4) assessing whether the app is easy to use; and 5) ascertaining whether data sharing and interoperability are built into the app.

SUMMARY

Smart devices, computer networks, and apps are here to stay and will become increasingly important clinical tools in the future as we find more sources of clinically relevant data to use as we work with our patients. In this chapter we have discussed the following topics:

- How clinicians can use new data, in addition to traditional forms of data, for assessment and treatment of patients. Such data can be reviewed with the patient during patient–clinician encounters.
- Two new types of data offered by new technologies for clinical use: passive data and active data.

  1. *Passive data* refers to information gathered without patients' active involvement, and with or without their knowledge or awareness. Passive data can be obtained from smartphones, smartwatches, wearable activity trackers, and other wearable devices. AR and VR headsets can also gather information about a patient's experiences. EHRs, EMRs, pharmacy records, and social media streams can provide further information. Passive data can also be obtained from experimental technologies such as voice recognition systems, motion detection devices, and eye-tracking systems.
  2. *Active data* refers to information that the patient knowingly submits to clinical systems or to the clinician directly. Active data can

TABLE 6–4. American Psychiatric Association app evaluation model

Step	Questions to ask
1—Gather background information	What is the business model? If the app is free, then how does it support its own development? Who is the developer? Does it claim to be medical? What is the cost? Does it require in-app purchases to unlock certain features? Is it free? Does it integrate advertising into its usability? On which platforms does it work (e.g., iOS, Android)? When was it last updated? How many updates have there been? What were the reasons for the updates (i.e., security updates; software glitches or bugs; improved functionality or added services)?
2—Risk/privacy and safety	Is there a privacy policy? What data are collected? Are personal data de-identified? Can you opt-out of data collection? Can you delete data? Are cookies placed on your device? Who are data shared with/What data are shared? Are data maintained on the device or the web (i.e., "the cloud")? Both? What security measures are in place? Are data encrypted on the device and server? Does it purport HIPAA compliance? Does it need to be HIPAA-compliant?

TABLE 6–4. American Psychiatric Association app evaluation model *(continued)*

Step	Questions to ask
3—Evidence	What does it claim to do vs. what does it actually do? Is there peer-reviewed, published evidence about tool or science behind it? Is there any feedback from users to support claims (App store, Web site, review sites, etc.)? Does the content appear of at least reasonable value?
4—Ease of use	Is it easy to access for the patient at hand (i.e., based on patient diagnosis or other factors)? Would it be easy to use on a long-term basis? Is the app or are features of the app customizable? Does it need an active connection to the Internet to work? What platforms does it work on? Is it accessible for those with impaired vision or other disabilities? Is it culturally relevant?
5—Interoperability	Who "owns" the data (i.e., patient, provider, developer)? Can it share data with the EHR? Can you print out your data? Can you export/download your data? Can it share data with other user data tools (e.g., Apple HealthKit, Fitbit)?

Source. Available at: https://www.psychiatry.org/psychiatrists/practice/mental-health-apps/app-evaluation-model. Accessed May 12, 2017.

include social media posts, text messages, smartphone app surveys, and smartphone app interactions with remote monitoring tools.

- Although consumer apps, devices, and technologies can be used for patient care, they must not be prescribed as a mandatory part of treatment unless the clinician's parent institution, insurance carrier, or other organization will take on liability if an app fails or suffers a privacy breach.
- When choosing among available apps, clinicians should bear in mind that these tools are not without unintended consequences and that even seemingly innocuous apps can have side effects—for instance, vertigo for virtual reality apps, or a breach of privacy in the case of social networking sites.
- Clinicians should be aware of the ethical dilemmas raised by new technologies and should follow recommended guidelines. They should avoid adding patients as connections to their social media accounts; refrain from interacting with patients via social media or unencrypted, non-HIPAA-compliant communication channels; and review electronic communications policies with patients early and often.

Clinical practice is rapidly changing, especially in this world of patient-centered health care, where patients themselves are increasingly presenting to physicians with data they have collected themselves or with requests to use apps and devices for self-monitoring. It is important that all mental health care professionals keep up to date with the ethical and clinical challenges that these new devices bring, and that they make good and appropriate use of these exciting technologies in daily practice.

REFERENCES

Adler-Milstein J: A Creative Plan That Could Help Providers Ineligible For Meaningful Use Not Get Left Behind In The Paper World. Health Affairs Blog, May 25, 2016. Available at: http://healthaffairs.org/blog/2016/05/25/a-creative-plan-that-could-help-providers-ineligible-for-meaningful-use-not-get-left-behind-in-the-paper-world/. Accessed July 16, 2017.

American Medical Association: THE CODE SAYS: The AMA Code of Medical Ethics' Opinions on Observing Professional Boundaries and Meeting Professional Responsibilities. AMA Journal of Ethics 17(5):432–434, 2015. Available at: http://journalofethics.ama-assn.org/2015/05/coet1-1505.html. Accessed April 6, 2017.

Ben-Zeev D, Brenner CJ, Begale M, et al: Feasibility, acceptability, and preliminary efficacy of a smartphone intervention for schizophrenia. Schizophr Bull 40(6):1244–1253, 2014 24609454

Ben-Zeev D, Scherer EA, Wang R, et al: Next-generation psychiatric assessment: using smartphone sensors to monitor behavior and mental health. Psychiatr Rehabil J 38(3):218–226, 2015 25844912

Ben-Zeev D, Scherer EA, Gottlieb JD, et al: mHealth for schizophrenia: patient engagement with a mobile phone intervention following hospital discharge. JMIR Mental Health 3(3):e34, 2016. Available at: https://www.ncbi.nlm. nih.gov/pmc/articles/PMC4999306/. Accessed April 6, 2017.

Bush NE, Skopp N, Smolenski D, et al: Behavioral screening measures delivered with a smartphone app: psychometric properties and user preference. J Nerv Ment Dis 201(11):991–995, 2013 24177488

Cepelewicz BB: Text messaging with patients: steps to avoid liability. Med Econ 91(10):42–43, 2014 25233752

Chan S, Torous J, Hinton L, et al: Mobile tele-mental health: increasing applications and a move to hybrid models of care. Healthcare (Basel) 2(2):220–233, 2014 27429272

Chan S, Torous J, Hinton L, Yellowlees P: Towards a framework for evaluating mobile mental health apps. Telemed J E Health 21(12):1038–1041, 2015 26171663

Clinton BK, Silverman BC, Brendel DH: Patient-targeted Googling: the ethics of searching online for patient information. Harv Rev Psychiatry 18(2):103–112, 2010 20235775

Fox S, Duggan M: Tracking for health. Pew Research Center's Internet and American Life Project, January 28, 2013. Available at: http://pewinternet.org/Reports/2013/Tracking-for-Health.aspx. Accessed September 8, 2016.

Genes N, Appel J: The ethics of physicians' web searches for patients' information. J Clin Ethics 26(1):68–72, 2015 25794296

Ginory A, Sabatier LM, Eth S: Addressing therapeutic boundaries in social networking. Psychiatry 75(1):40–48, 2012 22397540

Hill K: Facebook recommended that this psychiatrist's patients friend each other. Fusion, August 29, 2016. Available at: http://fusion.net/story/339018/facebook-psychiatrist-privacy-problems/. Accessed September 8, 2016.

Jones SP, Patel V, Saxena S, et al: How Google's "Ten Things We Know To Be True" could guide the development of mental health mobile apps. Health Aff 33(9):1603–1611, 2014. Available at: http://content.healthaffairs.org/content/33/9/1603.abstract. Accessed April 11, 2017.

Koh S, Cattell GM, Cochran DM, et al: Psychiatrists' use of electronic communication and social media and a proposed framework for future guidelines. J Psychiatr Pract 19(3):254–263, 2013 23653084

Lal S, Adair CE: E-mental health: a rapid review of the literature. Psychiatr Serv 65(1):24–32, 2014 24081188

McClernon FJ, Choudhury R: I am your smartphone, and I know you are about to smoke: the application of mobile sensing and computing approaches to smoking research and treatment. Nicotine Tob Res 15(10):1651–1654, 2013 23703731

Moore RC, Depp CA, Wetherell JL, Lenze EJ: Ecological momentary assessment versus standard assessment instruments for measuring mindfulness, depressed mood, and anxiety among older adults. J Psychiatr Res 75:116–123, 2016 26851494

Moran EK, Culbreth AJ, Barch DM: Ecological momentary assessment of negative symptoms in schizophrenia: relationships to effort-based decision making and reinforcement learning. J Abnorm Psychol 126(1):96–105, 2017 27893230

Most Famous Social Network Sites Worldwide as of August 2017, ranked by number of active users (in millions). Statista—The Statistics Portal. Available at: https://www.statista.com/statistics/272014/global-social-networks-ranked-by-number-of-users/. Accessed August 17, 2017.

Pew Research Center: Mobile Fact Sheet. January 12, 2017. Available at: http://www.pewinternet.org/fact-sheet/mobile/. Accessed July 30, 2017.

Pirelli G, Otto RK, Estoup A: Using Internet and social media data as collateral sources of information in forensic evaluations. Prof Psychol Res Pr 47(1):12–17, 2016. Available at: http://psycnet.apa.org/psycinfo/2016-00615-001/. Accessed April 11, 2017.

Puiatti A, Mudda S, Giordano S, et al: Smartphone-centred wearable sensors network for monitoring patients with bipolar disorder. Conf Proc IEEE Eng Med Biol Soc 2011:3644–3647, 2011 22255129

Rabbi M, Ali S, Choudhury T, et al: Passive and in-situ assessment of mental and physical well-being using mobile sensors, in Proceedings of the 13th International Conference on Ubiquitous Computing. New York, Association for Computing Machinery, 2011, pp 385–394

Roberts LW, Torous J: Preparing residents and fellows to address ethical issues in the use of mobile technologies in clinical psychiatry. Acad Psychiatry 41(1):132–134, 2016 27472934

Sabin JE, Skimming K: A framework of ethics for telepsychiatry practice. Int Rev Psychiatry 27(6):490–495, 2015 26493214

Satyanarayanan M: Pervasive computing: vision and challenges. IEEE Personal Communications 8(4):10–17, 2001. Available at: http://ieeexplore.ieee.org/document/943998/. Accessed April 11, 2017.

Snowdy CE, Shoemaker EZ, Chan S, et al: Social media and clinical practice: what stays the same, what changes, and how to plan ahead?, in e-Mental Health. Edited by Mucic D, Hilty DM. Cham, Switzerland, Springer International Publishing, 2016, pp 151–170

Torous J, Powell AC: Current research and trends in the use of smartphone applications for mood disorders. Internet Interventions 2(2):169–173, 2015.

Available at: http://www.sciencedirect.com/science/article/pii/ S2214782915000135. Accessed August 17, 2017.

Torous J, Staples P, Onnela J-P: Realizing the potential of mobile mental health: new methods for new data in psychiatry. Curr Psychiatry Rep 17(8):602, 2015 26073363

Torous J, Kiang MV, Lorme J, et al: New tools for new research in psychiatry: a scalable and customizable platform to empower data driven smartphone research. JMIR Ment Health 3(2):e16, 2016 27150677

Touchet BK, Drummond SR, Yates WR: The impact of fear of HIPAA violation on patient care. Psychiatr Serv 55(5):575–576, 2004 15128967

U.S. Department of Health and Human Services Office of Civil Rights: Text messaging and HIPAA. Health App Developers: Questions About HIPAA?, January 21, 2016. Available at: http://hipaaqsportal.hhs.gov/a/dtd/Text-messaging-and-HIPAA/135929-36899. Accessed September 6, 2016.

Vahia IV, Sewell DD: Late-life depression: a role for accelerometer technology in diagnosis and management. Am J Psychiatry 173(8):763–768, 2016 27477136

7

Clinical Documentation in the Era of Electronic Health Records and Information Technology

Daniel J. Balog, M.D.

Meera Narasimhan, M.D.

Jay H. Shore, M.D., M.P.H.

Clinical documentation is currently being transformed in the age of information technology. The leap to electronic health record (EHR) systems over the past decade across health systems and organizations will continue to affect and change the way psychiatrists engage with patients and practice medicine. This no-holds-barred transformation is inevitable and is being driven by funders and government mandates for billing, reimbursement, and regulation. Psychiatric providers are having to adapt to these mandates, which not only fundamentally change the process and content of documentation but also require changes and adaptation in the clinical workflow.

This chapter provides an overview of the foundations and forces behind clinical documentation and of how information technology and specifically EHRs are being implemented in clinical practice. This chapter is complementary to most of the chapters in this book but has special relevance to and overlaps with Chapter 5 ("Media Communication Skills and the Ethical Doctor–Patient Relationship") and Chapter 6 ("Data Collection From Novel Sources"), as well as with Chapter 8 ("Indirect

Consultation and Hybrid Care"), Chapter 9 ("Management of Patient Populations"), and Chapter 10 ("Quality Care Through Telepsychiatry: Patient-Centered Treatment, Guideline- and Evidence-Based Practice, and Lifelong Development of Professional Competencies and Skills"). On a pragmatic level, the modern EHR is the vehicle for the activities described in these other chapters.

We begin this chapter with an overview of forces impacting clinical documentation followed by a review of key principles, methods, and best practices in EHR documentation. We also explore how EHRs are interfacing with and being applied to emerging technology-enabled models of care such as patient portals and population management systems.

WHAT ARE THE HISTORICAL FORCES AND CURRENT DRIVERS IMPACTING CLINICAL DOCUMENTATION?

Clinical records, originally created for purposes of medical training and education, have grown significantly over the past two centuries. In the United States, the modern clinical record emerged from major teaching hospitals in the 19th century, with additional refinements made in the 20th century, when such records came into use for patient care in hospitals and outpatient clinics (Gillum 2013). The transition of medicine from the industrial age to the information age continues to drive the evolution of clinical documentation in all medical specialties, including psychiatry. The emergence of the EHR (or electronic medical record [EMR]) as the primary foundation is propelling transformation in documentation practices and in associated areas of quality, patient safety, coding/billing, and patient population management. Concurrent increases in prescriptive requirements dictating note content have had adverse effects on the daily workloads of physicians and other providers who carry the main burden of completing such notes. Many clinicians share the concern that the system's reliance on them as the primary recorders of an ever-increasing flow of clinical data has become a burden that is too great to bear alone. Without changes, the administrative burdens will only serve as a barrier to successful clinical relationships, and the technologies we rely on will only be seen as adding to rather than solving the problem. Before physicians can advocate for improvements in clinical documentation, they must first understand the various content drivers, which encompass five key domains (Ho et al. 2014):

1. *Clinical*—Support longitudinal care management, care coordination, and treatment planning.
2. *Administrative/billing*—Justify reimbursement.
3. *Legal*—Mitigate impacts of the for-profit legal industry.
4. *Research*—Support data collection and population data.
5. *Education*—Support growth and understanding among students and allied professionals participating in clinical care teams.

Additional forces affecting clinical documentation include mandated documentation of quality and population health–based measures to support value-based payment systems. Patient portals and the real-time medical records access they can provide to patients will also influence documentation practices, boundaries, and content. We explore some of the potential implications for clinical documentation, but the process is evolving, and physicians will need to influence the system at every level if they desire a result that preserves essential aspects of the physician–patient relationship and ensures that the personal computer does not become an entrenched barrier to that relationship.

WHY IS TECHNOLOGY CRITICAL FOR PATIENT-CENTERED CARE?

In its report *Crossing the Quality Chasm: A New Health System for the 21st Century,* the Institute of Medicine (2001) defined *patient-centered care* as care that is respectful of, and responsive to, an individual's preferences, needs, and values. Patient-centered care ensures that the patient's values guide all clinical decisions. Patient-centeredness must serve as the *basis of coordination,* and for this reason, the patient is a special member of the treatment team whose needs are a primary focus (Steichen and Gregg 2015).

Patient-centered, value-informed multispecialty care has long been an imperative in behavioral health, but as modern practice becomes further distributed, the system will increasingly rely on a health information framework that supports virtual integration, communication, and care coordination. In order to engage this framework, organizations will need to develop complementary clinical workflows, standardized documentation practices, and health information technology interoperability across organizations and settings where care is delivered (Steichen and Gregg 2015).

WHAT IS HIGH-VALUE CLINICAL DOCUMENTATION?

The primary goal of clinical documentation must be to support care delivery and improve patient outcomes. In consideration of the multiple drivers, this goal is not easily achieved. The conceptualization of clinical documentation as a static note generated by a physician during an isolated care transaction for the purpose of reimbursement must be expanded. Clinical documentation must be perceived and implemented as an essential care tool and process that enables multiple stakeholders to influence longitudinal care management across settings (Sequist 2015). To reach this goal of "high value" documentation, all care team members, including patients, need to be supported so that all appropriate skills are leveraged. Providing patients with the opportunity to directly enter their relevant history and symptoms prior to the clinical encounter, for example, would improve safety and efficiency. Expanding the documentation paradigm to include medication reconciliation, decision-support recommendations, and patient-reported outcome measures would provide additional and essential information on patient status. To achieve this vision of high-value documentation, it will be essential to design systems that can integrate data and describe whole-patient care from the perspective of multiple stakeholders (Sequist 2015).

The American College of Physicians has codified goals of high-value documentation and has further recommended that medical societies define professional standards for documentation; that EHRs should facilitate seamless patient care to improve outcomes and data collection; that structured data should be collected only when needed for care delivery or for quality assessment; that prior authorizations should be standardized; and that patient access to progress notes should be expanded as a means to improve quality through engagement (Kuhn et al. 2015).

HOW CAN HEALTH INFORMATION TECHNOLOGY SUPPORT CARE PLANS AND ADVANCE PATIENT-CENTERED CARE?

In an effort to advance the goals of high-value documentation, and in order to optimize safety and efficiency, the American Medical Informatics Association EHR-2020 Task Force promoted recommendations across five broad clinical areas: documentation, regulation, transparency, innovation, and person-centered care. The recommendations included reducing requirements that assign primary documentation burden to physicians; separating data entry from data reporting; improving data exchange and interoperability; focusing on outcomes (vs. data entry) for reimbursement; and integrating EHRs into the social context of care (Payne et al. 2015).

In order for EHRs to support patient-centered care in an environment that is increasingly distributed and partitioned, there needs to be a framework that standardizes data capture and provides key information both across levels of care and throughout clinical transitions. One such framework, the longitudinal care plan, presents information that is patient-centered, bidirectional, and targeted to an individual's health and wellness needs. Longitudinal care plans, also known as care plans, are multidisciplinary and are communicated, referred to, and updated across organizations and levels of care. Care plans require that EHRs assemble structured data from various elements and present these data in a format that is dynamic, targeted, and usable to members of the care team. These data provide actionable information that professionals reconcile during their specific care encounters in order to advance coordinated care and ultimately the patient's health and wellness goals.

Universal implementation of care plans remains an ideal that is not fully realized because of factors such as inconsistent definitions, practice and workflow challenges, and lack of agreement regarding longitudinal data elements (Dykes et al. 2014). Evolving requirements and efforts to clarify definitions represent steps toward more universal adoption of care plans. The Agency for Healthcare Research and Quality's Care Coordination Measurement Framework presented five broad approaches and associated activities, including creating a care plan, as a structure to advance care coordination (Agency for Healthcare Research and Quality 2014). The Standards and Interoperability (S&I) Framework within the Office of the National Coordinator for Health Information Technology (ONC) organizes care plans in a hierarchical structure wherein *treatment plans* refer to a single problem or health care concern, *plans of care* apply within a single discipline or setting, and *care plans*—assigned the highest level of complexity—exist across elements and are employed longitudinally. Following this framework, each patient has a single *care plan* that is composed of many *plans of care* and many *treatment plans* (S&I Framework 2013).

How Can Dashboards Improve Quality?

Dashboards have long been used in industry to summarize and integrate performance information across components and levels of an organization. Similar to how dashboards present performance metrics to assist industry leaders, clinical dashboards present clinical information to inform decisions and improve care. Dashboards capture data from multiple sources and present information that is visual, concise, and usable (Daley et al. 2013).

The incorporation of clinical and quality dashboards into clinical care environments is associated with improved care processes and patient outcomes (Dowding et al. 2015). Key dashboard characteristics include a visual display of quality or productivity metrics at the level of the patient or at the level of the health care professional, where practice data are compared with data from peers or a national benchmark. Dashboards employ various data visualization techniques (i.e., graphical displays, color-coded indicators, and other visual representations such as bar and pie charts) to facilitate information transfer and ease of use.

Although there is heterogeneity in settings where dashboards are used, there is some evidence that dashboards and other computerized decision support systems that provide information to clinicians can be associated with positive outcomes when they are presented and easily accessible at the point of care (Dowding et al. 2015; Kawamoto et al. 2005).

Clinical data registries similarly have emerged concurrently with EHRs and offer powerful tools for continuous improvement. Clinical data registries, which typically are maintained by specialty societies and accountable care organizations, have the potential to provide real-time data that are autonomously extracted from the EHR. Practice performance is further reinforced when clinicians see immediate results and when they are able to compare their performance with that of peers and with national benchmarks (Council of Medical Specialty Societies 2016).

What Methods and Formats Are Available for Entry of Data Into EHRs?

Typing remains the most common method of inputting data into an EHR, and while it has improved clarity and efficiency of data entry, it has also caused new problems relating to copying, pasting, and cloning of notes in the EHR. Copy/paste in particular, a function that allows the user to copy content and then easily place it electronically into multiple sections of the EMR, can create problems relating to note bloat, authorship attribution, inaccuracy, repetition, and overly inclusive notes that make it difficult for downstream users to discern relevant information. These issues have led a number of national organizations and systems to respond with policies and guidance for the use of copying and pasting in EHRs (Weiss and Levy 2014). When used properly, however, copy/paste or some similar manner of capturing data contained elsewhere in the EHR can greatly improve accuracy, completeness, and efficiency of documentation (Kuhn et al. 2015). A few guiding principles to support data integrity and quality documentation in inpatient settings include the following (Shoolin et al. 2013):

- EHRs should allow data to be entered once by an author and then used by others by reference (not as a copy).
- When specific elements of a patient's information or history do not change, these may be copied forward with an acknowledgment of the source, when applicable.
- Previously documented data elements that may be reasonably copied forward by reference include past medical/surgical/obstetric/psychiatric history, family history, social history, past reports with dates, and unique circumstances of the patient history.
- Specific sections that reflect the author's work product and that should not be carried forward include history of present illness, interim history of present illness, review of systems, physical examination, assessment, and plan.

Dictation is also a time-honored data-input method where psychiatrists and hospital systems employ services to transcribe dictated notes that are returned at a later time for editing, insertion, and signature. In order to improve the process, many EHRs have developed voice recognition functionality that inserts dictated notes into the medical record for immediate editing, review, and signature. Many transcription programs have robust medical language libraries that "learn" frequently used terms to minimize voice translation errors.

With respect to format, EHRs typically support free text data entry, structured data entry (e.g., in the form of templates), as well as hybrid approaches. All formats can be tailored to the type of note being written (see structured vs. flexible documentation section for further details). EHRs that support structured data importation can present these data (e.g., problem lists, medication lists, vitals/body mass index, screening measure results) in multiple formats and in ways that are targeted to a specific purpose (i.e., clinical note, insurance authorization).

CASE EXAMPLE: EXPERT NOTE: SHOULD TELEPSYCHIATRY SESSIONS BE RECORDED?[1]

A 40-year-old Aboriginal woman with depression who lives in an isolated outback community in Australia is referred for an assessment via telepsychiatry. After a fruitful session in which she discusses her situation in detail with the telepsychiatrist and speaks frankly about a number of personal matters, she asks whether it would be possible for her to have a video recording of her session. As was the usual practice, the session had not been recorded, and the patient is disappointed to learn this. She explains to the telepsychiatrist that she had enjoyed the session and wanted her friends to see her "on TV." She is not in the least concerned about confidentiality or privacy.

▌ KEY CONCEPT

Providers tend to be more concerned about privacy and confidentiality than do many patients. While lawyers used to always advise that telepsychiatry sessions not be recorded, in recent years many have given the opposite advice, noting that most physicians are competent and do not make egregious errors, so recording will generally support them if there is ever a lawsuit. Conversely, if physicians have made errors, then lawyers would often like to see those errors clearly demonstrated on video so that they can settle the case rapidly rather than become involved in expensive, drawn-out litigation.

WHO IS AUTHORIZED TO DOCUMENT CARE INTERACTIONS IN THE EHR?

EHRs can support simultaneous documentation by multiple professionals and by multiple members of the clinical team, including nurses, social workers, therapists, case managers, and medical assistants. EHRs can potentially receive digital information from sources including e-mail, text, portals, computers, mobile devices, wearable devices, and kiosks. In

---

[1]Case provided by Peter Yellowlees, MBBS, M.D.

order to optimally benefit from these capabilities, a number of medical specialties have leveraged their care teams to improve quality, timing, and efficiency of documentation. Primary care physicians, for example, employ medical assistants to support workflow and documentation requirements and as a result are improving productivity, quality, and interactions with their patients. These workflow changes also contribute to decreased physician burnout and improved work/life satisfaction (Shipman and Sinsky 2013). Although medical assistant–supported documentation has not yet become the norm in psychiatric practice, due in part to concerns about mental health care privacy and psychotherapeutic privilege, this practice represents a workflow that could one day reduce the documentation burden in outpatient clinics.

Despite many EHR enhancements, physicians continue to find themselves pressured to complete an inordinate number of administrative tasks that do not improve quality, clarify communication, or advance the care plan. In one study of emergency department physicians, the researchers found that 43% of physicians' time was spent entering data into EMRs, compared with 28% of their time spent in direct patient care (Hill et al. 2013). Interestingly, total mouse clicks per physician averaged almost 4,000 over 10 hours. Although psychiatry is usually considered to be a profession in which doctors have sufficient time to interact with their patients, mental health care is not immune to the pressures of productivity, documentation, and billing. In the context of these pressures, psychiatrists should learn from the experiences of other medical specialties as they work to preserve the primacy of their doctor–patient interactions, and they must continually remind themselves of, and advocate for, their right to practice in environments that leave them free to "treat the patient, and not the chart."

HOW CAN CARE TEAM MEMBERS COORDINATE THEIR DOCUMENTATION IN THE EHR?

Since EHRs enable documentation of care interactions that occur outside of the specific time-limited physician encounter, it is helpful to conceptualize patient care as existing in three broad time periods—preclinical, clinical, and postclinical. In each of these periods, specific documentation practices occur, and just as importantly, specific care plan advancements can take place.

In the preclinical period, if patients are presented with the opportunity to answer symptom/severity questions just prior to their clinical encounters (i.e., while they are at home or in the waiting room), then at least three important activities are occurring. First, patients are providing objective, structured information that will inform and improve their clinical encounters. Second, if the workflow is smartly designed, the structured information is entered into the EMR in a way that makes it immediately available for review by the psychiatrist prior to the clinical interaction. Additionally, if the EMR is smartly designed, the information is immediately available for subsequent downstream interactions that advance the care plan. Third, while patients are answering their questions and reflecting on their status, they are *priming and preparing for their clinical encounter.* During the preclinical period, most interactions, even those that occur during the process of collecting vitals/weights, are viewed as preparatory if they engage patients and encourage them to reflect on their status, refine their priorities, and prepare for their clinical appointments. During the clinical period, the psychiatrist, who is now less burdened with task of raw data entry, is able to move quickly to clarifying questions and to higher-order inquiry about meaning, impact, and etiology of confirmed symptoms. At the end of the clinical encounter, patients are returned to the medical assistant, who shepherds in the postclinical period, which includes educational, administrative, and clinical consolidation. The medical assistant actively engages with patients during this period and carries out specific tasks that advance the care plan. As medical assistants engage in their appropriate role during this period, they have ample opportunity to contribute and are more easily viewed as integral members of the care team. Similar to the status medical assistants achieve on inpatient psychiatric wards, medical assistants are experienced by patients as being very important in their care.

By conceptualizing care to be occurring in three broad repeating periods, time of care is seen as extended. Rather than focusing on the specific time-limited period of the clinical interaction, patients and professionals alike begin to understand work on the care plan as something that is ongoing, interactive, and cyclical. Once patients walk out the door, they reflect on their recent experiences and start to transition back to the preclinical phase over the subsequent days and weeks. In addition, this conceptualization of care as occurring in three connected phases facilitates creation of workflows and assignments and tracking of specific care team tasks.

- *Preclinical documentation:* Documentation done prior to the actual clinical encounter that includes information collected directly from the patient or by the medical staff. Self-report information can be obtained through patient portals, Web sites/apps, and questionnaires. Specialty tailored, cross-cutting symptom screens may be combined with severity measures covering specific diagnostic spectra. Other information collected in this period includes vital signs (e.g., temperature, blood pressure, pulse), body measurements (e.g., height/weight, abdominal circumference), and pain assessments.
- *Clinical documentation:* Documentation done during the clinical encounter, typically in a concurrent and collaborative style, that records relevant subjective information about the patient, including interim history, patient specifics, clarifying/confirming information on reported symptoms, pertinent negatives, subjective signs and symptoms supporting a diagnosis, objective information, assessment, clinical reasoning, and treatment plans.
- *Postclinical documentation:* Documentation occurring in the period right after the clinical period, including information relating to symptom monitoring, reporting, and administrative tasks as well as educational information on illness, treatments, and medications. Interactive communications via EHR, patient portals, or other electronic communications that reinforce treatment planning, reconcile medications, and confirm upcoming appointments should be documented postclinically. Patient portals and Web sites may facilitate and monitor patient status through scales, measures, and virtual therapy. This information should all feed into the EHR and facilitate patients' transition to "preclinical" preparation as their next clinical approaches.

A related area of focus is the fact that patients have increasing access to medical records via online portals and other means. Some health care systems print out a summary or even a full copy of each encounter as a matter of practice. Psychiatrists should be mindful of these evolving practices and, when documenting, should favor a neutral, factual style that minimizes risk of adverse impacts on the therapeutic relationship when patients review the notes.

What Types of EHR Notes Are Used in Psychiatry, and What Information Should Notes Contain?

The body of information to be gathered from a psychiatric interview may be termed "the psychiatric database." It is a variable set of data that is primarily focused on factors relating to the present state but necessarily includes information on development, early life, and relationships (Tasman et al. 2013). A number of factors influence what information is to be included in the database. Whose questions are to be answered (i.e., patient, family, or civil authority)? Who will have access to the data? What is the setting? Is this a one-time, an initial, or a follow-up assessment? In addition, answers rendered in certain areas will determine the depth of follow-on inquiry.

In active practice, psychiatrists determine how extensively each component of the comprehensive psychiatric history and mental status examination is explored and documented. The basic structure and expanded content of these examinations (e.g., psychiatric, developmental, sexual, mental status, thought, and cognitive) are well documented in clinical texts (American Psychiatric Association Work Group on Psychiatric Evaluation 2016; Sadock et al. 2014). EHR systems typically establish the formats of their standardized notes and increasingly will need to facilitate documentation of expanded inquiry when required by the clinical situation. Positive responses, for example, will drive additional inquiry, while negative responses in a sphere, coupled with a history of good occupational functioning, may preclude additional inquiry. Note formats are also being influenced by quality, organizational, and coding/billing requirements. An assortment of preformatted notes and treatment-planning templates are available, but in outpatient settings particularly, treatment plans often represent an administrative burden rather than a critical tool to advance patient-centered care.

Several broad categories of note types are used in psychiatry:

- *New-patient assessment/intake notes* focus on gathering a detailed new-patient history, formulating a psychiatric assessment, and often constructing biopsychosocially informed treatment recommendations.
- *Follow-up notes* are used for ongoing visits with patients for medication management and/or therapy treatment. These notes typically follow the subjective-objective-assessment-plan (SOAP) format.

- *Consultation notes* are used to provide specialty consultation to primary care physicians, providers, or other specialists who are managing a patient's care. These notes can follow a variety of formats, depending on the type of consultations being performed (e.g., collaborative care vs. forensic consultation). Consultation notes are often presented in the assessment-plan-subjective-objective (APSO) format (e.g., integrated care services) so that each note leads with the specialist's assessment and detailed plan in order to highlight the most important aspects of the consultation.

There exist a wealth of other materials that may be added to the medical record, but there is minimal ethical, policy, or professional guidance on their inclusion. The use of collateral information from family members, treatment providers, or other relevant parties is commonly documented, often without patient consent. What about inclusion of digital, social media, and other collateral sources? What about potential liability for reviewing and validating patient information that is readily available online? Should these activities, and the information revealed, be documented? The American College of Physicians and the Federation of State Medical Boards have issued a position paper advocating preservation of patient confidentiality while at the same time supporting the use of evolving technologies (Farnan et al. 2013).

Is Too Much Information Included in Present-Day EHR Notes?

The Association of Medical Directors of Information Systems (AMDIS) has addressed the modern documentation challenges of expanding documentation requirements, increased data volume, and proliferation of redundant content. Key to resolving this problem is the necessary recognition that EHR design *must **primarily** serve core needs of patients and health care professionals* and secondarily serve the needs of other stakeholders. It is telling that this truth even needs to be affirmed, but this understanding must drive the efforts of physicians and others who work to improve EHR design and the workflows that support care. Clinical notes that once existed as brief paper summaries of an episode of medical care have steadily evolved into a complex product that is expected to support clinical communication, rationale for decision making, quality metrics, outcomes measures, payment justifications, and legal defense. It was in this context of increased note bloat that AMDIS sounded the alarm and urged a return to clinical needs versus a focus on a complex web of administrative requirements targeting reimbursement. EHRs need to advance clinical efforts to make clinically relevant data easier to find. Additional guiding principles for electronic inpatient EHR documentation include documenting each encounter with the minimum data necessary and collecting and displaying the data in a way that meets the needs of users, supports integrity and quality, and ensures privacy and security (Shoolin et al. 2013).

WHAT ARE THE RELATIVE STRENGTHS AND WEAKNESSES OF STRUCTURED VERSUS FLEXIBLE DOCUMENTATION FORMATS?

One primary purpose of a clinical note is to create a text record of the patient–provider interaction at a particular point in time. Different types of notes may be created on the basis of setting, specialty, and the specific interaction being recorded, and because notes must meet a myriad of clinical, quality, safety, reimbursement, and government-driven requirements, there is a tension regarding how to best create these notes. How can clinicians ensure that all requirements are met while at the same time honoring a need for efficiency, accuracy, and usability? As EHR systems improve in their ability to capture structured data that are reusable and available for downstream processes, their designs will directly influence how clinicians review information, how they document clinical interactions, and how they conduct clinical reasoning. Clinical professionals have experienced collateral impacts in the battle between the push for standardization and the need for flexibility. In the end, notes need to be meaningful, sufficiently expressive, and an accurate depiction of the clinical interaction being documented.

In an effort to resolve this tension, a variety of computer-based documentation systems have been created in order to increase the availability of structured clinical data within an EHR. At one end of the spectrum, structured entry systems capture structured or standardized clinical data *during* the documentation process. These systems employ customized templates that work particularly well in specialty clinics and in settings where there is a more standard format (i.e., annual exams). These systems are also helpful in clinics where there are providers of different training levels, because they facilitate standardization, completeness, and quality. Checklist formats are particularly useful for specialists, but less experienced practitioners can devolve to a "laundry list" style of interviewing (Bajgier et al. 2012). In primary care practice settings, where clinical possibilities are exponentially increased, structured systems are experienced as more onerous as expanded interfaces slow users.

Post hoc text-processing algorithms produce structured data *after* the provider has recorded the care episode. In this setting, providers are free to employ their preferred, unstructured documentation approaches, and the transcribed notes subsequently undergo postproduction processing (Rosenbloom et al. 2011). In comparison with structured formats, text-processing approaches are less restrictive and allow more nuanced documentation of history and clinical impressions, but structured information is not typically available until after the note has been processed. These processing programs exist on a continuum ranging from programs that identify keywords to more complex systems that attempt to capture clinical concepts in their natural language context (Chapman et al. 2001; Friedman et al. 2004).

Because documentation methods often feature certain attributes at the expense of others (e.g., promoting narrative expressivity at the expense of formal note structure), it is recommended that health care providers be afforded a variety of methods to ensure that their documentation, data, and workflow needs are met. One value of this approach is that it focuses EHR development and implementation efforts on the primary task of clinical documentation and related issues of usability, efficiency, quality, and readability (Rosenbloom et al. 2011).

How Can EHR Systems Improve Clinician Efficiency?

Most EHR systems are optimized for documentation that is conducted as uninterrupted composition, but clinical documentation is fundamentally a synthesis activity where clinicians review available data from various sources and then summarize their impressions. This mismatch leads to fragmented clinical work and frequent task transitions (i.e., between the processes of reviewing data, documenting impressions, and updating plan of care). Ethnographic observations have shown a number of strategies that have been employed to reduce these transitions (e.g., handwritten notes, electronic templates, copy/pasting, reliance on memory, and prepopulating the EHR note prior to seeing the patient) (Saleem et al. 2013). Next-generation EHRs will need to consolidate the complex activities of data exploration, selective reading, annotation, clinical synthesis, and composition of notes as temporal structures (Mamykina et al. 2012).

HOW WILL POPULATION HEALTH AND VALUE-BASED CARE DRIVE FUTURE CHANGES IN EHRs AND CLINICAL DOCUMENTATION?

The Affordable Care Act of 2010 (ACA) and the more recent Medicare Access and CHIP [Children's Health Insurance Program] Reauthorization Act of 2015 (MACRA) have changed, and are changing, the health care landscape significantly, in part by introducing payment vehicles that encourage population health management approaches as defined by the Centers for Medicare & Medicaid Services (2010). As commercial payers began to focus on populations, their efforts included more coordinated chronic disease management and integrated care delivery strategies as well. The expectation was that stakeholders, including states and payers, could leverage quality metrics to advance the goals of cost-effective, patient-centric, and evidence-based population health management. This expanded focus offers potential returns for patients, providers, and payers alike (Meyer and Smith 2008). Improved data capture and integration of data from EHRs, scheduling modules, and patient portals could enable powerful datasets that empower patients to participate more actively in their own treatment, that enable providers to measure their performance against that of their peers, and that allow health systems to better manage covered populations. Prudent data-driven care that remains patient centric, individualized, and supportive of population-level assessments represents a growing priority in our evolving health care system (Meyer and Smith 2008).

Value-based care has similarly asserted itself as a driver as payers seek to scale resources and maximize quality. Value-based care can be employed in behavioral health care and other specialties where a proportion of the disease burden is already being covered in primary care settings. The drive to better integrate behavioral health care with medical care has never been stronger, and the result has been a variety of integrative and collaborative care approaches that scale resources, employ data, and improve team coordination to support primary care. In general, *collabora-*

tive models denote professions working together (i.e., collaborating) in the delivery of care, whereas *integrative models* denote professions working together and being subsumed into a single organizational framework. Integration requires collaboration, but collaboration does not require integration (Boon et al. 2009).

In contrast to traditional volume-based care, value-based care models incentivize and reimburse professionals in part based on performance metrics for covered populations. Critical to successful implementation of a value-based care system will be the development of meaningful metrics and improved population management practices. Collaborative care models have been shown to be particularly effective (Fortney et al. 2013) in that they maintain specialty separations while also efficiently integrating evidence-based behavioral health treatments into primary care environments. Patients who require specialty care will continue to have access to specialists, but collaborative models—which improve standardization, adherence to clinical practice guidelines, and integration—will increasingly deliver care appropriately provided in the primary care setting. Collaborative care models engage patients in real time, stratify groups by specific disease states, monitor utilization, and potentially reduce health care costs (Boyd et al. 2010; Centers for Medicare & Medicaid Services 2010). Integrated care models facilitate tracking of essential health outcome measures, such as the Healthcare Effectiveness Data and Information Set (HEDIS; National Committee for Quality Assurance 2017). Patient-centered medical homes and behavioral health homes, two effective integrated care models, allow for monitoring of mental health measures (e.g., Patient Health Questionnaire–9), physical health parameters (e.g., vital signs, body mass index, lipids, glucose), and findings from routine screenings (e.g., colonoscopy, mammography)

What Are the Overarching EMR Requirements for Successful Population-Based Care?

Chapter 9 ("Management of Patient Populations") focuses in detail on population-based care; here we address more specifically the pragmatic interface of population-based care with EMRs. In order to successfully engage in population-based care, professionals need to employ health information technology systems that create registries, collate data, and facilitate tracking of care data over time. These systems must have the capability to discriminate among particular conditions, characteristics, practice/provider groups, and other parameters. Professionals need to be supported by assigned staff that work to systematically assess, track, and manage the group's health conditions and treatment responses. They must proactively track the clinical outcomes, identify the care gaps, and address the urgent care needs of patients living with chronic disease.

DATA-DRIVEN CARE

Data-informed care is a critical element for successful population management. EMRs can create datasets of behavioral health measures (e.g., cross-cutting symptom measures, diagnosis-specific severity measures) and integrate these with other structured data (DSM-5, American Psychiatric Association 2013). EHRs can organize these data into defined subgroups and present registry data to facilitate communication and coordination of care between health care providers and across organizations. Data can be sorted by provider and/or by practice to enable organizations to assess and improve performance. Interactive patient registries and analytics can be combined to advance efficiency, effectiveness, and outcomes. Clinical data and payer databases can also be organized into various registries and seamlessly shared to inform treatment (Fitzgerald 2015). Datasets that include extracts from both claims data and EMR data can provide information on cost and quality.

CARE MANAGEMENT

Care management is an essential aspect of population management, particularly when considered in the context of value-based contracts. Care managers, for example, can use data to identify patients with high utilization of avoidable services (e.g., emergency departments). Care management can be conducted face to face, via telephone, or via video teleconferencing (Darkins et al. 2008; Reid et al. 2011). The care managers or navigators build relationships with patients and then meet with the clinical team to advocate for interventions that improve care, advance quality, and reduce costs.

Population management is also critical for other aspects of health homes, including the following health home services specifically defined in the Affordable Care Act (Centers for Medicare & Medicaid Services (2010):

- *Comprehensive care management*—Identifying high-risk/high-use patients, assessing needs, and monitoring adherence to population health guidelines.
- *Care coordination*—Creating customized treatment plans in partnership with the patient, community, and long-term services.
- *Health promotion*—Advancing health in the community via health education and stakeholder engagement.
- *Comprehensive transitional care/follow-up*—Facilitating transition from inpatient care to other settings and ensuring follow-up.
- *Patient, family, and community support services*—Working with authorized representatives, community referrals, and social support services.

How Can Psychiatrists Actively Influence the Evolution of Clinical Documentation?

The use and purpose of clinical documentation will continue to evolve as technology and care practices evolve. Psychiatrists should expect continually changing methods, processes, and standards for clinical documentation, and to the degree that they are able, they should act to influence the evolution of these standards. A primary method of exerting influence is through active advocacy in an organization's clinical documentation improvement program (Arrowood et al. 2015). The clinical challenge of the day is to work to ensure that information technologies remain tools that advance clinical relationships (as opposed to acting as barriers to those relationships). In addition, physicians should

- *Educate themselves about their organization's EHR and clinical documentation systems.* Beyond a basic orientation, they should seek out clinical information technology champions and become familiar with the range of options, configurations, short cuts, and supports offered by the EHR. These efforts can pay dividends in the long run by increasing efficiency and the practitioner's ability to maximize available features.
- *Learn to benefit from the many process efficiencies afforded by the EHR,* such as automatic templating and data importation.
- *Consider adoption of new models or methods of documentation as these become available,* such as working with medical assistants or voice recognition technologies.

- *Practice patient-focused, concurrent documentation* so as to be able to serve the treatment needs of patients and also ensure completion of most documentation requirements by the end of the clinical encounter.

SUMMARY

Despite the disruptions and challenges that EHR adaptations can create for systems and individual providers, the EHR affords opportunities for psychiatrists to increase their efficiency of practice, to better track and manage patients, and to enhance communication across teams and organizations in care. Important topics covered in this chapter include the following:

- Physicians need to be aware of the content drivers of clinical documentation, which encompass five domains: *clinical, administrative/billing, legal, research, and education.*
- Psychiatrists should understand the capabilities and functions of their organization's EHR in order to best tailor and customize their content and processes to maximize efficiency in documentation and communication. To accomplish this goal, they should adhere to best practices in documentation (e.g., use of standards/templates, cut/paste guidelines). Psychiatrists should also track and stay abreast of emerging models (e.g., use of medical assistants, scribes, dictation technology) that support efficiency of EHR documentation.
- Psychiatrists need to remain current with emerging population health care management tools that incorporate clinical registries and understand how these can be implemented in their individual practices.
- Ultimately, the EHR and clinical documentation exist to provide the best possible care and treatment for each patient. Clinicians must strive to balance clinical documentation and management needs against the primary care of the patient. They should always bear in mind the imperative to "treat the patient, not the chart" as a guiding principle for navigating the challenges faced by physicians in this era of information technology.

REFERENCES

Agency for Healthcare Research and Quality: Chapter 3: Care coordination measurement framework, in Care Coordination Measures Atlas Update. Rockville, MD, Agency for Healthcare Research and Quality, 2014. Available at:

http://www.ahrq.gov/professionals/prevention-chronic-care/improve/
coordination/atlas2014/chapter3.html. Accessed June 22, 2017.

American Psychiatric Association: Diagnostic and Statistical Manual of Mental Disorders, 5th Edition. Arlington, VA, American Psychiatric Association, 2013

American Psychiatric Association Work Group on Psychiatric Evaluation: Practice Guidelines for the Psychiatric Evaluation of Adults, 3rd Edition. Arlington, VA, American Psychiatric Association, 2016

Arrowood D, Bailey-Woods L, Easterling S, et al: Best practices in the art and science of clinical documentation improvement. J AHIMA 86(7):46–50, 2015 26642623

Bajgier J, Bender J, Ries R: Use of templates for clinical documentation in psychiatric evaluations—beneficial or counterproductive for residents in training? Int J Psychiatry Med 43(1):99–103, 2012 22641933

Boon HS, Mior SA, Barnsley J, et al: The difference between integration and collaboration in patient care. J Manipulative Physiol Ther 32(9):715–722, 2009 20004798

Boyd C, Leff B, Weiss C, et al: Faces of Medicaid: Clarifying Multimorbidity Patterns to Improve Targeting and Delivery of Clinical Services for Medicaid Populations. Hamilton, NJ, Center for Health Care Strategies, 2010. Available at: http://www.chcs.org/media/Clarifying_Multimorbidity_for_Medicaid_report-FINAL.pdf. Accessed April 6, 2017.

Centers for Medicare & Medicaid Services: Health Homes for Enrollees with Chronic Conditions (letter, November 16, 2010). Available at: https://downloads.cms.gov/cmsgov/archived-downloads/smdl/downloads/smd10024.pdf. Accessed June 22, 2017.

Chapman WW, Fizman M, Chapman BE, et al: A comparison of classification algorithms to automatically identify chest X-ray reports that support pneumonia. J Biomed Inform 34(1):4–14, 2001 11376542

Council of Medical Specialty Societies: CMSS Primer for the Development and Maturation of Specialty Society Clinical Data Registries: For Specialty Societies and Organizations Developing and Advancing Clinical Data Registries, 1st Edition. Chicago, IL, Council of Medical Specialty Societies, January 2016. Available at: https://cmss.org/wp-content/uploads/2016/02/CMSS_Registry_Primer_1.2.pdf. Accessed June 22, 2017.

Daley K, Richardson J, James I, et al: Clinical dashboard: use in older adult mental health wards. The Psychiatrist Online 37(3):85–88, 2013. Available at: http://pb.rcpsych.org/content/37/3/85. Accessed April 6, 2017.

Darkins A, Ryan P, Kobb R, et al: Care Coordination/Home Telehealth: the systematic implementation of health informatics, home telehealth, and disease management to support the care of veteran patients with chronic conditions. Telemed J E Health 14(10):1118–1126, 2008 19119835

Dowding D, Randell R, Gardner P, et al: Dashboards for improving patient care: review of the literature. Int J Med Inform 84(2):87–100, 2015, 25453274

Dykes PC, Samal L, Donahue M, et al: A patient-centered longitudinal care plan: vision versus reality. J Am Med Inform Assoc 21(6):1082–1090, 2014 24996874

Farnan JM, Snyder Sulmasy L, Worster BK, et al: Online medical professionalism: patient and public relationships: policy statement from the American College of Physicians and the Federation of State Medical Boards. Ann Intern Med 158(8):620–627, 2013 23579867

Fitzgerald M: When health care gets a healthy dose of data: how Intermountain Healthcare is using data and analytics to transform patient care. MIT Sloan Management Review (June):3–17, 2015. Available at: http://sloanreview.mit.edu/case-study/when-healthcare-gets-a-healthy-dose-of-data/. Accessed April 6, 2017.

Fortney JC, Pyne JM, Mouden SB, et al: Practice-based versus telemedicine-based collaborative care for depression in rural federally qualified health centers: a pragmatic randomized comparative effectiveness trial. Am J Psychiatry 170(4):414–425, 2013 23429924

Friedman C, Shagina L, Lussier Y, et al: Automated encoding of clinical documents based on natural language processing. J Am Med Inform Assoc 11(5):392–402, 2004 15187068

Gillum RF: From papyrus to the electronic tablet: a brief history of the clinical medical record with lessons for the digital age. Am J Med 126(10):853–857, 2013 24054954

Hill RG Jr, Sears LM, Melanson SW: 4000 clicks: a productivity analysis of electronic medical records in a community hospital ED. Am J Emerg Med 31(11):1591–1594, 2013 24060331

Ho YX, Gadd GS, Kohorst KL, Rosenbloom ST: A qualitative analysis evaluating purposes and practices of clinical documentation. Appl Clin Inform 5(1):153–168, 2014 24734130

Institute of Medicine, Committee on Quality of Health Care in America: Crossing the Quality Chasm: A New Health System for the 21st Century. Washington, DC, National Academy Press, 2001. 25057539

Kawamoto K, Houlihan CA, Balas EA, Lobach DF: Improving clinical practice using clinical decision support systems: a systematic review of trials to identify features critical to success. BMJ 330(7494):765, 2005 15767266

Kuhn T, Basch P, Barr M, et al: Clinical documentation in the 21st century: executive summary of a policy position paper from the American College of Physicians. Ann Intern Med 162(4):301–303, 2015 25581028

Mamykina L, Vawdrey DK, Stetson PD, et al: Clinical documentation: composition or synthesis? J Am Med Inform Assoc 19(6):1025–1031, 2012 22813762

Meyer J, Smith B: Chronic Disease Management: Evidence of Predictable Savings. Lansing, MI, Health Management Associates, 2008. Available at: https://www.healthmanagement.com//wp-content/uploads/Chronic-Disease-Savings-Report-Nov-2008.pdf. Accessed August 29, 2014.

National Committee for Quality Assurance: Healthcare Effectiveness Data and Information Set (HEDIS). Healthcare Effectiveness Data and Information Set (HEDIS). Available at: http://www.ncqa.org/hedis-quality-measurement. Accessed June 22, 2017.

Payne TH, Corley S, Cullen TA, et al: Report of the AMIA EHR-2020 Task Force on the status and future direction of EHRs. J Am Med Inform Assoc 22(5):1102–1110, 2015 26024883

Reid SC, Kauer SD, Hearps SJ, et al: A mobile phone application for the assessment and management of youth mental health problems in primary care: a randomized controlled trial. BMC Fam Pract 12:131, 2011 22123031

Rosenbloom ST, Denny JC, Xu H, et al: Data from clinical notes: a perspective on the tension between structure and flexible documentation. J Am Med Inform Assoc 18(2):181–186, 2011 21233086

Sadock BJ, Sadock VA, Ruiz P: Kaplan and Sadock's Synopsis of Psychiatry: Behavioral Sciences/Clinical Psychiatry, 11th Edition. Philadelphia, PA, Lippincott Williams & Wilkins, 2014

Saleem J, Adams S, Frankel R, et al: Efficiency strategies for facilitating computerized clinical documentation in ambulatory care. Stud Health Technol Inform 192:13–17, 2013 23920506

Sequist TD: Clinical documentation to improve patient care. Ann Intern Med 162(4):315–316, 2015 25581123

Shipman SA, Sinsky CA: Expanding primary care capacity by reducing waste and improving the efficiency of care. Health Aff (Millwood) 32(11):1990–1997, 2013 24191091

Shoolin J, Ozeran L, Hamann C, et al: Association of Medical Directors of Information Systems consensus on inpatient electronic health record documentation. Appl Clin Inform 4(2):293–303, 2013 23874365

Steichen O, Gregg W: Health information technology coordination to support patient-centered care coordination. Yearb Med Inform 10(1):34–37, 2015 26293848

S&I Framework: HL7 Implementation Guide for CDA Release 2: Consolidated CDA Templates for Clinical Notes Vol.1, Section 1.1.2—Care Plans, 2013. Available at: http://www.hl7.org/implement/standards/product_brief.cfm?product_id=435. Accessed August 17, 2017.

Tasman A, Kay J, Ursano R: The Psychiatric Interview: Evaluation and Diagnosis. Chichester, West Sussex, United Kingdom, John Wiley & Sons, Ltd, 2013. Available at: http://onlinelibrary.wiley.com/book/10.1002/9781118341001. Accessed June 22, 2017.

Weiss JM, Levy PC: Copy, paste, and cloned notes in electronic health records: prevalence, benefits, risks, and best practice recommendations. Chest 145(3):632–638, 2014 24590024

8

Indirect Consultation
and Hybrid Care

Peter Yellowlees, MBBS, M.D.

Shazia Shafqat, M.D., M.S.

Kathleen Myers, M.D., M.P.H., M.S.

In this chapter we focus on psychiatrists who are increasingly practicing in a hybrid manner—meeting with patients both in person and online. Hybrid practices utilize a wide range of technologies, such as electronic program applications ("apps"), patient registries, and indirect (or asynchronous) consultation, to treat both individual patients and populations of patients. The psychiatrist in a hybrid practice may treat patients individually or as part of team-based care (Fortney et al. 2015; Katon et al. 2012). This approach will become increasingly common in the future and will change the traditional doctor–patient relationship. This relationship will inevitably become a hybrid one—both in-person and online—with the possibility of around-the-clock availability along with the creation of new boundary issues that such on-demand availability creates. In this hybrid environment, the doctor–patient relationship may need to be more formalized than in the past, with the introduction of new guidelines to allow psychiatrists to maintain ethical practice standards while also maintaining a reasonable work–life balance.

This chapter outlines novel approaches that integrate technology into hybrid practice to provide both direct and indirect consultations and to include psychotherapy as an essential part of this hybrid care. Technology-based hybrid practice facilitates the inclusion of genetics, evidence-based treatment, multiple apps, and online programs to customize treatment to individual need—a medical model frequently referred to as *precision medicine* (also see Chapter 9, "Management of Patient Populations").

The psychiatrist as part of a team and the approaches, training, and skills needed to work in this type of environment, especially where population-based reviews and indirect consultations are involved, are examined, as is the potential for asynchronous consultations to occur across languages and to thereby enhance our cultural understanding of our patients. The chapter concludes with sections describing how to conduct indirect consultations, using both video and text/e-mail, which is a clinical area predicted to experience a dramatic expansion of interest and activity in the future. We believe that this increase in asynchronous consultations will lead to extensive changes to psychiatric work practices over the next decade, with psychiatrists increasingly working in team-based environments, spreading their skills and expertise, all of which will have a positive impact on the current workforce shortages the profession is facing.

Why Do Psychiatrists Need to Adopt Hybrid Models and Change the Way They Practice?

There is a dearth of psychiatrists and allied mental health care professionals in the United States, in spite of the rising demand for their services (Hankir and Zaman 2015). Between 2008 and 2013, the nation's population increased from 304 million to 315 million, with an increase of 3.7% in the total number of physicians. However, the same increase did not hold true for psychiatrists, despite the fact that psychiatrists are needed even more than before to fulfill the growing demands of the rising population, to cover the increased number of baby boomers and the millions more Americans who have become eligible for mental health care coverage under the Affordable Care Act. Rural areas bear the brunt of the shortage, as most practicing psychiatrists are concentrated in urban areas, with more than half of all counties in the United States not possessing a single psychiatrist.

An additional problem is that the number of psychiatry residents in the United States has remained essentially unchanged over the past one and a half decades (Association of American Medical Colleges 2016), while there has been a steadily increasing number of medical students nationally, resulting in a proportional decrease in the number of medical students choosing careers in psychiatry. Currently, less than 5% of U.S. medical students choose psychiatry for residency training, and the number of psychiatrists entering the field is not expected to increase in the near future. Inadequate reimbursement of mental health care services from government and private insurance plans, high administrative burdens imposed by Medicare and private insurance companies, the stigma attached to mental diseases and the associated job stress, as well as the perception of a relatively low index of satisfaction among practitioners have made the field of psychiatry less desirable as a specialty for many medical students.

Research has shown that although more women than men pursue psychiatry for their residency training, female psychiatrists practice the profession less actively once they have graduated from residency. In 2015, 54% of psychiatry residents were female, but only 38% of psychiatrists in active practice were female (Association of American Medical Colleges 2016). Female psychiatrists work on average 7 hours less than male psychiatrists per week, and therefore see fewer overall patients than their male counterparts. This lighter workload has been attributed to women's historically higher share of responsibility for parenting and family caregiving.

Psychiatrists are also aging. Out of the estimated 37,736 active psychiatrists in the United States in 2016, 22,777, or 60%, were older than 55 years (Association of American Medical Colleges 2016). These aging psychiatrists tend to work fewer hours than their younger colleagues and are likely to retire in the next 10–15 years. Once again, this effect is more pronounced in the case of female psychiatrists, who either resort to part-time work or reduce work hours with age. In addition, 32% of psychiatrists ages 65 years or older tend to work only part-time, which further reduces their capacity to see patients. In summary, it is expected that more psychiatrists will leave the specialty than will enter it over the next decade, further exacerbating current psychiatrist shortages.

The U.S. Health Resources and Services Administration has estimated that the United States needs 25.9 psychiatrists for every 100,000 individuals. Based on the U.S. Census Bureau's 2010 Census of Population, the total population of the United States as of July 2015 was estimated at 321 million, suggesting an ideal estimate of about 83,000 psychiatrists. Currently, the nation has about 38,000 full-time practicing psychiatrists (Association of American Medical Colleges 2016), which according to these calculations leads to an estimated shortage of 45,000 psychiatrists. Most shortage estimates are less dramatic than this figure; shortages of 10,000–15,000 psychiatrists are more frequently quoted numbers that may relate better to the large number of psychiatrist vacancies around the United States.

The introduction of electronically mediated indirect consultations and team-based work into usual psychiatric practice could substantially increase the numbers of patients that can be seen and treated by psychiatrists (as will be discussed later in this chapter). Using the example of the notional 30-hour clinical working week (described later in this chapter), we believe that the widespread incorporation of indirect consultations into hybrid integrated care and team-based models could lead to between 20% and 30% more patients being effectively seen and treated by psychiatrists nationally—a substantial contribution to amelioration of current and future shortages of psychiatrists.

What Is Hybrid Psychiatry, and How Will It Be Practiced in the Future?

Hybrid providers are clinicians who interact with patients both in person and online, so that their doctor–patient relationships cross both environments. The addition of interactions via videoconferencing, e-mail, text messaging, and telephony leads to improved access and interactions at times and places not possible when care is restricted to the in-person venue. This hybrid practice is becoming a preferred model of care for many physicians as secure messaging is incorporated into electronic medical record (EMR) systems. It is especially relevant to telepsychiatry because a range of video technologies, text-based systems, and apps can readily complement in-person care, depending on the psychiatrist's and patient's preferences (Yellowlees et al. 2015). The incorporation of online models of care into practice can strengthen the doctor–patient relationship by increasing empathy and forming a trusting therapeutic bond.

What will all this mean for psychiatrist–patient relationships of the future? It is worthwhile taking a brief look at the current process of that relationship using an informatics perspective (Yellowlees et al. 2015). There are three core components to any doctor–patient interaction:

- *The history, physical examination, and information gathering*—or, in informatics terms, "data collection."
- *Formulating a diagnosis from this information*—or, in the informatics field, "data analysis."
- *Creation of a treatment plan*—or, in informatics, "project implementation."

The separation of these three components is a phenomenon of long standing in several medical specialties, such as pathology and radiology, in which data collection (e.g., x-rays, blood work) typically is not done by radiologists or pathologists. Such separation is now occurring in asynchronous telepsychiatry approaches, where recording of a diagnostic interview by a physician extender at one time, then interpretation of the interview by a psychiatrist at another time, is later followed by implementation of the psychiatrist's recommendations by the primary care practitioner (PCP). The evolution of more mobile, team facilitated, and asynchronous environments will enable further separation of the components of the traditional in-person psychiatric consultation to allow more highly trained and paid psychiatrists to focus on the more difficult analytic and planning components of patient care.

The implications of these changes are twofold. The hybrid doctor–patient relationship of the future will still be based on the gold standard in-person consultation that establishes an immediate trusting interaction as the foundation for support and healing. This traditional relationship will be improved by multiple online interactions that can be more patient focused by providing more frequent and convenient access to care, anytime and anywhere. Providers should also find the hybrid relationship advantageous, particularly through their use of the virtual space during videoconferencing, when they engage as intimate participants while also serving as objective observers (Figure 8–1), as discussed in Chapter 5 ("Media Communication Skills and the Ethical Doctor–Patient Relationship"). The online component allows psychiatrists to work from home at preferred times, freeing them from the typical business week practice.

A potential downside to this "always on" hybrid relationship concerns the need for psychiatrists to ensure that appropriate professional bound-

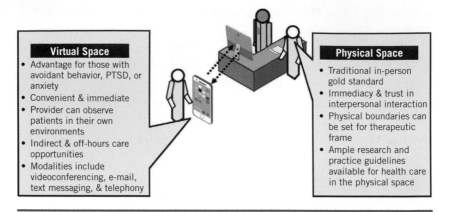

FIGURE 8–1.   The hybrid doctor–patient relationship.

Source.   Diagram and illustrations by Steven Chan, M.D., M.B.A. Used with permission.

aries—ethical, physical, technical, and time related—are maintained. Psychiatrists must establish simple "rules" of communication and engagement in their practices. Sharing such policies with patients ensures that both parties have the same expectations of the relationship and respect each other's privacy.

INTEGRATION OF PSYCHOTHERAPY AND TELEPSYCHIATRY— WHAT DOES CURRENT EXPERIENCE SHOW?

In this section we discuss integration of the major enabling principles of short-term therapies into online practice. Clinical use of the virtual space in videoconferencing-based consultation is discussed in Chapter 5.

Psychotherapeutic approaches established in traditional psychiatric practice—for example, the development of rapport and empathy—are readily incorporated into online therapies. A solid evidence base has established the advantages of psychiatric treatment delivered through videoconferencing and telephony, beyond increasing access to care. Both patients and providers endorse high satisfaction ratings, while the online delivery of cognitive-behavioral therapies has the strongest evidence base of all available psychotherapies. Empirical studies, including large randomized controlled trials, have demonstrated the efficacy of treatment provided through telepsychiatry (Bashshur et al. 2016). Multiple trials of online brief therapies, particularly cognitive-behavioral approaches, have shown outcomes equivalent to those of in-person psychiatric care, while online delivery of prolonged exposure therapy for veterans with posttraumatic stress disorder (PTSD) has been associated with better outcomes than in-person therapy (Fortney et al. 2015). Younger patients often prefer telepsychiatry over in-person encounters and will commonly discuss intimate issues more readily with telepsychiatrists than with in-person providers (Yellowlees et al. 2015). Telepsychiatry also offers opportunities for more ecologically valid observations of patients' lives than is possible in the clinic setting, such as observing an elderly patient in the nursing home or a child disrupting the classroom. Patients with paranoia, social anxiety, or PTSD often prefer services delivered to their homes (Chan et al. 2015).

Psychotherapists, especially analytically oriented practitioners, have been using telephony with patients for more than 50 years, and many have moved to using videoconferencing in recent years. Thousands of patients have benefited through receiving brief psychotherapy via videoconferencing, and numerous studies using telephony, Internet-enabled programs, and videoconferencing support their integration into hybrid models of care. A number of key issues are now explored.

What Are the Indications for and Contraindications to Online Psychotherapy?

The main indication for conducting psychotherapy online is the same as in person, namely that the patient wishes to have therapy for a specific purpose, and the therapist is qualified and willing to provide it. The telepsychiatry literature and guidelines of care (Turvey et al. 2013) are clear in indicating the types of patients that can be treated online—anyone, with any disorder.

Patients with anxiety, depressive, and substance-related disorders are those most likely to be treated online with short-term psychotherapy, but patients with psychoses and major mood disorders are also appropriate for online supportive therapy.

The only absolute contraindications to online therapy are patient refusal and patient aggression or self-harm at the time of the consultation. Nonetheless, online therapy may be the only option for some patients living in distant communities or unable to access available care. Safety and crisis management are crucial to treatment planning for patients who participate in online therapy, as is discussed in Chapters 3 ("The Business of Telepsychiatry") and 5 ("Media Communication Skills and the Ethical Doctor–Patient Relationship").

Finally, sparse information is available regarding online psychotherapy with patients diagnosed with DSM Cluster 2 personality disorders (i.e., antisocial, borderline, histrionic, and narcissistic personality disorders). Such patients may be more difficult to manage in the hybrid environment, in which the psychotherapeutic relationship is more fluid. Safety planning must take into account the possibility that increased access will lead to more splitting or impulsive acting out. The psychiatrist should address potential boundary violations and enactment of conflicts with the patient when discussing the policy regarding the "rules" of communication and engagement.

How Might the Hybrid Environment Lead to Improved Psychotherapeutic Outcomes?

The clinical and research literature on telepsychiatry suggests that some psychotherapeutic outcomes for telepsychiatry may be better than those for in-person therapy, so combining both approaches makes sense. Among the many factors that contribute to patient satisfaction with online care, patients often note the empathic connection they feel with their online providers, as discussed in Chapter 5. Inexperienced telepsychiatrists frequently report surprise at the intensity of emotion that can be experienced during video consultations. Other factors cited by patients include reduced anxiety from being able to receive care close to their homes or their PCP's clinic, as well as the savings in reduced travel time and cost.

A more subtle issue concerns the power relationship between provider and patient, as described in Chapter 5. In the in-person relationship, the therapist typically has a position of authority and the psychological advantage of being in his or her clinic. In contrast, patients tend to feel more "in control" during video consultations and can potentially "switch off" the therapist and leave the consultation without any embarrassment. In most situations, the online relationship has the potential to be more egalitarian and patient focused than the relationship established during traditional in-person care (Hilty et al. 2013; Shore 2013).

Another significant advantage of video consultations over traditional in-person consultation is that it facilitates therapists' collaboration across disciplines with local providers and specialists, as well as with patients and their families (Fortney et al. 2015; Hilty et al. 2013). Fortney et al. (2015) demonstrated that the addition of online cognitive-behavioral psychotherapy to usual care could improve in-person care and showed that psychotherapy for PTSD was conducted with better fidelity and was more effective when delivered online versus in person.

CASE EXAMPLE 1: PTSD TREATMENT IN A SINGLE TELEPSYCHIATRY SESSION[1]

Matt, a 45-year-old National Guard veteran with a clear history of PTSD from his past tours in Iraq was referred for assessment. Matt was married, with two children, and since his return from his last tour had been isolating himself, was irritable, was having difficulty at his work and in his marriage, and had started drinking heavily. His PCP had been appropriately treating him with antidepressants and had referred him to the U.S. Department of Veterans Affairs (VA) for group therapy. P.Y. had a good interactive telepsychiatry session with him and focused on educating him about PTSD, on motivational interviewing for his drinking, and on suggesting a series of behavioral activation and lifestyle changes. He was seen only once, and recommendations for follow-up were sent to his PCP.

Six months later, P.Y. was interviewing a 40-year-old married beautician who, after 10 minutes of the interview, admitted that she did not have any psychiatric concerns herself but was, in fact, Matt's wife, and that she had made the appointment to meet and thank the person whom she credited with completely turning her husband's life around in one session. She recounted how Matt had come home from the session energized and optimistic, talking about how this "expert from afar" seemed to be able to understand him and had set up a plan for him to follow. Her husband had since minimized his drinking, started a fitness regimen, and improved his relationships with his family and at work, while still attending group therapy at the VA and following up with his PCP. His wife was delighted and said that she felt more positive about the future than she had for several years.

▌KEY CONCEPT

Powerful relationships can be formed through videoconferencing and can be used to implement treatment recommendations that may have long-lasting therapeutic effects.

---

[1]Case provided by Peter Yellowlees, MBBS, M.D.

How Do Core Outcome Variables Differ for Telepsychiatry Versus In-Person Psychotherapy?

All three core psychotherapeutic factors that have been described as affecting patient outcomes—patient variables, relationship factors, and placebo, hope, and expectancy—are altered through telepsychiatry and in the hybrid relationship.

Patient variables were discussed earlier and include high satisfaction with telepsychiatry, improved engagement, and capacity to form strong, and perhaps more intimate, relationships with their therapists online than in person.

The most interesting issues of relevance here are the placebo, hope, and expectancy effects and the likelihood that these also may be enhanced in some patients who are treated online. The power of an "expert" being "beamed in" from a distance, hence increasing the likelihood of an enhanced placebo effect, is the most obvious example. Patients also frequently attribute to their PCP increased importance when observing them interact collegially through videoconferencing with expert psychiatrists, who historically have tended to be based at academic medical centers. Indeed, this perception is a well-known motivator for some PCPs to become involved in telemedicine programs. For those patients receiving hybrid care, the distance of a videoconsultation itself may make a well-known therapist appear more powerful, thereby increasing the hope and expectancy effect that increases psychotherapy effectiveness.

Finally, there are many studies in the human–computer interaction literature that describe humans' greater honesty and lower embarrassment when responding to questions about stigmatized topics on a computer compared with an in-person interview or a supervised questionnaire (Yellowlees 2008). This factor is particularly important for cognitive-behavioral therapies that require questionnaire and remote data monitoring in conjunction with therapist interactions.

CASE EXAMPLE 2: IN-HOME PARENT–CHILD THERAPY DELIVERED VIA TELECONFERENCING[2]

Susan, an 8-year-old girl living with her family in a rural city (population of 45,000) approximately 2 hours away from the nearest metropol-

---

[2]Case provided by Donald M. Hilty, M.D., and Erica Z. Shoemaker, M.D.

itan area academic health center, had been taken to the emergency department several times by her parents when her behavior became severely disruptive. The main symptoms were "talking back to us," striking out at her mother, and throwing objects at home and at school. It was not feasible for Susan's family to travel from their rural setting to obtain therapy and support for their daughter. Susan was diagnosed with depression, oppositional defiant behavior, and attention-deficit/hyperactivity disorder (ADHD); her mother also had depression and was receiving treatment.

Videoconferencing was set up in Susan's home using a mobile unit to allow the delivery of Parent–Child Interaction Therapy (PCIT) in the home context. PCIT is a parent training modality in which a therapist coaches a parent in real time through the use of a two-way mirror and "bug-in-the-ear" technology. PCIT is generally split into two parts, with the first half focused on helping the parent to develop a warm and responsive parenting style by training the parent to be an enthusiastic and responsive play partner, and the second half focused on coaching the parent to train the child in being compliant with parent commands. Six weekly sessions of 1.5 hours each were conducted by a therapist and a child and adolescent psychiatrist. Susan's behavior improved gradually (as measured by quantity of verbal outbursts and times throwing objects [parental assessment]), and the parents' confidence was also self-reported as being improved.

I KEY CONCEPTS

Expert services delivered in the family home via telepsychiatry may have an advantage over expert services delivered in a clinic, in that this setting enables the clinician to observe baseline parent and child behavior in a familiar environment.

PCIT is an evidence-based treatment that can be delivered via videoconferencing, replacing the office technology of the two-way mirror with a webcam, an in-room omnidirectional microphone, and a Bluetooth-based earbud worn by the parent.

WHAT PROVIDER CHALLENGES ARE ASSOCIATED WITH ADOPTION OF HYBRID MODELS OF PSYCHOTHERAPY?

It has been widely documented that the main challenge posed to the broad dissemination of hybrid models of psychotherapies relates to therapists' acceptance of the hybrid model of care. Although patients give very high satisfaction ratings to telepsychiatry, providers assign lower satisfaction ratings to the modality (approximately 20% lower than patients' ratings). This disparity is not surprising, given that it is providers who must make changes to their practices, learn current technologies, master new skills, and deal with the extra administrative complications associated with treating patients online. However, provider attitudes toward these new models of care may be changing as patients increasingly demand better access to their providers and more choices of therapies and psychiatrists, and other providers increasingly incorporate online psychotherapy into their practices. Provider groups especially in favor of hybrid models of practice include young parents who wish to spend more time at home, older clinicians who seek more flexibility as they approach retirement, and individuals who prefer to work nontraditional hours in order to pursue alternative interests.

HOW ARE TEAM-BASED AND COLLABORATIVE CARE MODELS CHANGING THE PRACTICE LANDSCAPE IN MENTAL HEALTH CARE?

Health care models are changing and becoming more focused on making efficient use of medical resources to serve the greatest public good. Such models emphasize team-based care. Psychiatrists and other mental health care professionals have long worked in teams—for example, in community mental health care environments, on inpatient units, and for research and education. The University of Washington's Advancing Integrated Mental Health Solutions (AIMS) Center has defined five core principles embodied in the collaborative care model that underlie team-based care (AIMS Center 2017):

1. *Patient-Centered Team Care* in which primary care and behavioral health care providers collaborate effectively using shared care plans that incorporate patient goals.
2. *Population-Based Care* in which a care team shares a defined group of patients tracked in a registry to ensure that no one "falls through the cracks."
3. *Measurement-Based 'Treatment to Target"* in which each patient's treatment plan clearly articulates personal goals and clinical outcomes that are routinely measured by evidence-based tools. If patients are not improving as expected, treatments are actively changed until the clinical goals are achieved.

4. *Evidence-Based Care* in which patients are offered treatments with credible research evidence supporting their efficacy in treating the target condition.
5. *Accountable Care* in which providers are accountable and reimbursed for quality of care and clinical outcomes, not just for the volume of care provided.

The structure of this collaborative care model is shown in Figure 8–2. A team of professionals with complementary skills work together to care for a population of patients with the same mental conditions, such as depression or anxiety. This shift from current medical practice to team-based collaborative care creates new workflows and adds two new roles— the care manager and the psychiatric consultant—to the traditional practice of "one patient, one provider." Here psychiatrists focus on panels and populations of patients that they manage in collaboration with PCPs, who maintain primary responsibility for the patients (as also discussed in Chapter 9).

CASE EXAMPLE 3: WORKING WITH THE FAMILY AND THE PRIMARY CARE PRACTITIONER TO TREAT A MANIC PATIENT[3]

Harry is a 20-year-old single male who was diagnosed with bipolar I disorder after he had his first severe manic episode requiring involuntary hospitalization at age 18 years. He, and his family (consisting of his mother and two sisters), had been traumatized by the process of this illness and hospitalization, which had involved the police and a humiliating and very public and embarrassing forced removal from his small rural community. He was seen several times via telepsychiatry following this admission, but he eventually stopped taking his mood stabilizers, resorted to regular cannabis use, and then became manic again. At this stage, his telepsychiatrist was asked to see him urgently. Harry was floridly manic, with multiple grandiose delusions in the setting of insomnia, hyperactivity, and excitement, but he retained a small amount of insight and was terrified of being forcibly sent to the hospital. The psychiatrist met on video with Harry, his mother, his sisters, and his PCP. It was agreed that Harry would be looked after at home as long as he was not a danger to himself or to others. His family would make sure that he took any prescribed medications and would monitor his sleep and activities,

---

[3]Case provided by Peter Yellowlees, MBBS, M.D.

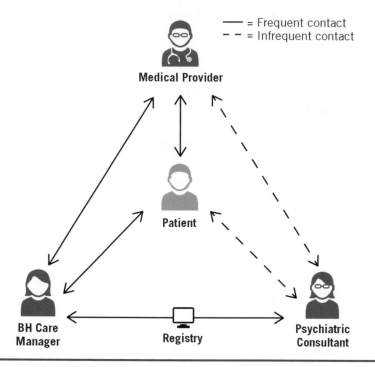

FIGURE 8–2.   Collaborative care team structure.

BH=behavioral health.

Source.   Reprinted from AIMS (Advancing Integrated Mental Health Solutions) Center Web site (http://aims.uw.edu/collaborative-care/team-structure), Division of Population Health, Department of Psychiatry & Behavioral Sciences, University of Washington School of Medicine, Seattle, WA, 2017. Copyright 2017, University of Washington. Used with permission.

while he agreed that he would not leave the family home without a family member with him and that he would see the telepsychiatrist or his PCP at least once a week. Harry was restarted on his previous mood stabilization regimen, and over the next 6 weeks gradually settled. His family worked in shifts to look after and monitor him and were present at the weekly consultation Harry had with the telepsychiatrist and/or his PCP. At follow-up over the next year, Harry gradually accepted the need for long-term medication and remained well.

▌KEY CONCEPT

A collaborative partnership—with the patient, his or her family, his or her PCP, and the telepsychiatrist working as a team in an

> integrated care model—can enable even floridly psychotic pa-
> tients to be treated at home instead of requiring hospitalization.

Synchronous and asynchronous technologies and modern technological infrastructures in health care have fueled opportunities for adoption of
collaborative care models. Psychiatrists can spread their knowledge by
participating in the care of patient populations and strengthening the skills
of their teammates, particularly PCPs, who maintain responsibility for
overall patient management. Team members' shared access to asynchronous EMRs and patient registries ensures their mutual participation in patient treatment plans, helps minimize the risk of patient dropouts from
treatment, and allows monitoring of patient adherence to treatment plans,
including plan modifications if patient conditions are not improving.

HOW ARE VIDEO, PHONE, E-MAIL, AND TEXT USED IN INDIRECT ASYNCHRONOUS E-CONSULTATIONS?

Asynchronous consultations are already in common use in psychiatric
practice on fixed and mobile devices via e-mail, telephony, or texting. In
recent years, asynchronous (commonly called store-and-forward) videoconferencing e-consultation—also known as asynchronous telepsychiatry (ATP)—has been developed and has shown effectiveness in
collaborative care settings (Yellowlees 2008; Yellowlees et al. 2010) in
which psychiatrists work within a primary care network to provide a
wide range of asynchronous e-consultations.

All of these types of asynchronous e-consultations involve capture of
data (video, voice, or text) by a referring provider and subsequent asynchronous transmission of these clinical data, sometimes with enhancements (e.g., language interpretation), to an expert clinician who assesses
the data and provides an opinion, typically in the form of a report with a
diagnostic assessment and treatment plan. This is essentially the same
process that occurs in a "curbside consultation" but with the addition of
valuable video clips or written descriptions of the patient. For example,
in an ATP consultation, a referring clinician records a semistructured interview or obtains representative audio/visual clips of the patient and
transmits this information via e-mail or Web applications to a distant
psychiatrist, who will review the data at a later time and generate an expert opinion regarding diagnosis and treatment planning. In this type of

care, the psychiatrist does not evaluate the patient directly, but instead guides the PCP regarding the treatment of the patient. If the consulting psychiatrist is uncertain of the diagnosis (which in our experience occurs in 5%–10% of cases), the patient can be referred for an in-person or synchronous videoconference appointment as part of the ATP recommendations. In the ATP collaborative care model, the referring PCP and the psychiatrist share the responsibility for the patient's care, minimizing medicolegal liability (Bland et al. 2014).

Similar indirect clinical processes and workflows occur with text and e-mail and recorded audio or voicemail. In the future, such consultations will include other technologies, such as virtual reality, imaging (e.g., incorporating facial- or movement-recognition software), and mobile smartphone data streams.

What Are the Advantages and Disadvantages of Indirect Care From Provider and Patient Perspectives?

The delivery of technology-enabled indirect psychiatric care is particularly welcomed by younger generations, popularly known as the "digital natives" (Yellowlees et al. 2015), who are keen to receive their health care in a more accessible and convenient mode than traditionally available. In addition, in this era of patient-centered care, they wish to be engaged in their treatment and to share major health care decisions.

Indirect technology-enabled psychiatric consultations enable improved access to mental health care providers at times and places not previously possible, thereby helping to alleviate the geographic and numeric maldistribution of psychiatrists. While in-person encounters between physicians and patients will continue as the gold standard of care for most types of consultations, use of indirect technologies frequently facilitates more productive and efficient interactions between patients and physicians without necessitating an office visit and may help overcome the reluctance to seek psychiatric care. Indirect consultations facilitate hybrid approaches to care. For example, patients may receive in-person core therapy services that are augmented with secure messaging within an EMR system to provide supplemental guidance regarding drug dosages, medical protocols, and side effects. Using these systems, referring providers, consulting psychiatrists, and patients are all able to monitor the patients' response to treatment, with multiple check-ins potentially reducing the need for office visits while at the same time strengthening the bond between patients and their health care providers. The technology-enabled hybrid model of care especially benefits patient populations that face challenges to traditional in-person care, such as the elderly, the poor, and those with disabilities. However, despite the fact that e-mail and text messaging are inexpensive, widely available, and convenient, these technologies are most likely to be used by young, middle-class patients. The growth of health and digital literacy will help to rectify this disparity in the future (Atherton et al. 2013).

Indirect technology-based care also includes stand-alone services, especially in communities and populations that lack access to traditional mental health care services (Wodarski and Frimpong 2013). In particular, asynchronous videoconferencing offers the advantage of patient observation by an expert psychiatrist while reducing challenges to patients and health care workers of travel, time, office schedules, costs, and administrative supports. These advantages may be especially appreciated by patients who are anxious, avoidant, shy, or paranoid or simply prefer the distance from the provider.

Such digital encounters may also be favored by providers who prefer the distance of asynchronous care, such as in correctional environments, or those who appreciate the flexibility of services delivered on their own schedules, anytime and anywhere (Yellowlees et al. 2010).

Certain patient populations are probably not suitable for asynchronous consultations as the only form of care. These include patients with acute psychiatric disorders and those requiring emergency interventions, including those with suicidal ideation. A small number of patients refuse to cooperate with any data-collection process, such as filming. In our experience, reasons for objecting to filming may be either clinical or legal. Some patients are paranoid or have incorporated technology into their delusional systems. Most commonly, patient refusal is due to legal situations in which the recordings may be discoverable, as with a patient who is an undocumented immigrant or involved in a worker's compensation action. Other individuals may simply refuse to be recorded as a matter of principle.

In What Types of Scenarios Might Indirect Consultations Be Most Clinically Useful?

Indirect consultations have the potential to be just as useful as direct video consultations in improving the accessibility, consistency, and quality of mental health care delivered to hard-to-serve populations such as youth, the elderly, persons with disabilities, immigrants, and inmates in correctional institutions. Therapists and PCPs can strengthen their skills by using indirect consultations with specific patients or by training in specific disorders, such as through Project ECHO (Extension for Community Healthcare Outcomes; http://echo.unm.edu/initiatives/community-health-workers/). Group-format indirect consultations can help to build a community of providers who learn to support each other's practices.

LONG-TERM MANAGEMENT OF CHRONIC PSYCHIATRIC AND COMORBID CONDITIONS

Many and perhaps most patients with a primary chronic illness, whether medical or psychiatric, have comorbid disorders. Indirect consultations can assist in these patients' long-term management in a primary care integrated environment. Indirect consultations are increasingly being used at the University of California (UC) Davis within the primary care network of 17 clinics spread throughout Northern California, all accessible through one EMR and Web-based videoconferencing system. A team of psychiatrists, health coaches, and case workers are teaching patients and their caregivers preventive strategies, offering remote monitoring, maintaining surveillance, and promoting mental health by delivering biological, psychological, and social therapies in a hybrid model more efficiently and effectively than is possible in traditional models of care (Bashshur et al. 2016; Chan et al. 2015).

CORRECTIONAL FACILITIES

There are about 2.3 million prisoners in the United States, of whom half are estimated to have a major psychiatric or substance use disorder (Wagner and Rabuy 2017). Correctional institutions have long used direct telepsychiatry consultations for initial treatment evaluations, crisis intervention, medication management, and patient education. The delivery of direct telepsychiatry services not only is cost effective but also is safe for providers and patients inside the facilities and has a high rate of acceptance among inmates, their families, and prison staff (Manfredi et al. 2005). Consequently, a major expansion into indirect consultations seems inevitable.

MILITARY PERSONNEL AND VETERANS

The VA has been a leader in technology-enabled health care, as described in Chapters 4 ("Clinical Settings and Models of Care in Telepsychiatry: Implications for Work Practices and Culturally Informed Treatment") and 9 ("Management of Patient Populations"). In 2016, 133,500 unique veterans utilized telemental health care services in a total of more than 400,000 encounters, an increase of 16% from 2015 (Comstock 2016). ATP could be used to treat veterans who have PTSD with consultations supported through the VA's nationally available electronic records system, Vista.

PEDIATRIC PATIENTS

In 2016, there were 8,300 clinicians specializing in child and adolescent psychiatry in the United States, a number far lower than the projected need of 20,000 pediatric-certified psychiatrists (American Academy of Child and Adolescent Psychiatry 2016). As a consequence, only 42% of the estimated 20% of American youth with psychiatric disorders receive mental health care services. Direct telepsychiatry is well accepted by families and referring PCPs and is increasingly implemented in both clinic and naturalistic settings (Myers et al. 2007, 2015). Indirect psychiatric consultations could be utilized as one solution to this need and for many young people could prove preferable to videoconferencing encounters. An estimated 81% of youth find it easier to open up to providers about their lives in encounters online, in virtual psychiatric clinics, and via mobile devices than through traditional office-based, in-person communications (Ben-Zeev et al. 2013).

Indirect consultations could be used to diagnose psychiatric and developmental disorders in young people (Myers et al. 2007). Child psychiatry telephony consultation programs across the country have demonstrated their acceptability to PCPs, their successful integration into primary care, and their ease of augmentation with direct videoconferencing for more challenging clinical situations (National Network of Child Psychiatry Access Programs: http://nncpap.org/).

ELDERLY POPULATIONS

In 2013, 14.1% of the U.S. population (44.7 million individuals) were older than 65 years. By 2060, this population is expected to double. Outcomes for assessments and cognitive interventions, as well as patient satisfaction ratings, have been found to be similar or slightly higher for direct telepsychiatry consultations than for in-person services (Choi et al. 2014), without the hurdles of immobility, stigma, and geographical isolation associated with attendance at in-person sessions (Bashshur et al. 2016). Several ongoing studies in elderly residents in nursing homes who have depression, dementia, or bipolar disorder are demonstrating the effectiveness of indirect consultations in reducing the need for transfers to general hospitals and the use of psychotropic medications, while saving time and costs (see "Pilot Study of Asynchronous and Synchronous Telepsychiatry for Skilled Nursing Facilities" [ClinicalTrials.gov Identifier: NCT02537093] and "Comparison of Asynchronous Telepsychiatry vs. Synchronous Telepsychiatry in Skilled Nursing Facilities" [ClinicalTrials.gov Identifier: NCT03264560]; available at: https://clinicaltrials.gov).

PATIENTS WITH RARE DISEASES

Patients with rare diseases, such as Huntington's disease and other genetically caused disorders, face unique challenges in accessing expert care. Indirect consultations allow them and their PCPs to secure opinions and treatment from the few specialists in their disorder. Many such patients already belong to social media networks and closed online social groups that often include physicians and other specialty providers. Medical opinions are frequently rendered using e-mail or secure messaging, although increasingly will be assisted by adding video, which will especially aid care for patients with movement disorders or similar physical impairments (Yellowlees et al. 2015).

HOW DO OUTCOMES OF INDIRECT CONSULTATIONS DIFFER FROM THOSE OF DIRECT IN-PERSON OR VIDEO CONSULTATIONS?

ATP allows for the equitable delivery of patient-centered care and puts the PCP and specialist in close communication while increasing access to, and the quality of, care. ATP overcomes cost and distance barriers in some of the most underserved populations and reduces language barriers that can limit access because the ATP datasets can be reviewed by a provider tailored to each patient's language and specialty expertise needs.

The only study currently being undertaken to compare clinical and economic outcomes of ATP with real-time telepsychiatry started at UC Davis in 2013 and will finish in 2018 (see "A Controlled Trial of Patient Centered Telepsychiatry Interventions" [ClinicalTrials.gov Identifier: NCT02084979]; available at: https://clinicaltrials.gov). In this randomized trial, 200 primary care patients referred for psychiatric assessment and monitoring are being re-evaluated every 6 months via either ATP or synchronous telepsychiatry for a period of 2 years, so that each patient will have a total of five consultations. At the time of this writing, halfway through the study enrollment, the outcomes of both groups have not been analyzed, but anecdotally they seem to be reasonably similar. About 20 PCPs are continuing to refer patients to the study, and their initial feedback has been positive with respect to the treatment of patients in both arms of the study (Yellowlees et al., in press). It is hoped that the results of this study will establish an initial evidence base supporting the use of ATP in integrated care systems.

Other indirect consultations using e-mail and messaging have shown positive results in small trials in various setting, such as nursing homes (G. L. Xiong, M.D., personal communication, July 2017). As is the case for most technology-enabled care, more research with a focus on comparative effectiveness is needed to establish the role of indirect consults in hybrid and collaborative models of care.

CASE EXAMPLE 4: MEDICATION ASSESSMENT AND MONITORING PROVIDED VIA ASYNCHRONOUS TELEPSYCHIATRY[4]

Philip, a 63-year-old man with a history of bipolar disorder and several inpatient hospitalizations, was referred, after some persuasion, by his PCP to a telepsychiatry study for symptoms of depression and anxiety and was randomly assigned to receive asynchronous telepsychiatry consultations. Philip made it clear that he had not had "good experiences" with psychiatrists and did not consider psychiatry to be "a very good industry," noting that in his view, psychiatrists were expensive and "ask you very little, but you have to go." After reviewing his recorded baseline

---

[4]Case provided by Alvaro D. González, M.A., M.F.T.I.

telepsychiatry consultation video conducted by a trained clinician interviewer, Philip's psychiatrist recommended increasing his paroxetine dosage to help with his depressive symptoms and starting quetiapine for bipolar spectrum depression, as well as a number of other behavioral activation interventions. Philip met with his PCP following the ATP consultation, and the treatment plan was implemented. In two subsequent ATP consultations after 6 and 12 months, Philip's medications were monitored and adjusted, and he reported a decline in his depressive and anxious symptoms. On his patient satisfaction survey, Philip noted that he preferred the asynchronous visit over an in-person visit with a psychiatrist and indicated that he would recommend a virtual visit to a friend or family member.

▌ KEY CONCEPTS

For some patients, ATP is preferable both to in-person psychiatry and to live telepsychiatry.

ATP assessments can be integrated into primary mental health care and can enable PCPs to better manage their patients.

HOW IS INTERVIEWING CONDUCTED IN AN ASYNCHRONOUS (STORE AND FORWARD) TELEPSYCHIATRY CONSULTATION?

ATP consultations consist of video-recorded 20- to 30-minute interviews performed by an expert clinician who obtains a psychiatric history and interacts with the patient to allow the reviewing psychiatrist to objectively assess the patient's mental status. The following guide to setting up and implementing an ATP consultation was developed over time by Yellowlees and his colleagues at UC Davis (Figure 8–3). The ATP completion steps are outlined in Table 8–1.

HOW CAN ASYNCHRONOUS CONSULTATION EFFECTIVELY SUPPORT CROSS-CULTURAL COMMUNICATION?

In the U.S. Census Bureau's 2010 Census of Population, 4.7% of U.S. respondents reported speaking a language other than English in their homes, with 15% of that group rating their English-speaking ability as "not well" and 7% rating their ability as "not at all." Language plays a fundamental role in diagnosis, assessment, and treatment of patients, particularly in psychiatric care (Bauer et al. 2010). Thought disorders can lead to disorganized, nonsensical speech, which could represent a psy-

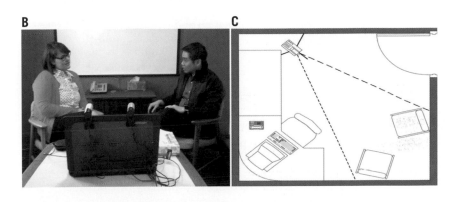

FIGURE 8–3. Guide to setting up and implementing an asynchronous telepsychiatry (ATP) consultation.

A, ATP workflow. HIPAA=Health Insurance Portability and Accountability Act; PCP=primary care provider. **B,** Recording an ATP in-office interview (interviewer on left; patient on right). **C,** Typical room setup for ATP in-office interview showing how patient and interviewer are recorded.

Source. Courtesy of Peter Yellowlees, MBBS, M.D. Used with permission.

chotic disorder in one person or a culture-bound syndrome or an "attack of nerves" in another. Mood disorders can lead to slowed speech (depression) versus rapid, pressured speech (mania); however, rapid speech may be very normal for languages of low information density per syllable, such as Japanese. Cultural differences can make it difficult for even someone who speaks the same language to understand certain cultural concepts, so that cursing can also be considered a cultural nuance, as

---

TABLE 8–1.   Completion of the ATP consultation

Consulting psychiatrist

- Completes consultation evaluations on any computer with a secure network connection. Setup may vary according to preference. The most efficient setup is to use three computer screens—one to watch video, one to review EMR and any pre-collected data, and one to write report while observing the recorded consultation.

- Uploads interview video and clinical histories.

- Reviews video interview, data collection set, and any additional documentation and completes the telepsychiatry consultation note.

- Uploads this note (diagnostic evaluation and treatment plan) and sends to PCP on any computer with a secure network connection.

PCP

- Downloads evaluation and modifies the patient's treatment.

PCP and psychiatrist

- May need to clarify one or two patient issues via secure messaging after the consultation.

Note.   EMR=electronic medical record; PCP=primary care provider.

---

such words can convey multiple definitions and emotive connotations in different contexts. In all of these situations, a straight word-for-word translation may therefore provide the wrong meaning.

Patients who do not speak English have been shown to receive substandard care, to undergo excessive tests, to experience more medical errors, and to have longer hospital stays. Thus, expert language interpretation is critical when an interpreter joins the doctor and the patient during the clinical encounter. Live medical interpreters are considered the gold standard for interpretation; however, there are few studies examining the accuracy of their interpretations, and many clinicians question the accuracy of their interpretations on occasion. Furthermore, interpreters are sometimes not available. Often-used (but not recommended) alternatives include interpretation by family members or by assisting health care staff.

What Alternatives to Direct In-Person Language Interpretation Are Available for Use in Telepsychiatry?

Videoconferencing technologies have long been used to provide live interpreters on demand. They enable interpreters to see patients' affect and movements and assist the provider in interpreting nonverbal cues, increasing the interpreters' role as cultural brokers. This approach has been preferred in several studies comparing in-person, video, and telephonic medical interpretation. Using videoconferencing can decrease delays in acquiring interpreter services because no travel time is required, and online interpretation across health care networks has led to decreased delays and increased efficiency of interpreters, with several reports in the literature of substantial economic savings.

Computerized interpretation systems offer another approach to translation and interpretation, such as Google Translate and similar systems from Microsoft and IBM, among others. Although these commercially available technologies are widely used around the world, their levels of accuracy have not been established and are not generally considered sufficient for medical standard work.

A promising area in medical interpretation is the combination of automated speech recognition (also called text-to-speech or voice dictation) and machine translation technologies—collectively known as *automatic simultaneous translation apps.* Chan et al. (2015) have proposed that such apps be added to asynchronous telepsychiatry consultations so that (for example) an English-speaking psychiatrist can review a patient being interviewed in Spanish with the aid of automated subheadings placed in the video file in near real time. Without a doubt, psychiatrists will in the future be using these technologies to help them communicate with patients from differing cultural and language backgrounds, and trials of automated translation technologies in asynchronous telepsychiatry consultations have already commenced at UC Davis in California (see "Telepsychiatry crosses language barriers" 2017).

How Should Communication by Secure E-Mail, Texting, and Messaging Occur?

Increasingly, physicians are communicating online with their patients using written language via three modalities—e-mail, texting, and messaging. There are many ways to communicate online using secure software compliant with the Health Insurance Portability and Accountability Act (HIPAA) on phones, tablets, and computers, either as independent programs or apps or as part of an EMR package in which patients have access to parts of their records. Many clinicians are reluctant to communicate with these technologies because they are concerned that patients will overuse the communications. They continue to communicate with patients via telephone, with its attendant frustration of "phone tag." There are now effective technology-enabled approaches that can be integrated into routine patient care to improve the efficiency of doctor–patient communication.

There are two issues to address initially. The first is the need to develop basic guidelines covering the scope of the communications, and the second is the need to communicate effectively in writing. The rules for communication are covered in the American Medical Association's ethical guidelines, section 2.3.2 (www.ama-assn.org/go/codeofmedicalethics), summarized here:

- Electronic communication involves the same ethical responsibilities as other clinical encounters, especially involving privacy, security, and integrity of patient information.
- E-mail correspondence should not be used to establish a patient–physician relationship, but to supplement other more personal encounters.
- Patients should be informed of the inherent limitations of electronic communication—such as breaches of privacy or confidentiality, difficulty in validating identities, and delays in response.
- Physicians should obtain consent for use of such communication and should present information professionally.

When using social media, the following added points are noted to be important:

- Appropriate privacy settings should be used, and the boundaries of the patient–physician relationship should be maintained as in any other context, which may mean separating personal and professional content.

- Physicians should routinely monitor their own Internet presence and identity to ensure that information about them is accurate and appropriate.
- If physicians see content posted by colleagues that appears unprofessional, they have a duty to bring that to the attention of the individual and must recognize that their actions online and content posted may negatively affect their reputations and may have consequences for their medical careers, as well as undermine public trust in the medical profession.

So, in brief, providers should ensure that their patients understand that e-mail or text messaging should be used only for nonurgent, short communications that are primarily administrative. Most EMR messaging systems allow providers to set a maximum number of characters permissible per patient message. In addition, these systems allow providers to have an "out of office" message sent automatically in response to every patient message for nonurgent matters and to inform patients of how rapidly they can expect a response.

How, then, should you write your messages to patients? Malka et al. (2015, p. 28) suggested the following guidelines for use of e-mail-style communication in the professional medical setting:

1. Proofread each e-mail for proper spelling, grammar, and punctuation.
2. Use a meaningful subject line that is descriptive of e-mail content.
3. Avoid background colors, patterns, all capitals, and unusual fonts.
4. Avoid humor that may be misinterpreted.
5. Don't send an e-mail to the wrong person; be especially careful with reply all and mass forwarding.
6. Don't send emotionally charged e-mails; instead, consider a direct conversation for complex or sensitive topics.
7. Transmit protected patient data cautiously using a private or secured computer or handheld device via an encrypted, secured network. Avoid sending such data to or from a public e-mail service such as Gmail, Yahoo, or Hotmail.

Using these simple guidelines on writing messages and discussing the scope of online communication directly with patients should make the use of these helpful technologies easy and professional and should improve provider–patient relationships.

WHAT OTHER TYPES OF ASYNCHRONOUS E-TOOLS MAY ASSIST IN HYBRID MODELS OF CARE?

Four other types of asynchronous e-tools currently show promise in promoting hybrid models of care: 1) patient registries and tracking systems, 2) mHealth devices, 3) self-administered e-therapies, and 4) remote training. These e-tools target the roles of psychiatrists, PCPs, and other mental health care staff collaborating in treatment planning, such as in a medical home model of care, as described in Chapter 4.

PATIENT REGISTRIES AND TRACKING SYSTEMS

Patient registries and tracking systems identify populations of patients in a practice with a specific psychiatric disorder diagnosis, track selected health variables, tabulate relevant health services, and graphically display patient responses to treatment (also see Chapter 9). Patient registries help psychiatrists and PCPs to know their population of patients with selected disorders, document their decision making, and establish trackable treatment plans (Ratzliff et al. 2016). Staff can enter dates of anticipated completion of a test or a follow-up appointment. Patients complete rating scales at designated times and submit results through secure portals for entry into the registries (Myers et al. 2015). At a glance, providers can note patients' scores on physiological tests or rating scales and coordinate their scores with medication use or other interventions. The registry then provides a quick assessment of patients' progress that guides modification of the treatment plan. If adherence and improvement are not adequate, supporting staff can proactively contact patients to ascertain adherence to the treatment plan or to return to the clinic.

Registries encourage the delivery of evidence-based care, documentation of which is increasingly required by accountable care organizations and tied to emerging reimbursement models. Patient registries and tracking databases have been used predominantly in integrated models of care, with demonstrated effectiveness in improving patient care and outcomes (Ratzliff et al. 2016). Systems are now commercially available and may be included in an electronic medical record.

MHEALTH DEVICES

mHealth devices capture samples of patients' behavior in naturalistic settings to aid in diagnostic assessment and treatment planning (also see Chapter 6, "Data Collection From Novel Sources"). Recordings of patient interviews that are later viewed remotely can facilitate diagnostic assessment for sites without access to traditional psychiatric expertise. This asynchronous technology can also be used to capture samples of patients' behaviors in naturalistic settings to aid medical decision making and treatment planning. A mobile device records a behavioral episode, and the recording is then uploaded to a secure Web site for later review (Nazneen et al. 2015). For example, a child's behavior in the classroom during free unstructured time may optimally demonstrate teachers' concerns about a developmental or behavioral disturbance. A fragile adult in a nursing home may show behavioral changes that suggest illness progression versus medication complications.

By capturing a sample of patients' behaviors in naturalistic settings, providers obtain primary data demonstrating their patients' needs and response to treatment, rather than having to rely on third-party reports or observing the patient in the artificial clinic environment, and caregivers at the patients' sites may participate in these sessions. Recording and downloading videos to a secure Web site allow the provider to efficiently review the clinical data, update the treatment plan in collaboration with staff at the patient's site, and potentially save the patient a later clinic or emergency department visit. Disadvantages of remote recordings are the requirements for the providers' time outside of usual clinic hours, technical support, and addressing family and staff endorsements of the value of such an approach. Remote behavioral recordings have demonstrated effectiveness in diagnosing autism spectrum disorder in children (Nazneen et al. 2015).

SELF-ADMINISTERED E-THERAPIES

Self-administered e-therapies are nonpharmacological interventions delivered to patients in a convenient setting on their preferred device (also see Chapter 6). E-therapies are increasingly being developed as an alternative, or complement, to traditional in-person treatment. Psychiatrists may include an e-therapy to complement pharmacotherapy, or PCPs may "prescribe" e-therapy as a first step in treatment. For some patients who eschew clinic visits, a fully self-administered approach using an on-line cognitive-behavioral program with no therapist involvement may be tried, although telephone or online support improves patient adherence to these types of self-driven therapies (Melville et al. 2010) as well as their efficacy (Andersson and Cuijpers 2009). Alternatively, patients may alternate e-therapy sessions on their phones, tablets, or computers with in-person sessions, thereby promoting patients' continuing work between sessions to boost their own productivity.

Certain populations may be especially appropriate for self-administered e-therapies—for example, teenagers may find e-therapy less stigmatizing than attending a clinic. Other advantages include e-therapies' inherent fidelity in content delivery and patients' access to sessions at their convenience, at their own pace, and in privacy. A number of capabilities of such programs are associated with success, including scheduled reminders to engage in therapeutic exercises; point of performance support; individually tailored information; real-time symptom assessment; and readily accessible asynchronous communication (Whiteside 2016). E-therapies have a robust evidence base supporting their effectiveness, particularly with adults reporting depression or anxiety disorders (Andersson and Cuijpers 2009), and several studies also suggest their effectiveness with teens in clinical and educational settings (Stasiak et al. 2016). Support from real-time staff online, by telephone, or via text improves outcomes.

REMOTE TRAINING

Remote training involves digitized recordings of sessions conducted by experts that can be viewed and studied by therapists seeking to improve and update their skills. In particular, remote training can be of immense benefit to mental health care providers practicing in underserved communities, who have historically been trained without evidence-based skills in selected disorders across the age spectrum. Psychiatrists consulting to a practice may make their own recordings to demonstrate specific techniques (McCarty et al. 2015). Remote training can enable therapists to increase their skills without compromising their productivity by taking time away from the clinic, and recordings may be viewed repeatedly or in groups to consolidate skills.

What Are the Potential Efficiency Gains of Asynchronous E-Tools for Individual Providers, and How Will They Affect Psychiatric Practice?

Patient registries and secure portals facilitate timely follow-up and interventions geared toward preventing further morbidity, limiting urgent visits, and containing costs of a higher level of care. In evolving accountable care organizations, such benefits will be rewarded. Given the ubiquity of mobile devices, remote behavioral monitoring and e-therapies may be an attractive means of obtaining information in naturalistic settings and of disseminating evidence-based interventions. There is some evidence that e-therapies save both money and time, but these efficiencies may be best realized by organizations providing population-based care with a large, well-defined patient population, so that costs are offset by delivery to a large number of patients, with incentives to providers for improving outcomes. Partnering with commercial companies and/or insurers will likely be needed to ensure financial sustainability for individual providers.

Absences from the office are costly for individual providers or agencies and jeopardize productivity. Asynchronous trainings can be completed at providers' convenience and with lower costs than required for continuing education at distant sites. Furthermore, multiple training sessions may be efficiently accessed through digitized recordings.

Asynchronous e-tools will affect psychiatric practice and workforce development, and the recent proposal by the Centers for Medicare & Medicaid Services (CMS) to reimburse for collaborative models of care will encourage the sustainability of collaborative models and this change in practice. Finally, patient demand will converge with ongoing technological developments to further determine the role for asynchronous e-tools in mental health care that facilitate a positive experience of psychiatrists, PCPs, and patients.

How Can Indirect Consultations Make Psychiatrists More Efficient?

Indirect consultations mediated through telephony, e-mail, text, or videoconferencing, especially in a team-based environment integrated into primary care, can reach a far greater number of patients than traditional in-office consultations, making it more effective from a population health perspective, especially for patients living in underserved areas where there is a major lack of psychiatric providers.

Telephone consultations, e-mails, and text messaging for status updates and patient queries can often take just minutes to effect and can leave mental health care providers with more time to devote to more complicated patients. In addition, a psychiatrist can complete one ATP teleconsultation in about 30 minutes (Butler and Yellowlees 2012), which is much shorter than the standard 1-hour in-person consultation for a new patient. Studies have shown that the number of patients who can be seen by a psychiatrist in a collaborative care setting can be as high as four to six patients per hour (up to 20 patients per hour in reviewing a case load registry) (Raney 2015).

In the United States, patients fail to show up for about 10%–20% of their scheduled psychiatric and behavioral health appointments, almost twice the rate in other medical specialties, and up to 50% of patients who miss their appointments drop out of scheduled care (Mitchell and Selmes 2007). It is also estimated that 20%–57% of missed appointments occur at the first clinical appointment itself (Aeby et al. 2015). Environmental factors such as distance from the clinic, weather, time of day and date of the appointment, long waiting times, and costs of transportation and child care can contribute to missed appointments and can affect everything from patient attendance to treatment. Conversely, synchronous telepsychiatry appointments are generally more likely to be kept and less likely to be canceled or not attended, because these appointments are devoid of such barriers, as is also the case for asynchronous appointments. Additionally, no-shows represent a missed opportunity to provide care for other patients who could have been seen in the unused appointment intervals.

It is self-evident that if psychiatrists begin to increase the number of indirect consultations they perform, they will assess and oversee greater numbers of patients than traditionally seen. This approach would also add flexibility to patient scheduling processes, thus allowing consultations to be performed during "down time" created by no-shows. U.S. psychiatrists work an average of 40 hours per week. Of these 40 weekly hours, 10 are dedicated to administrative work, including teaching and research, which is normally unpaid, while the remaining 30 are utilized for patient care (Grisham 2017). It may be instructive to examine how this notional 30-hour clinical week might be used in two different scenarios:

1. *Current scenario with traditional in-person psychiatric consultations:* Out of the 30 total patient-care hours, 3 hours are lost due to the average no-show rate of 10%. With 27 hours left for patient care, a psychiatrist can examine up to 40 patients per week. In this notional average practice, these comprise 4 new patients (1-hour consultation for each) and 36 follow-up patients (10 patients at 1 hour each [i.e., 10 hours] and 26 patients requiring 1 half-hour each of the psychiatrist's time [i.e., 13 hours]).

2. *Proposed scenario with hybrid/indirect care:* Out of the 30 work hours per week, 15 hours are dedicated to standard in-person consultations with the same ratio of patients seen as in the traditional scenario (20 patients—2 new and 18 follow-up). The remaining 15 hours are dedicated to asynchronous or indirect consultations via telephone, e-mail, text, or videoconferencing, with a total of 60 patients receiving assessment or treatment monitoring. In this time, 20 new patients may be assessed on ATP for half an hour each (10 hours) and 20 follow-up patients reviewed via collaborative team-based care (5 hours of collaborative care at 4 patients per hour). No time is lost to no-shows, because all of this time can be used for indirect ATP consultations.

This proposed change to psychiatrists' work practices has the potential to increase psychiatrists' efficiency by roughly 50% and can aid in managing the supply and demand crisis of mental health care prevalent in the United States today. For this model to work, there must be changes to payment policies—a move away from fee-for-service to a volume-based model of care and a population–based reimbursement model, which, as of 2016, CMS has opted to introduce over the next few years (as discussed in Chapter 9). This reimbursement model will greatly incentivize team care, and although nonpsychiatric practitioners and physician extenders—including social workers, behavioral health specialists, and licensed mental health counselors—cannot replace psychiatrists, they can augment their work by increasing their efficiency, thereby providing a partial solution to the psychiatrist shortage, working alongside psychiatrists, who will increasingly be spreading their skills further than in the past via this variety of indirect team-based consultations.

Summary

In this chapter we have reviewed the collaborative care model of integrated mental health care and described how—with the advent of a range of indirect or asynchronous consultations conducted by psychiatrists working in teams and facilitated by a number of technologies—the severity of effects from the impending shortage of psychiatrists can be at least in part reduced. Specific topics discussed include the following:

- The new role of psychiatrist as hybrid mental health practitioner, who will be able to work more efficiently in collaborative teams performing indirect consultations using video, phone, e-mail and messaging. Advantages and disadvantages of this form of indirect care from both provider and patient perspectives were also examined.
- Indications for and contraindications to the use of online psychotherapy, as well as provider challenges associated with delivering online psychotherapy.
- How the process of providing consultation to referring clinicians through asynchronous (store and forward) telepsychiatry works, as well as principles governing good-quality communication with patients by secure email and text and messaging.

It is essential that psychiatrists begin practicing in a hybrid manner, working not just with individual patients but also increasingly in multidisciplinary teams with populations of patients, using a wide variety of apps, devices, patient registries, and communication systems, including text, e-mail, telephony, and video.

References

Aeby VG, Xu L, Lu W, et al: Evidence-based social work interventions to improve client attendance in rural mental health: an overview of literature. Psychology and Cognitive Sciences 1(2):39–45, 2015. Available at: http://openventio.org/Volume1_Issue2/Evidence_Based_Social_Work_Interventions_to_Improve_Client_Attendance_in_Rural_Mental_Health_An_Overview_of_Literature_PCSOJ_1_106.pdf. Accessed April 6, 2017.

AIMS Center: Principles of Collaborative Care. Seattle, WA, University of Washington School of Medicine, Department of Psychiatry & Behavioral Sciences, Division of Population Health, 2017. Available at: https://aims.uw.edu/collaborative-care/principles-collaborative-care. Accessed May 3, 2017.

American Academy of Child and Adolescent Psychiatry: Workforce issues. Last updated February 2016. Available at: https://www.aacap.org/aacap/resources_for_primary_care/Workforce_Issues.aspx. Accessed August 17, 2017.

Andersson G, Cuijpers P: Internet-based and other computerized psychological treatments for adult depression: a meta-analysis. Cogn Behav Ther 38(4):196–205, 2009 20183695

Association of American Medical Colleges: 2016 Physician Specialty Data Book. Washington, DC, Center for Workforce Studies, Association of American Medical Colleges, 2016. Available at: https://www.aamc.org/data/workforce/reports/457712/2016-specialty-databook.html. Accessed August 17, 2017.

Atherton H, Pappas Y, Heneghan C, et al: Experiences of using e-mail for general practice consultations: a qualitative study. Br J Gen Pract 63(616):e760–e767, 2013 24267859

Bashshur RL, Shannon GW, Bashshur N, Yellowlees PM: The empirical evidence for telemedicine interventions in mental disorders. Telemed J E Health 22(2):87–113, 2016 26624248

Bauer AM, Chen C-N, Alegría M: English language proficiency and mental health service use among Latino and Asian Americans with mental disorders. Med Care 48(12):1097–1104, 2010 21063226

Ben-Zeev D, Davis KE, Kaiser S, et al: Mobile technologies among people with serious mental illness: opportunities for future services. Adm Policy Ment Health 40(4):340–343, 2013 22648635

Bland DA, Lambert K, Raney L, et al: Resource document on risk management and liability issues in integrated care models. Am J Psychiatry 171(5):1–7, 2014 24788296

Butler TN, Yellowlees P: Cost analysis of store-and-forward telepsychiatry as a consultation model for primary care. Telemed J E Health 18(1):74–77, 2012 22085113

Chan S, Parish M, Yellowlees P: Telepsychiatry today. Curr Psychiatry Rep 17(11):89, 2015 26384338

Choi NG, Hegel MT, Marti N, et al: Telehealth problem-solving therapy for depressed low-income homebound older adults. Am J Geriatr Psychiatry 22(3):263–271, 2014 23567376

Comstock J: How telemedicine is helping the VA address its access crisis. MobiHealthNews, May 17, 2016. Available at: http://www.mobihealthnews.com/content/how-telemedicine-helping-va-address-its-access-crisis. Accessed August 17, 2017.

Fortney JC, Pyne JM, Turner EE, et al: Telepsychiatry integration of mental health services into rural primary care settings. Int Rev Psychiatry 27(6):525–539, 2015 26634618

Grisham S: Medscape Psychiatrist Compensation Report 2017. Medscape, April 12, 2017. Available at: http://www.medscape.com/slideshow/compensation-2017-psychiatry-6008585. Accessed August 17, 2017.

Hankir A, Zaman R: Global strategies targeting the recruitment crisis in psychiatry: the Doctors Academy Future Excellence International Medical Summer School. Psychiatr Danub 27 (suppl 1):S130–S135, 2015 26417748

Hilty DM, Ferrer DC, Parish MB, et al: The effectiveness of telemental health: a 2013 review. Telemed J E Health 19(6):444–454, 2013 23697504

Katon W, Russo J, Lin EH, et al: Cost-effectiveness of a multicondition collaborative care intervention: a randomized controlled trial. Arch Gen Psychiatry 69(5):506–514, 2012 22566583

Malka ST, Kessler CS, Abraham J, et al: Professional e-mail communication among health care providers: proposing evidence based guidelines. Acad Med 90(1):25–29, 2015 25162617

Manfredi L, Shupe J, Batki SL: Rural jail telepsychiatry: a pilot feasibility study. Telemed J E Health 11(5):574–577, 2005 16250821

McCarty CA, Vander Stoep A, Violette HD, Myers K: Interventions developed for psychiatric and behavioral treatment in the Children's ADHD Telemental Health Treatment Study. J Child Fam Stud 24(6):1735–1743, 2015. Available at: https://link.springer.com/article/10.1007/s10826-014-9977-5. Accessed April 6, 2017.

Melville KM, Casey LM, Kavanagh DJ: Dropout from Internet-based treatment for psychological disorders. Br J Clin Psychol 49(Pt 4):455–471, 2010 19799804

Mitchell AJ, Selmes T: Why don't patients attend their appointments? Maintaining engagement with psychiatric services. Adv Psychiatr Treat 13(6):423–434, 2007. Available at: http://apt.rcpsych.org/content/13/6/423. Accessed April 6, 2017.

Myers KM, Valentine JM, Melzer SM: Feasibility, acceptability, and sustainability of telepsychiatry for children and adolescents. Psychiatr Serv 58(11):1493–1496, 2007 17978264

Myers K, Vander Stoep A, Zhou C, et al: Effectiveness of a telehealth service delivery model for treating attention-deficit/hyperactivity disorder: a community-based randomized controlled trial. J Am Acad Child Adolesc Psychiatry 54(4):263–274, 2015 25791143

Nazneen N, Rozga A, Smith CJ, et al: A novel system for supporting autism diagnosis using home videos: iterative development and evaluation of system design. JMIR Mhealth Uhealth 3(2):e68, 2015 26085230

Raney LE: Integrating primary care and behavioral health: the role of the psychiatrist in the collaborative care model. Am J Psychiatry 172(8):721–728, 2015 26234599

Ratzliff A, Unützer J, Katon W, Stephens KA: Integrated Care: Creating Effective Mental and Primary Health Care Teams. Malden, MA, John Wiley & Sons, 2016. Available at: http://onlinelibrary.wiley.com/book/10.1002/9781119276579. Accessed April 6, 2017.

Shore JH: Telepsychiatry: videoconferencing in the delivery of psychiatric care. Am J Psychiatry 170(3):256–262, 2013 23450286

Stasiak K, Fleming T, Lucassen MF, et al: Computer-based and online therapy for depression and anxiety in children and adolescents. J Child Adolesc Psychopharmacol 26(3):235–245, 2016 26465266

"Telepsychiatry crosses language barriers," Behavioral Health Center of Excellence at UC Davis, 2017. Available at: http://behavioralhealth.ucdavis.edu/docs/innovate-series/telepsychiatry-innovate-yellowlees.pdf. Accessed September 1, 2017.

Turvey C, Coleman M, Dennison O, et al: ATA practice guidelines for video-based online mental health services. Telemed J E Health 19(9):722–730, 2013 23909884

Wagner P, Rabuy B: Mass Incarceration: The Whole Pie 2017 (press release). Northampton, MA, Prison Policy Initiative, March 14, 2017. Available at: https://www.prisonpolicy.org/reports/pie2017.html. Accessed August 17, 2017.

Whiteside SPH: Mobile device-based applications for childhood anxiety disorders. J Child Adolesc Psychopharmacol 26(3):246–251, 2016 26244903

Wodarski J, Frimpong J: Application of e-therapy programs to the social work practice. J Hum Behav Soc Environ 23(1):29–36, 2013. Available at: http://www.tandfonline.com/doi/abs/10.1080/10911359.2013.737290. Accessed April 6, 2017.

Yellowlees P: Your Health in the Information Age: How You and Your Doctor Can Use the Internet to Work Together. Bloomington, IN, iUniverse, 2008

Yellowlees PM, Odor A, Parish MB, et al: A feasibility study of the use of asynchronous telepsychiatry for psychiatric consultations. Psychiatr Serv 61(8):838–840, 2010 20675845

Yellowlees P, Richard Chan S, Burke Parish M: The hybrid doctor–patient relationship in the age of technology—telepsychiatry consultations and the use of virtual space. Int Rev Psychiatry 27(6):476–489, 2015 26493089

Yellowlees P, Parish MB, Gonzalez A, et al: Asynchronous telepsychiatry: a component of stepped integrated care. Telemed J E Health (in press)

9

Management of Patient Populations

John Luo, M.D.

Peter Yellowlees, MBBS, M.D.

Managing populations of patients involves much more than just managing the patients in a private practice, group practice, or health system. It is the 10,000-foot level looking at the needs of specific diagnostic groups of patients, across providers, and even across facilities to address the group's specialized needs to ensure the best quality of care. Health care reform is helping to drive this change as the fee-for-service model is transitioning toward a pay-for-performance and value-based care model. Without a doubt, technology plays a significant role as electronic health records (EHRs) enable identification of these patients and provide the tools to address and coordinate patient care, as well as engage patients in this process; health networks and interoperability initiatives allow physicians and electronic medical records (EMRs) to communicate; and multiple apps and devices are increasingly being used to collect individual and aggregated data.

WHY IS POPULATION-BASED CARE NEEDED?

Public health and population health perspectives trace their roots back to ancient civilizations, who recognized that the health of the entire civilization was dependent on policies, procedures, plans, laws, and regulations. Even though exact understanding of the disease state or etiology was not clear, citizens learned that data gathering and management was essential to survival and prosperity. For example, in England, improvements in standards of living, especially dietary quality, led to improvements in health following the medieval Black Death (circa 1347–1351), which killed tens of millions of Europeans (DeWitte 2014). Today, with many modern tools, such as EHRs, registries, and a discipline devoted to public health, maintenance and improvement of health quality and safety have become easier despite the increasing threats of new diseases and the challenges of keeping pace with the evolving landscape of health management.

Early public health disease management involved the use of patient registries. Today, patient registries—defined as "organized system[s] for the collection, storage, retrieval, analysis, and dissemination of information on people who share a disease or risk factor" (Gliklich et al. 2014)—remain a vital mechanism for evaluating health outcomes. A classic example of such systems is an immunization registry, which does not track outcomes but does maintain significant information on the management of diseases that may potentially impact a population. As many of us have experienced in our personal lives, immunizations required to enter school vary by state; however, they typically include hepatitis B, diphtheria, tetanus, pertussis, polio, measles, mumps, rubella, and chickenpox. Much of this information is stored at the local level of students and their schools. One ongoing challenge is how to capture this information at a higher level, such as the school district and county level, where it can then be used to identify gaps in immunizations as well as to facilitate an understanding of why certain outbreaks occur. For example, in 2015, there was a large measles outbreak in multiple states linked to an amusement park in California (Clemmons et al. 2015). The majority of people who got measles were unvaccinated, and the outcry regarding this outbreak eventually led to changes in vaccination exemptions in California. The California Immunization Registry (www.cairweb.org) is a private–public partnership of immunization registries that facilitates the secure electronic exchange of immunization information to support elimination of vaccine-preventable diseases. This registry provides an exchange infrastructure to sponsor automatic uploading of immunization records from various EMR systems as well as manual uploading of data from physician practices. It helps providers and organizations to disseminate public health information and meet meaningful use and other incentives regarding EHR use (as is reviewed later in this chapter). The California Department of Public Health, with its public health informatics program, is able to mine the data in this registry as part of its mission to improve the health of the public in California. From a mental health care perspective, this immunization registry may eventually play a role of great importance by confirming current data showing that certain immunizations do not cause children to have autism, as has been erroneously suggested by some in recent years. The registry may also be able to be linked to, say, longer-term epidemiological studies of patients with schizophrenia to examine whether early infections and a lack of immunization may make certain individuals more vulnerable to this disease in later life, as has been found in some British studies correlating influenza in pregnant women with an eventual increased prevalence of schizophrenia in their children.

Surveillance is another public health function that involves the continuous collection and analysis of data, along with timely dissemination of that information for the prevention and control of disease and injury (Jamison et al. 2006). Surveillance can be either active or passive, in that agencies can actively seek out the appropriate reportable information or just receive it from hospitals, providers, or other sources. The essential benefit of public health surveillance is that it produces the information needed for analysis and interpretation to then generate an appropriate intervention. A relevant example of such surveillance is the organized response of public health institutions to the recent outbreaks of Zika virus, an acute infectious disease that can have dire consequences for women of childbearing age. The potential risks of epidemic microcephaly in newborns and of Guillain-Barré syndrome in adults has created a shift in research as well as funding resources to combat this problem. Education and dissemination of outbreak information, including travel advisories, have been important interventions to decrease the incidence and spread of Zika and its related consequences. The World Health Organization's weekly Zika report (www.who.int/emergencies/zika-virus/situation-report/en/) is issued as part of its emergency response to international disease concerns.

In response to this and other initiatives in population health, the National Institute of Mental Health in 2016 updated its research priorities, and as part of Research Strategy 3.3—"Test interventions for effectiveness in community practice settings"—added the following:

1. Performing effectiveness studies in community practice settings that systematically examine heterogeneity in representative patient populations—including standardized collection of core data to promote data integration, sharing, and pooled analysis—in the service of identifying mediators/moderators and informing more prescriptive approaches.
2. Testing modular or stepped-care approaches for matching intervention intensity and components to illness severity and specific functional impairments.
3. Testing the utility of novel applications of technology that could generalize across indications, target populations, and operating platforms, for facilitating the delivery of research-supported strategies in a manner that both enhances the reach of evidence-based interventions and boosts their therapeutic value over and beyond standard delivery approaches.

All three of these strategies focus on, and are supported by, the need to collect, share, and analyze data to improve population health, whether the target group is children with autism spectrum disorder or attention-deficit/hyperactivity disorder (ADHD), adults with schizophrenia or depression, or seniors with dementia or delirium.

One of the challenges in public health surveillance is the use of data standards to ensure that data captured over time, with different approaches, and even across multiple countries can be appropriately compared. The Centers for Disease Control and Prevention (2016) have developed Epi Info™, a public-domain tool for public health researchers and practitioners to facilitate data capture and analysis with statistics, maps, and graphs. Data gathering also includes monitoring of hospitals for incidence of specific diseases, such as severe acute respiratory syndrome (SARS), which has prompted many hospital EHR systems to modify their triage forms to ensure proper documentation of recent travel to specific countries where outbreaks have been recently reported. Sharing this information via registries as well as reporting to local and regional public health entities helps the community determine whether more resources may need to be directed to prevent further spread of disease. In particular, when local hospitals share best practices and information, especially when they are on the same EMR vendor, coordination and communication is timely and more effective.

Traditional health care funding in America has used the fee-for-service model. In many ways, this payment model reflects the American spirit of entrepreneurship, wherein those who work harder, who provide more complex or skilled services, or who work in locations with lower densities of providers receive greater financial rewards for their services. However, despite the advent of various health insurance models such as health maintenance organizations, preferred provider networks, and independent practice associations along with employer-subsidized health insurance, America today is spending more of its domestic gross national product on health than all other countries in the world, but without good returns on its investment, in that our population has lower life expectancies compared with populations in many other countries (see Figure 1–3 in Chapter 1 of this volume). The current obesity and drug epidemics have been implicated as in part contributing to a reduction, in 2016—for the first time in two decades—in the potential average life span of an American person (National Center for Health Statistics 2017). These issues, along with the rising costs in the unsustainable fee-for-service model, have driven health care in the United States to adopt new funding models that emphasize incentives and reimbursement for preventive care at a population health level. The fee-for-service model will gradually be extinguished over the next decade or so as payment for population-based care becomes the norm, as discussed in Chapter 1 ("Psychiatric Practice in the Information Age").

One of the major health outcomes policy goals of the American Recovery and Reinvestment Act of 2009 (ARRA) was to improve population and public health, and it was predicted that this goal could be achieved if more professionals and hospitals adopted, implemented, or upgraded to certified EHR systems. In order to help increase the EHR adoption rate and promote innovation, incentive payments to individuals and hospital systems were created by the Centers for Medicare & Medicaid Services (CMS). These incentive payments ranged up to $44,000 over 5 years for Medicare providers as they met the criteria for different stages of meaningful use. Participation in the CMS Medicare incentive program was optional; however, if eligible providers or hospitals failed to start by 2015, they would begin to have annual reductions of 1% in their Medicare/Medicaid fees, with reductions of up to 3% by 2017 (Centers for Medicare & Medicaid Services 2017).

The Patient Protection and Affordable Care Act (ACA) of 2010 ("Obamacare") marked a significant sea change in health care financing (www.hhs.gov/healthcare/about-the-law/read-the-law/), as discussed in

Chapter 1. It mandated that all U.S. citizens purchase health insurance so that all Americans could have access to health care. By reducing premium costs via tax relief, capping out-of-pocket expenses, and requiring coverage of preventive care without out-of-pocket expenses, the ACA made access to health insurance more affordable for Americans and ensured that they could no longer be denied insurance because of preexisting medical conditions. It was thought that guaranteeing insurance and access to preventive care would result in a healthier population that in turn would use fewer services and decrease costs, helping to sustain the fiscal viability of the Medicare system while linking payments to improved quality and efficiency in health care.

Integrated care has become the new trend in care delivery for many of the reasons described here, as well as in Chapters 4 ("Clinical Settings and Models of Care in Telepsychiatry: Implications for Work Practices and Culturally Informed Treatment") and 8 ("Indirect Consultation and Hybrid Care"). *Integrated care* refers to the provision of behavioral health care in primary care settings as well as the provision of primary care in behavioral health settings, both delivered in an integrated manner. There are logical reasons for both models in integrated care. Many mild to moderate behavioral health problems are prevalent in primary care settings, such as anxiety, depression, and substance abuse in adults and ADHD, anxiety, and behavioral problems in children. Early intervention before conditions worsen and require inpatient and higher-level services is just one reason why behavioral health care in primary care settings makes sense. In addition, many medical conditions are associated with comorbid mental disorders, such as depression in heart disease, and it has been shown in numerous studies that by addressing both problems, worse outcomes and higher costs can be avoided. Improved access is yet another reason that mental health care services should be made available in primary care settings so as to serve populations in rural areas with limited availability of mental health care clinics due to shortages of providers, as well as populations whose cultural beliefs and attitudes may make going to a such clinics difficult.

For similar reasons, sharing of tasks across teams (Hoeft et al. 2017) and embedding of primary care practitioners (PCPs) in mental health care settings also make sense. Patients with severe behavioral health problems are often taking medications that place them at higher risk for diabetes, dyslipidemia, obesity, and hypertension, and because many in this population smoke, cardiovascular disease and the risk of stroke are also quite high. Access to primary care services for patients with mental disorders is also limited, often due to lack of transportation, absence of perceived need, and financial difficulties. However, integrated care goes beyond mere collocation of services—it requires true collaboration between primary care and behavioral health care providers. Real collaboration involves coordination of care, including collegial discussions about patients and exchange of information, and in this context, shared access to the same EMR system is particularly helpful (Coleman et al. 2017; Fortney et al. 2015).

HOW ARE MENTAL HEALTH INFORMATICS AND TECHNOLOGY-FOCUSED APPROACHES USED TO SUPPORT POPULATION-BASED CARE?

The care of populations is supported by, and completely dependent on, multiple health technologies. To meet the needs of integrated health systems, data must not only be exchanged but also collected, organized, analyzed, and acted upon in a systematic way to achieve the desired quality outcomes, such as those outlined in the ACA and the Medicare Access and CHIP [Children's Health Insurance Program] Reauthorization Act of 2015 (MACRA) (Centers for Medicare & Medicaid Services 2016). Large datasets, commonly referred to as "big data," have become the key to identifying new and subtle associations in medical conditions as well as aiding in medical decision making. This approach—wherein information from large datasets on populations will in the future be used to customize care by taking into account individual variability in genes, environment, and lifestyle for each person—has been called "precision medicine."

The University of California's **Re**search e**X**change, known as UC ReX (www.ucrex.org), is an initiative of the five University of California medical campuses that has combined and de-identified data from more than 15 million patient records. The data have been extracted from each institution's clinical data warehouse and transformed into an i2b2 (Informatics for Integrating Biology and the Bedside) common data representation format to allow for searches of demographics, diagnosis, procedures, laboratory values, medications, visit details, vital signs, and vital status. Query tools can be used to analyze information, so that (for instance) a physician can identify the number of patients on antipsychotic medication who also have a diagnosis of diabetes and who receive ongoing monitoring by endocrinologists at each medical center to determine whether there are enough patients at each center to justify the addition of a new protocol that prompts physicians to start metformin for any patient showing elevated blood glucose levels at three consecutive measurements. In the future, when genomic NLP data are included in the database, these data will allow physicians to determine, on the basis of clinical outcomes of thousands of other patients in the same database, which antipsychotic medication is most likely to be clinically effective for an individual patient in accord with his or her genotypic and phenotypic data. These data are also searchable with natural language-processing queries, so that even the "free text" medical information from patient visits can be mined for associations and patterns.

How Are Machine Learning and Natural Language Processing Used as Analytical Tools to Manage Population Data?

Data analysis, especially on a large scale, requires multiple analytic tools to achieve the desired outcomes in managing populations of patients. *Machine learning* is the science of teaching computers how to learn without explicit programming. It is a type of artificial intelligence that teaches itself to grow and change with new data. It is very similar to *data mining;* however, the key difference is that in data mining, the system looks for patterns of trends and relationships to help humans understand the data, whereas in machine learning, the system uses data analysis to adjust its own programming. Examples of machine-learning software include those used to run self-driving cars and speech-recognition programs. Supervised machine learning takes what has been learned in the past and applies it to new data, whereas unsupervised machine learning develops inferences from specific datasets. Machine learning techniques allow systems to sift through extremely large datasets to build an understanding of trends and relationships in the data, and these techniques are increasingly being used to improve the language-interpretation capacity and accuracy of automated translation and interpretation systems.

Natural language processing (NLP) is the ability of a computer to understand human speech and to translate it into the appropriate actions.

This type of artificial intelligence is important, because unlike computer programming languages, human speech is neither precise nor unambiguous, and its linguistic structure encompasses multiple variables, including slang, social context, and regional pronunciation differences. NLP bridges the communication gap between humans and computers by taking verbal questions and converting them into computer-based queries. NLP capabilities are important for analysis of EMRs because data are kept in both unstructured (e.g., free-text prose of admission notes, progress notes, and discharge summaries) and structured (e.g., repeated laboratory values) formats.

IBM'S WATSON

Watson, a massively multistrategy artificial intelligence system developed by IBM to answer questions posed in natural language, provides a dramatic example of what can be accomplished by a computer with machine learning capability. In 2011, Watson competed against Ken Jennings, the man who had the longest winning streak on the *Jeopardy!* game show, and Brad Rutter, who had earned the biggest prize pot on the show. The machine handily beat its two human competitors on the game show, winning the million-dollar prize, and it now spends its time analyzing health care data to help physicians make difficult cancer care decisions. In 2013, IBM partnered with Memorial Sloan Kettering Cancer Center to analyze medical literature, medical journals, medical textbooks, and treatment strategies to create Watson for Oncology (www. watson/health/oncology), a system that can analyze a patient's medical record, identify potential evidence-based treatment options, and provide supporting evidence from several sources. More recently, Quest Diagnostics has forged a partnership with Memorial Sloan Kettering and IBM Watson Health that will offer IBM Watson Genomics to Quest's network of cancer centers and hospitals to advance the concept of precision medicine and combine genomic tumor sequencing with cognitive computing ("Bringing Precision Medicine to Community Oncologists" 2017).

EPIC STAR DATA WAREHOUSE

Health care systems utilize separate databases for financial and clinical purposes; however, clinical knowledge is often gleaned from analysis of both types of data. Epic, one of the many large-enterprise EMR companies, has a data warehouse module called Cogito, which takes data from the Epic Chronicles database of clinical information and combines it with non-Epic data, such as financial transaction data or patient satisfaction data. This information is then combined into a simplified reporting database, called a "Star Schema Data Warehouse," that users can query without needing to learn new tools to create and run reports (Oberteuffer ND). This database facilitates collaboration with other Epic customers, so that all five University of California health systems can combine their information beyond what is available in UC ReX. These tools are used to analyze data on a population level to determine changes needed for value-based care as well as other quality measures.

HOW ARE CLINICAL DECISION SUPPORT SYSTEMS, DOCUMENTATION TEMPLATES, AND OTHER EMR TOOLS USED TO IMPROVE OVERALL POPULATION HEALTH?

Another way that EMRs can improve population health is through use of tools that allow providers to optimize their treatment of individual patients. There are multiple approaches that help the provider make decisions—a functionality known as *decision support*. One simple decision-support tool is an alert system, such as drug alerts. These alerts come in all types, including drug interaction, drug dosage, indications for use, alternate drug therapies, and drug allergy. Despite what may appear to be the obvious benefit of incorporating medication alerts in the EHR, they are also one of the more challenging decision support tools to set up properly. If alerts are too frequent and therefore become manually overridden to get through a workflow such as ordering medications, they create an atmosphere of "alert fatigue" such that the user will become habituated into ignoring alerts in the system. Setting the drug alert level is not an easy process. It involves the engagement of physician leadership, especially those with a clinical informatics background, as well as the pharmacists to reach an agreement, because not all drug–drug interactions or drug dosages have clinical ramifications. Drug alerts are especially challenging because certain specialties such as psychiatry may prescribe medications at higher dosages than the U.S. Food and Drug Administration recommendation, especially in patients who are treatment refractory or who may be fast metabolizers of the cytochrome P450 enzyme system that breaks down the medication.

Not all alerts are medication related. There can also be alerts based on medical conditions on the problem list that trigger an alert to the provider to decide on a specific order, so that, for example, if on the problem list of medical conditions, a patient has bipolar disorder and is taking lithium, the EMR can prompt the provider to order a lithium level if one has not been ordered in the past 6 months. Alerts can also be location based, in that if the patient is in a specific clinic or hospital ward, the EMR can trigger an alert if an action has not been completed, such as an assessment of "suicidality" for patients with severe depression and prior suicide attempts on a psychiatric ward or intensive outpatient clinic.

On a related note, if there are condition-specific documentation templates that physicians in population health management are required to use, the system can automatically call up a condition-specific order set— a panel of orders, such as admission orders, that facilitate the admission of a patient with a specific condition by ensuring that all of the necessary orders—such as those specified in clinical guidelines—are implemented. For example, for a patient with bipolar disorder who is on a mood stabilizer with regular monitoring of drug levels to determine compliance, the order set would recommend that a baseline drug level be ordered, along with other tests as appropriate. That way, patients on lithium would have lithium levels ordered on admission along with a basic metabolic panel to measure thyroid and kidney function, which can be adversely affected by prolonged lithium use. A condition-specific order set or subpanel may also be invoked when clozapine is prescribed, to ensure that weekly, twice-weekly, or every-4-week white blood counts are ordered. Condition-specific order sets and documentation templates make good sense but can be a challenge to implement, because the mapping of these templates needs to be appropriately linked to a cluster of related *International Classification of Diseases, Tenth Revision, Clinical Modification* (ICD-10-CM; National Center for Health Statistics 2016) diagnoses.

Along with condition-specific order sets and documentation templates, an EMR system should be able to provide focused patient data reports and summaries to help providers manage conditions across differing populations. Specific population health management tools are available in most enterprise-level EHR systems to remind providers that (for instance) a patient is due for both a colonoscopy and an influenza shot. Likewise, these tools can create a registry of all patients with depression and then determine which of these patients have not received a

Patient Health Questionnaire–9 (PHQ-9) screening recently. The population health manager is then able to send the PHQ-9 to the patient portal or queue a reminder to the provider or clinic to screen the patient at his or her next outpatient visit. These tools require that the data elements be in a "data warehouse," as described previously, and typically these queries are on such a large scale that they are run as a daily batch report versus on demand due to time constraints. Another key issue to enable these processes is not technological in nature. Policies must be in place in the health system to utilize protocols for population management as well as privilege the population health manager to take action. In addition, patients need to be informed by their providers that their condition is also being managed at a system or population health level, so that patients are not surprised when they receive specific orders and questionnaires.

Finally, the best care of patients is a challenge without the right diagnosis. Simply by using an EMR, all clinical information is available in one place to be reviewed at one time so that the current diagnosis can be confirmed or modified. There may also be paper-based information from other providers and health systems to be reviewed, and most EMR systems provide access to that information in the form of an Adobe PDF. Specific items on the problem list can trigger consultation order suggestions to help the provider take advantage of the resources in the health system, such as perhaps a psychiatric referral following a high PHQ-9 score. In addition, many EMR systems provide contextually relevant reference information in the form of hyperlinks to educational resources, such as UpToDate (www.uptodate.com), so that providers can read more about medications and conditions, including workup and management of these diseases. These tools help ensure that both individual patients and populations of patients receive the best possible care.

WHAT ARE SOME CURRENT EXAMPLES OF POPULATION-BASED CARE IN ACTION?

Population health strategies in mental health care are beginning to become the norm rather than the exception, and several are detailed in Chapters 4 and 8. Populations are very diverse and can include people living in specific geographic regions (e.g., nations, states, or communities such as a city or a region), employees (e.g., a large company or health system), racial/ethnic groups (e.g., Native Americans), people with a disability (e.g., deaf or blind), and patients enrolled in a health care system (typically defined by insurance status or access capacity). In order to provide effective care for any population, an intervention needs to both reach as many individuals as possible and be as effective as possible. This dual need is where telepsychiatry is of such importance, because the various technologies discussed in this book, incorporating remote measurement in differing workflows and through various connected devices, have the potential to geographically redistribute specialty mental health care services, thereby increasing equity in access as well as capacity and producing a population-level impact (Fortney 2015).

COLLABORATIVE INTEGRATED PRIMARY CARE–MENTAL HEALTH CARE MODEL

The most heavily researched and described example of population-based care is the collaborative care model of integrated mental health care into primary care developed by Wayne Katon, M.D., and Jurgen Unützer, M.D., over the past two decades at the University of Washington, Seattle, which was described in detail in Chapter 8. This form of care is highly evidence based, is supported by more than 80 clinical trials, and is now being implemented in numerous U.S. health care systems. Collaborative mental health care usually has a strong informatics and telepsychiatry focus, so that teams of mental health care professionals, including psychiatrists, can review panels of patients and provide a range of therapies, directly and indirectly, in person and online, using what is increasingly called "stepped care" approaches. Here individual patients receive differing levels of intervention according to their needs. One patient may just have their history and medications reviewed by a collaborative care team, with a secure message being sent to their PCP suggesting some extra labs or a change of medication, while the next patient may have an individual consultation using telepsychiatry arranged urgently to prevent a possible hospital admission. A range of therapeutic choices is available to the team, and these choices are individually matched to the needs of a panel of patients being reviewed both as a population (e.g., all patients may receive depression screening tests) and as individuals (e.g., specific patients may receive differing levels of mental health care consultations—direct, indirect, online, in person, messaging, e-mail, telephony, or videoconferencing—and support in association with any care being provided by their PCPs). The collaborative care model is very different from the traditional mental health care options available for PCPs to offer to their patients—an in-person referral to a psychiatrist or therapist being the only choice.

U.S. DEPARTMENT OF VETERANS AFFAIRS TELEPSYCHIATRY INITIATIVES

Now let us examine some of the other current and potential clinical settings in which population health care is incorporating telepsychiatry and other health technology solutions. The U.S. Department of Veterans Affairs (VA) has been a leader in providing population-based health care, and the various studies of posttraumatic stress disorder (PTSD) treatment from John Fortney, Ph.D., and his team (described in Chapter 4) have been leading examples. In their 2013 study, Fortney et al. (2013) described how collaborative care management in the VA setting, using a multidisciplinary depression care team, can also provide guideline-driven depression treatment in the primary care setting at multiple sites, with more fidelity to the treatment program than in-person providers. Peter Shore, Psy.D., another innovative VA psychologist, has had a long-standing focus on the provision of care in the home using videoconferencing, thereby extending the reach and access of treatment for veterans. In the case example that follows, Dr. Shore describes how the development of safety protocols and their policy implementation has led to substantially improved levels of population-based care for veterans.

CASE EXAMPLE 1: MEETING VETERANS "WHERE THEY'RE @": IN-HOME TELEMENTAL HEALTH CARE MADE POSSIBLE BY A SAFETY NET[1]

Combat veterans who live in remote rural locations due to a preference for isolation—particularly those who find it distressing to leave their homes and go out in public—are resistant to traveling to a clinic for PTSD treatment. Up until December 2009, there was no answer to this dilemma. Then a psychologist and a small number of his existing patients decided to try something different: treatment delivered via a webcam and a personal computer in the patient's own home. The VA leadership was worried that there would be no safety net if a veteran be-

---

[1]Case provided by Peter Shore, Psy.D.

came suicidal. What would happen if a veteran decompensated? How would he get help? What if veterans recorded their sessions and put them on YouTube? In collaboration with his small group of veterans, the psychologist developed a plan, and the patient support person (PSP)—an individual identified by the veteran patient whom the psychologist could contact in case of an emergency—concept was born. The PSP served as the psychologist's eyes and ears. Having the "insurance" of the PSP gave the VA leadership the confidence they needed to approve a pilot study. A standard operating procedure manual and subsequent policy were developed. For the next couple of years, approximately 80% of all enrolled veterans receiving behavioral health care at home via webcam and personal computer in this pilot indicated that they would not have received any mental health treatment if this modality had not become available. The veterans receiving PTSD treatment became socialized to the treatment, experienced early successes, and many ultimately also became engaged in in-person care. As of February 2017, more than 6,000 veterans nationally have received mental health care in their homes via webcam and personal computer or tablet. So far in this program, a PSP has never been utilized for a situation of emergency, but many veterans have expressed increased comfort in knowing that "someone would be there" if an emergency occurred.

▌ KEY CONCEPT

Mental health care in the home extends the reach of providers to a fragile population of veterans with PTSD and is safe as long as safety policies are followed.

Another excellent example from the VA of population-based care is the long-standing cross-cultural program for rural Native American veterans provided by Jay Shore, M.D., and his team at the University of Denver. This program has been extensively described in the literature (Shore et al. 2008, 2012) and over a period of about 15 years has led to a greatly increased understanding of how to provide culturally appropriate care to isolated veterans.

CASE EXAMPLE 2: CROSS-CULTURAL TELEMENTAL HEALTH CARE FOR RURAL NATIVE AMERICAN VETERANS[2]

Native American veterans serve in the military at the highest rate per capita of any ethnic group, disproportionately suffer the consequences of

---

[2]Case provided by Jay H. Shore, M.D., M.P.H.

military service, are the most rural veterans, and have significant barriers to accessing care. In response to these needs, the VA, in collaboration with the University of Colorado, developed a series of videoconferencing-based clinics to provide VA mental health care services for Native American veterans living on or near rural reservations in the Western United States. The clinics employ a model of culturally centered care by bringing together mental health care services combined with cultural facilitation and care coordination enabled through technology. The clinics utilize culturally knowledgeable providers who work with onsite tribal outreach workers. These outreach workers are often veteran tribal members who logistically support the clinic at the patient site, educate providers about cultural and community issues, and help to facilitate linkage with local services, including traditional healing. These clinics offer a full range of evidence-based services via videoconferencing, including pharmacological management, individual psychotherapy, group and family therapy, case management, crisis management, and care coordination. This model builds trust, rapport, and engagement with a target patient population to overcome barriers found when interfacing with Western health care systems. The clinics have used an ongoing evaluation process to create a growing body of evidence delineating their clinical model and supporting their effectiveness.

❙ KEY CONCEPT

Telepsychiatry services can be developed and tailored to provide culturally centered care for underserved populations with chronic and complex conditions, improving both access and quality of care.

U.S. DEPARTMENT OF DEFENSE TELE-BEHAVIORAL HEALTH SYSTEM

Another important population requiring innovative health care delivery approaches is active-duty soldiers, especially those who are on tours of duty in combat zones, where it is very difficult to provide specialized mental health care services at the best of times, and where soldiers are commonly under great stress, resulting, ultimately and tragically too often, in suicides and withdrawal from deployment. The U.S. Department of Defense, as described in the following case example, has actively used technologies to assist troops in combat zones and, as in many other areas of health care, has combined best clinical practices, research, and innovation to support the care of individuals who serve in the armed forces.

CASE EXAMPLE 3: MENTAL HEALTH SERVICES
DELIVERED VIA VIRTUAL HEALTH TECHNOLOGIES
FOR SOLDIERS IN COMBAT MILITARY OPERATIONS[3]

In early 2010, the Army's Telemedicine and Advanced Technology Research Center (TATRC) was directed to develop and support a Tele-Behavioral Health (TBH) system for soldiers in combat zones. Soon, during the height of combat operations, 87 operational remote TBH sites were established in Afghanistan and Iraq. An internal public health command survey revealed that TBH provided approximately 20% of all mental health patient encounters (1,900 visits annually), from 2012 to 2015; more than 72% of the soldiers stated that they would not have sought behavioral health care if virtual TBH had not been available, and 43% of providers reported 1–3 days saved per encounter. TBH services were provided in a timely manner using secure, synchronous, bidirectional video technology and overcoming weather challenges and dangerous travel risks in combat-related conditions. Soldiers far forward on the battlefield benefited from services including teleconsultations between soldiers and providers and between providers to confirm a diagnosis; recommendations on medication management and treatment options; and telecoaching. The most common uses of TBH in Afghanistan included provision of psychodynamic therapy (69%) and management of medications (23%). As of August 2016, there remain 10 active TBH sites in Afghanistan supporting two regional combat support hospitals and one combat operational stress command. The Afghanistan successes generated two additional TBH programs, and now 4 sites are functional in Kuwait with outreach to the Sinai, and 10 in Iraq. TATRC continues to coordinate monthly teleconferences with the deployed medical units throughout central command.

▌ KEY CONCEPT

Providing timely virtual mental health care services to soldiers in combat reduces travel risks and improves outcomes through rapid therapeutic intervention.

SOUTH CAROLINA EMERGENCY DEPARTMENT TELEPSYCHIATRY INITIATIVE

Another setting in which it is difficult to access psychiatrists is the emergency department (ED). As described in Chapter 1, psychiatric beds have been dramatically reduced throughout the United States in the past 30

---

[3]Case provided by Francis Leo McVeigh, O.D., M.S.

years, and this, combined with the continuing high prevalence of substance abuse—especially opiates and stimulants—has resulted in increased numbers of patients presenting to EDs throughout the country. While many psychiatrists do work in EDs, there are simply not enough of them available nationally, and increasingly patients are primarily treated by ED staff in conjunction with other mental health care professionals, such as social workers. The problem with this is that study after study has shown that psychiatrists, with their higher level of training, are much more likely to make earlier, more effective treatment decisions than alternative providers and overall are highly cost-effective because they are more likely to avoid unnecessary admissions and to discharge patients earlier. Not surprisingly, telepsychiatry in EDs is booming, because it has been realized that a small group of telepsychiatrists can service multiple hospitals. Only one state, however, has really taken the next step and created a statewide emergency telepsychiatry service. The state? South Carolina, led by Meera Narasimhan, M.D. (Narasimhan et al. 2015), at the University of South Carolina, as described in the following case example.

CASE EXAMPLE 4: A STATEWIDE EMERGENCY DEPARTMENT TELEPSYCHIATRY INITIATIVE[4]

The South Carolina statewide telepsychiatry initiative has proved to be a promising strategy for improving care and clinical and cost outcomes of mental health ED visits by increasing access to emergency psychiatric consultation, leading to reduced lengths of stay in the hospital and better treatment (Narasimhan et al. 2015). The program started in 2009 and gradually expanded, so that by February 2017, telepsychiatry consultations had been provided at 23 EDs (rural and urban), with more than 30,000 patients served. The program provides emergency psychiatric care access 24 hours a day, 7 days a week via a group of dedicated university-based telepsychiatrists who deliver assessments and recommendations for initial treatment and work closely with ED doctors to identify resources in the community to help patients with follow up care—a necessity that reduces the risk of rehospitalization and improves quality of life for both patients and their families. The hospital EDs fax relevant information to a toll-free server at the South Carolina Department of Mental Health (DMH), and all of the telepsychiatrists work from the same queue, with access to a statewide Health Information Exchange (HIE). When telepsychiatrists in the queue become available to

---

[4]Case provided by Meera Narasimhan, M.D.

see their next patient, information from the hospital is displayed on their monitors, and if the patient has ever been served by the HIE, physicians can see dates, diagnoses, and locations of services, including both inpatient and outpatient for episodes of care. They can also view all clinical notes in the EMR for outpatients from 2007 to the present. Consults are wholly electronic and are completed in the EMR, so that when psychiatrists apply their signatures to consults, an electronic ticket appears that automatically initiates e-faxing of the consult to the requesting hospital from the DMH server, so there is no "paper" to manage or file.

▌ KEY CONCEPT

Statewide emergency telepsychiatry services can increase patients' access to psychiatrists in emergency settings, leading to improved clinical and cost outcomes. Technologies such as EMRs and HIEs enable this workflow.

WHAT DOES THE FUTURE HOLD FOR POPULATION-BASED CARE?

The examples of population-based care strategies described in the previous sections could be used in many different populations and settings. There are, however, a number of population-based care approaches and methods that offer opportunities to help patients in ways beyond those possible today, and that will undoubtedly be used in the future. These generally depend on "big data," or at least data sources that we do not traditionally equate with mental health diagnosis or monitoring. In Chapter 6 ("Data Collection From Novel Sources"), the use of smartphone-related data sources, such as geographic tracking devices, activity monitors, photographs, and social networks, is discussed. Some studies (e.g., Kahr et al. 2016) have demonstrated a correlation between depression and obesity in inner-city females, poverty, and the close geographic proximity of fast-food outlets, using data from geographic information systems, mapping and tracking devices, social networks and photographs, and epidemiological and depression-screening data. What this potentially leads to is identification of a population of individuals who might be helped by changes in their shopping, exercise, and eating habits; the introduction of better-quality food in their neighborhoods; and a community program aimed at increasing meaningful training, community development, and leadership opportunities, hence preventing the development of depression at a later age.

The use of data from areas we have not typically thought of using in health care could very well lead to interesting and innovative approaches to detecting depression but could still incorporate conventional mental health therapies as required. Examples of such innovative data use include an exploratory study in 2014 that analyzed postings on Twitter to monitor community attitudes about depression and schizophrenia (Reavley and Pilkington 2014) and a study in 2017 that collected and examined a representative sample of content related to deliberate self-injurious cutting on three popular social media platforms: Twitter, Tumblr, and Instagram (Miguel et al. 2017). Currently, most of these studies focus on possible methods to be developed and used and have little clinical significance, but as we continue to develop more sophisticated data analysis capabilities, the massive datasets that make up Twitter and Facebook, for instance, will undoubtedly be increasingly mined in the future. It is important to note that the use of social networks is not all positive, as these social media have already been blamed for spreading suicidal ideation and cyberbullying within networks of young, vulnerable individuals and school populations.

This idea of early detection of disease using data collected at the network level has also been demonstrated by Google with Google Flu Trends. Using the frequency of searches for flu and related conditions, this software was able to predict an uptick in flu cases in 2008, 2 weeks before the traditional reporting methods of the U.S. Centers for Disease Control and Prevention were able to demonstrate the same increasing trend. Unfortunately, the algorithm was later determined to be flawed because it missed the 2013 influenza peak, which ultimately brought an end to the project (Lazer and Kennedy 2015). However, Google Flu Trends demonstrated how analysis of big data could yield surveillance information of immense public benefit as well as how changes in the search behavior of individuals over time could cause algorithms to fail. The follow-up to this program demonstrated how data sources can change with changing social behavior; the app Sick Weather (www.sickweather.com) also analyzes big data, but in this case, it monitors social media networks such as Facebook and Twitter for public disclosures that people are sick, in addition to seeking direct reports from users of the Sick Weather smartphone app. The vendor claims that the app is able to detect trends for illness conditions such as allergies, food poisoning, chicken pox, and influenza weeks ahead of traditional surveillance methods and can send alerts with information as detailed as the "street level" where they are occurring. It will be interesting to see whether the capabilities of such apps might eventually encompass detection of trends in mental disorders such as depression and anxiety.

So where is this all leading us? The use of large datasets combined with the potential to predict population-level changes and to provide customized stepped care to individuals brings us to what may be the largest health threat facing the world in 2017. Human-caused climate change, with global warming, is occurring. Heat waves are more intense and last longer, and floods and storms are more frequent, as the world's temperatures and sea levels rise. Much has been written about the potential health impacts of extreme weather events around the world, such as through infectious diseases, but the impact of climate change on the mental health of individuals and populations is possibly even greater. A recent review of this topic (Every-Palmer et al. 2016) concluded that extreme weather events such as floods, droughts, heat waves, wildfires, and storms will markedly increase the prevalence of PTSD, depression, anxiety, and substance use disorders. More significant indirect effects were also described, primarily from damage to land, infrastructure, and community functioning, leading to migration, armed conflict, and other violence. These effects will likely be unevenly distributed and will disproportionately affect disadvantaged peoples and communities, placing those with chronic mental illness at greater risk than the rest of the population.

Following Hurricane Katrina, for example, the floodwaters left many impoverished, chronically mentally ill patients literally stranded without shelter, food, or medication, and EMRs and medication monitoring systems were developed on the fly to help them. This is a common and classic use of telemedicine that has been lifesaving in many disaster situations over the past 50 years around the world and will continue to be lifesaving. We know that both acute and chronic disaster situations will occur worldwide with increasing frequency in the future. There will therefore be a need, through the use of population-based EMRs, videoconferencing consultations, indirect consultations supporting first responders, and virtual pharmacies, to develop much better-planned and flexible mental health care services that can cross national boundaries if we are to help affected individuals and assist in preventing mass disaster migrations in the years to come.

SUMMARY

Population-based care is gaining recognition as an area of critical importance, and in the mental health care field, growing numbers of practitioners are learning the skills and knowledge required to deliver such care. New health care funding models increasingly require that individual practitioners focus on panels of patients and delivery of quality and value across these panels, not just to individuals. Issues discussed in this chapter have included the following:

- Population-based care depends on the foundation provided by health information technology, which requires the use of large datasets, patient registries, and the tools of "precision medicine" to customize grouped knowledge for individuals.
- These multiple data sources and data streams are frequently too complicated for individual physicians to manage, so decision support tools of many varieties are being developed and introduced.
- A wide range of populations with various mental health needs are being treated with telepsychiatry and a range of other preventive and therapeutic approaches. Such populations include patients in collaborative integrated primary mental health care systems, Native American veterans, active-duty soldiers, and patients in emergency departments.

The greatest health challenge of the future will undoubtedly be global warming, with both chronic/slow and acute/rapid changes in weather conditions occurring across countries and continents. To meet this challenge, the field of mental health care needs to incorporate many more population-based technologies for prediction, prevention, and pre- and postdisaster management.

REFERENCES

Bringing precision medicine to community oncologists. Cancer Discov 7(1):6–7, 2017 27864232

Centers for Disease Control and Prevention: Epi Info™. Atlanta, GA, CDC Division of Health Informatics & Surveillance, Center for Surveillance, Epidemiology & Laboratory Services, updated September 13, 2016. Available at: https://www.cdc.gov/epiinfo/index.html. Accessed June 22, 2017.

Centers for Medicare & Medicaid Services: CMS Quality Measure Development Plan: Supporting the Transition to the Merit-based Incentive Payment System (MIPS) and Alternative Payment Models (APMs). Baltimore, MD, Centers for Medicare & Medicaid Services, May 2, 2016. Available at: https://www.cms.gov/Medicare/Quality-Initiatives-Patient-Assessment-Instruments/Value-BasedPrograms/MACRA-MIPS-and-APMs/MACRA-MIPS-and-APMs.html. Accessed May 5, 2017.

Centers for Medicare & Medicaid Services: 2017 Medicare Electronic Health Record (EHR) Incentive Program Payment Adjustment Fact Sheet for Eligible Professionals. Baltimore, MD, Centers for Medicare & Medicaid Services, July 3, 2017. Available at: https://www.cms.gov/Regulations-and-Guidance/Legislation/EHRIncentivePrograms/Downloads/PaymentAdj_EPTipsheet.pdf. Accessed August 17, 2017.

Clemmons NS, Gastanaduy PA, Fiebelkron AP, et al: Measles—United States, January 4–April 2, 2015. MMWR Morb Mortal Wkly Rep 64(14):373–376, 2015 25879894

Coleman KJ, Magnan S, Neely C, et al: The COMPASS initiative: description of a nationwide collaborative approach to the care of patients with depression and diabetes and/or cardiovascular disease. Gen Hosp Psychiatry 44:69–76, 2017 27558107

DeWitte SN: Mortality risk and survival in the aftermath of the medieval Black Death. PLoS One 9(5):e96513, 2014 24806459

Every-Palmer S, McBride S, Berry H, Menkes DB: Climate change and psychiatry. Aust N Z J Psychiatry 50(1):16–18, 2016 26553219

Fortney J: Harnessing the Power of Measurement and Technology. Keynote address presented at the American Psychological Association "Global Approaches to Integrated Health Care" Summit, Washington, DC, November 4, 2015. Available at: https://www.youtube.com/watch?v=dHAfz51XQHc. Accessed August 17, 2017.

Fortney JC, Enderle MA, Clothier JL, et al: Population level effectiveness of implementing collaborative care management for depression. Gen Hosp Psychiatry 35(5):455–460, 2013 23725825

Fortney JC, Pyne JM, Turner EE, et al: Telepsychiatry integration of mental health services into rural primary care settings. Int Rev Psychiatry 27(6):525–539, 2015 26634618

Gliklich RE, Dreyer NA, Leavy MB (eds): Registries for Evaluating Patient Outcomes: A User's Guide, 3rd Edition (2 vols; AHRQ Publ. No. 13(14)-EHC111). Rockville, MD, Agency for Healthcare Research and Quality, April 2014. Available at: https://www.ncbi.nlm.nih.gov/books/NBK208643/. Accessed April 6, 2017.

Hoeft TJ, Fortney JC, Patel V, Unützer J: Task-sharing approaches to improve mental health care in rural and other low-resource settings: a systematic review. J Rural Health Jan 13, 2017 [Epub ahead of print] 28084667

Jamison DT, Breman JG, Measham AR, et al (eds): Disease Control Priorities in Developing Countries, 2nd Edition. New York, Oxford University Press, The International Bank for Reconstruction and Development, and The World Bank, 2006. Available at: https://www.ncbi.nlm.nih.gov/books/NBK11728/. Accessed June 22, 2017.

Kahr MK, Suter MA, Ballas J, et al: Geospatial analysis of food environment demonstrates associations with gestational diabetes. Am J Obstet Gynecol 214(1):110.e1–110.e9, 2016 26319053

Lazer D, Kennedy R: What we can learn from the epic failure of Google Flu Trends. Wired, October 1, 2015. Available at: https://www.wired.com/2015/10/can-learn-epic-failure-google-flu-trends/. Accessed June 22, 2017.

Miguel EM, Chou T, Golik A, et al: Examining the scope and patterns of deliberate self-injurious cutting content in popular social media. Depress Anxiety 34(9):786–793, 2017 28661053

Narasimhan M, Druss BG, Hockenberry JM, et al: Impact of a telepsychiatry program at emergency departments statewide on the quality, utilization, and costs of mental health services. Psychiatr Serv 66(11):1167–1172, 2015 26129992

National Center for Health Statistics: International Classification of Diseases, Tenth Revision, Clinical Modification (ICD-10-CM), 2016 Edition. Hyattsville, MD, National Center for Health Statistics (under authorization by the World Health Organization), 2016. Available at: https://www.cdc.gov/nchs/icd/icd10cm.htm. Accessed May 5, 2017.

National Center for Health Statistics: Table 15 (Life expectancy at birth, at age 65, and at age 75, by sex, race, and Hispanic origin: United States, selected years 1900–2015), in Health, United States, 2016: With Chartbook on Long-Term Trends in Health. Hyattsville, MD, National Center for Health Statistics, 2017, p 116. Available at: https://www.cdc.gov/nchs/data/hus/hus16.pdf#015. Accessed August 17, 2017.

National Institute of Mental Health: Priorities for Strategy 3.3. Updated September 2016. Available at: https://www.nimh.nih.gov/about/strategic-planning-reports/strategic-research-priorities/srp-objective-3/priorities-for-strategy-33.shtml. Accessed June 22, 2017.

Oberteuffer R: Epic Star Data Warehouse. Baltimore, MD, The Johns Hopkins Institute for Clinical and Translational Research, ND. Available at: http://ictr.johnshopkins.edu/clinical/clinical-resources/clinical-research-informatics-core/epic-cogito-data-warehouse/. Accessed June 22, 2017.

Reavley N, Pilkington PD: Use of Twitter to monitor attitudes toward depression and schizophrenia: an exploratory study. PeerJ 2:e647, 2014 25374786

Shore JH, Brooks E, Savin D, et al: Acceptability of telepsychiatry in American Indians. Telemed J E Health 14(5):461–466, 2008 18578681

Shore J, Kaufmann L J, Brooks E, et al: Review of American Indian veteran telemental health. Telemed J E Health 18(2):87–94, 2012 22283396

10

Quality Care Through Telepsychiatry

Patient-Centered Treatment, Guideline- and Evidence-Based Practice, and Lifelong Development of Professional Competencies and Skills

Donald M. Hilty, M.D.

Carolyn Turvey, Ph.D., M.S.

Tiffany Hwang, M.D.

Patient-centered care—a health care reimbursement model suggested as far back as the early 1990s by the National Research Council—focuses on quality, affordability, and timeliness of health care (Institute of Medicine 2001) and has recently expanded to embrace a more holistic approach to patient care. The patient-centered care model competes with fee-for-service and other models of reimbursement (e.g., accountable care organizations and value-based care) that are driven by health care funding systems from the Centers for Medicare & Medicaid Services (CMS) and the Affordable Care Act of 2010 (ACA). There is still a healthy tension between the idea of health care as a preference determined by a market economy versus a social justice perspective that health care is a right.

The evidence base for telepsychiatry is growing, as are the methods used to determine its effectiveness. The majority of the studies have been conducted as part of formal research projects, with methods for these studies often including randomization of patients and strict protocols around how providers may engage with patients. However, many telepsychiatry practitioners would like to evaluate the effectiveness of their treatments and the provider–patient experiences without engaging in formal research. Although high-quality evaluation does not require randomization of patients or a strict clinical protocol, there are agreed-upon methods that providers can adopt to demonstrate the value of the care they provide.

Competency is best considered on a continuum of lifelong learning, as providers in practice and trainees need to stay current with rapidly evolving technologies, telepsychiatry research findings, and policies. Foremost, providers should assess their own clinical competence in providing care for patients both in general and in the face of pressures to increase access to services to underserved populations. Traditionally, there was an emphasis on knowledge acquisition, even though in its early years the knowledge base for telepsychiatry was not robust (Hilty et al. 2013a). The field of education emphasizes skills (e.g., interviewing, assessment) and key attitudes that ensure quality care (e.g., appropriate model, legal standards, privacy). Both residents and other young practitioners have significant interest in telepsychiatry at a time when there is a growing demand for telepsychiatrists.

One map to telepsychiatry competencies has been contextualized using the training milestones set forth by the Accreditation Council of Graduate Medical Education (ACGME). The ACGME map uses a template with domains of patient care, medical knowledge, practice-based learning and improvement, interpersonal and communication skills, professionalism, and systems-based practice (Accreditation Council on Graduate Medical Education et al. 2016). A technology competency and systems-based practice components on administration, culture, and community engagement were added recently (Hilty et al. 2015a).

This chapter will help clinicians to

1. Evaluate new technology options in preparation for selecting appropriate tools for use in their practices to set goals, achieve quality outcomes, and maintain good clinical care.

2. Focus on skill development in telepsychiatry, comparing and contrasting the use of real-time interactive video versus asynchronous methods and teaching others (e.g., trainees) to adapt their clinical approaches to technology.
3. Apply the growing telemedicine literature—including guidelines, practice parameters, policies, and evidence-based articles—to their own practices in order to maintain and enhance the quality of the care they provide.

HOW IS VALUE-BASED PAYMENT REFORM AFFECTING CLINICAL RESEARCH AND EVALUATION AND DRIVING THE ADOPTION OF TELEPSYCHIATRY?

Nonresearch evaluation of clinical practice has become increasingly important in light of payment reforms that tie reimbursement to providers' performance on quality metrics. Federal insurance programs such as Medicare and Medicaid are evolving toward a payment system that bases reimbursement on both the provision of a service and the demonstration of quality care and improved patient health outcomes. For example, the Physician Quality Reporting System provides incentives to report data on quality measures for Medicare Part B services. Behavioral health care measures include metrics such as suicide risk assessment, depression screening (with provision of follow-up plans for those who screen positive), alcohol screening, counseling, and initiation of treatment. The most recent manifestation of payment reform is the Medicare Access and CHIP [Children's Health Insurance Program] Reauthorization Act of 2015 (MACRA) discussed in Chapter 1 ("Psychiatric Practice in the Information Age"). Although the programs promoting value-based reimbursement will change over time, it is widely acknowledged that in the future, provider reimbursement for both federally and privately insured patients will require providers to demonstrate the quality of their care. Providers will need to know the specific agreed-upon metrics required by insurers and be able to collect this information without disrupting their clinical workflows or overburdening patients.

Another quality trend has been the growing proliferation of clinical guidelines. In addition to clinical guidelines targeting treatment of specific disorders such as major depressive disorder or schizophrenia, there are guidelines for the optimal practice of telepsychiatry. The American

Telemedicine Association (ATA) offers several guidelines on telepsychiatry practice, as do other professional organizations (e.g., the American Psychological Association). Metrics based on guidelines can demonstrate how a clinical practice can maintain quality while providing care via telemedicine.

Despite the many challenges of implementing value-based reimbursement, telepsychiatry should benefit from this development in two key areas. First, telepsychiatry has spurred the widespread deployment of communications technology in health care settings, most obviously electronic health records (EHRs). Second, telepsychiatry facilitates high-value care relative to in-person care by improving access to care; improves quality of care by facilitating specialist consultation; and reduces costs to both patients and providers. In short, telepsychiatry brings value to standard practice in ways that value-based reimbursement will measure and reward.

How Is Information Technology Being Leveraged to Evaluate Health Care Quality?

In telepsychiatry clinical services, discussions of technology most often focus on videoconferencing software and the quality of communication devices. However, in evaluation, technology can be deployed to efficiently and unobtrusively collect data that can be used to demonstrate the quality of care. To date, most quality metrics have focused on outcome and process. An *outcome metric* is one that reflects the clinical goals the patient and provider are trying to attain. Most of the technology deployed to assess quality has focused on *process metrics,* although insurers are asserting that value-based reimbursement will increasingly be dependent on demonstrated improvements in outcome metrics. In short, providers will need to demonstrate that they are helping their patients get better.

For a good example of outcome metrics, consider the treatment of depression, for which the primary outcome metric is reduction in depressive symptoms. The official CMS Electronic Clinical Quality Measures (eCQMs) metric "Depression Remission at 12 Months (CMS159v5)" is defined as follows: "Patients age 18 and older with major depression or dysthymia and an initial Patient Health Questionnaire—9 (PHQ-9) score greater than 9 who demonstrate remission at 12 months (±30 days after an index visit) defined as a PHQ-9 score less than 5" (Centers for Medicare & Medicaid Services 2017). In substance abuse treatment, the outcome metric might be number of contiguous days sober. By contrast, a process metric reflects behavior of the health care organization, provider, and/or patient that by definition must occur in order to accomplish the outcome metric. For example, depression screening and follow-up must occur in order to collect data that demonstrate a reduction in overall depression in a target population.

Moving forward, providers evaluating their clinical practices should collect both process and outcome metrics to evaluate whether providers are meeting agreed-upon standards of care and whether patients are improving on key clinical outcomes.

ELECTRONIC HEALTH RECORDS

Meaningful use is a federal program that provides incentives for the adoption and meaningful use of EHRs (as described in Chapter 7 ["Clinical Documentation in the Era of Electronic Health Records and Information Technology"] and Chapter 9 ["Management of Patient Populations"]). Many of the program's guidelines are aimed at preparing clinical practices for reporting within the new health care delivery and payment models. Although the initial adoption of EHRs was controversial, with providers complaining about spending more time looking at the computer screen than at patients, the value of EHRs in facilitating evaluation and defining the analytics of practice is irrefutable.

Providers adopting EHRs benefit from choosing more common technologies that have demonstrated the ability to "talk well" with other EHRs or health information technologies. Most vendors are well aware of current quality metrics and can assist providers in implementing standard reports on these metrics generated by the EHR. As stated earlier, these initial metrics tend to focus on process. For example, providers document each time they conduct a depression screen and provide documentation of a follow-up plan.

PATIENT PORTALS

With the growing emphasis on outcome metrics, technologies supporting evaluation must develop the capability to assess clinical outcomes. A patient portal is a secure electronic Web site that gives patients access to parts of their electronic health information stored within a provider's

EHR. Through these portals, current EHRs now have the capability to administer patient questionnaires and surveys that then become a permanent part of the provider's EHR. Portals provide a bridge between patients and their health care organizations that allows for streamlined assessment and integration of patient-reported outcomes. In our ongoing example, at both the initial visit and the 12-month follow-up for a depressed patient, the provider can administer the PHQ-9 through the portal, and the resulting screening scores are easily extractable for quality reporting because they are stored directly in the provider's EHR.

KIOSKS AND TABLETS

Not all providers have EHRs with portals that can conduct assessments. Moreover, not all patients are interested in or able to use patient portals due to inexperience with technology or limited access to high-speed Internet. A popular alternative is to provide kiosks within the reception area of the practice where patients can easily complete targeted outcome metrics using a touch screen. Tablets with touch-screen assessments are also widely used and allow greater mobility to better accommodate impaired patients.

MOBILE APPS

Conducting assessments through mobile applications has yet to be adopted widely in standard clinical practice; however, the functionality is available, as described in Chapter 6 ("Data Collection From Novel Sources"). The benefits of mobile apps include their ease of use and widespread accessibility wherever the patient is located. These have relatively higher adoption rates than do patient portals among younger cohorts and patients of lower socioeconomic status.

WEARABLE DEVICES

Even less widely disseminated than mobile apps are wearable devices such as the Fitbit or Apple Watch, which have generated a lot of excitement. Data captured via the enclosed accelerometers provide a range of health information, such as sleep patterns or activity levels, as well as vital statistics such as heart rate or temperature. Although these are not typical psychiatric outcome measures, functionality continues to develop, and some standard assessments can be conducted via these devices. Assessments performed with data collected from wearable devices can be synchronized with the EHR, so that these devices essentially serve as wearable patient portals. Such practices have yet to be disseminated widely, but the functionality is within reach for most EHRs from established vendors. If proven valid and reliable, this type of data may eventually lead to tracking for value-based reimbursement.

How Should Telepsychiatrists Approach the Task of Incorporating Evaluation Protocols Into Their Practices?

Evaluation presumes that the provider will conduct standardized assessments to measure target concepts such as depression severity, psychotic symptom intrusiveness, or substance use. For better or worse, there are an infinite number of potential domains one can assess to evaluate a typical telemedicine practice.

We now face the dilemma that our potential to collect data is exceeding our ability to analyze the data and translate the results into improvements in clinical practice. Although patient portal– or kiosk-delivered assessments have the potential to revolutionize patient engagement, shared decision making, and personalized medicine, patients who take the time to complete these assessments seldom receive feedback about them. It is critical that providers generate a manageable subset of assessments that efficiently capture core concepts relevant to the quality of their clinical care and that can be used to shape clinical decision making without unnecessarily overburdening patients.

The first step in evaluation is to identify domains or targets to assess. Available frameworks to guide selection of domains include the Dartmouth Hitchcock Medical Center's Value Compass and the Institute for Healthcare Improvement's Model for Improvement (www.ihi.org/resources/Pages/HowtoImprove/default.aspx). Also available are standard quality-reporting metrics, such as those from the CMS Web Interface (https://qpp.cms.gov/docs/QPP_CMS_Web_Interface_Fact_Sheet.pdf) and the National Quality Forum (NQF; www.qualityforum.org/measuring_performance/measuring_performance.aspx). Finally, clinical guidelines are available both for specific conditions and for the practice of telemedicine. Each of these resources provides potential metrics to choose from based on the goals of your clinical practice.

How Should Providers Approach the Task of Selecting Measures for Use in Assessments?

Patients are currently being inundated with assessments, yet the value of these assessments in truly improving clinical care has yet to be realized. Therefore, efficient design of evaluation methods is needed.

1. CHOOSE A STANDARD MEASURE OF A TARGET OUTCOME THAT IS ALREADY WIDELY USED

Measure development is a science requiring specialized training in item development, testing, and evaluation of reliability, validity, and sensitivity to change. The process, when well done, can take years, so providers should not simply write up their own measures based on what they think should be assessed, nor should they modify existing measures. A change in question wording in a validated questionnaire, such as the Beck Depression Inventory, may seem minor, but if it alters how patients understand the question and thereby alters their answers, the total score will ultimately diverge from the standard threshold provided by the original measure developer.

2. ANTICIPATE REGULATORY AND PAYER METRICS

Health care and its reimbursement are in the middle of a radical shift, wherein providers are becoming more accountable for the quality of their care, with payment determined by this quality. Being aware of the quality metrics of national organizations, such as those of CMS or NQF, and adopting some of these metrics in their practices will prepare providers for the gradual shift to value-based reimbursement. These national quality organizations recognize that the unchecked proliferation of quality metrics places a heavy burden on clinicians and consequently are in the process of streamlining their measures, so that (for example) providers will be able to choose just one depression screening metric or just one tobacco cessation metric. Similarly, if providers wish to anticipate value-based reimbursement, they should review these metrics first and aim to not duplicate their content in any additional metrics they choose to measure.

3. USE A MEASURE ONLY IF IT WILL DIRECTLY SHAPE QUALITY EVALUATION OR CLINICAL DECISION MAKING

Although many providers are initially reluctant to conduct standard assessments in conjunction with their clinical practice, it is remarkable how many providers, once they start, add everything but the kitchen sink to their assessments. Although, in the abstract, one can think of many domains to assess, it is important to weigh patient burden and carefully consider whether the metric truly improves quality. Appropriate design of a metric scheme is imperative, or patients and staff will not complete the assessments. Moreover, we owe it to our patients to make good use of their time.

4. PROVIDE CLINICIANS AND PATIENTS IMMEDIATE ACCESS TO THE RESULTS OF THEIR ASSESSMENTS

Patients need to understand why assessments are being done and how they benefit from the time they put into them. A recent review of the impact of patient-reported outcomes on quality of clinical care found that the procedures used for patient self-assessments involved a range of workflows (Krägeloh et al. 2015). Some practices were doing the assessments and providing the results to neither provider nor patient; others were providing assessment results to providers only; and still others were presenting results to both patient and provider with a standard protocol for results review. Only the latter option demonstrated any improvement in the quality of care. Although this conclusion may seem self-evident, most current practices simply conduct the assessments, and patients and providers meet in complete unawareness of the results of those assessments. Needless to say, this strategy will not yield any value.

5. HELP PATIENTS AND PROVIDERS IDENTIFY THE DOMAINS MOST MEANINGFUL TO THEM

If patients and providers will be using these assessments as part of their clinical decision making, it makes sense that they should participate in the process of selecting key outcomes. Engagement will go a long way toward ensuring both provider and patient adoption. This recommendation may seem to conflict slightly with prior recommendations where selection is guided by national payer metrics or standardized widely used measures. Patients may come up with a broad range of constructs they want to assess that do not coincide with these prior recommendations. However, providers can provide patients with a range of possible metrics and allow them to choose the ones that most closely reflect their valued treatment goals. For example, many patients value functioning over symptom reduction. There are a range of well-developed functional measures that patients can choose from. Provider review of patients' self-assessments on selected functional measures can be used to guide treatment decisions and can positively influence patient perceptions of treatment effectiveness.

WHICH METRICS ARE WELL MATCHED WITH TELEPSYCHIATRY?

In addition to the metrics just described, which would apply to any evaluation of psychiatric services, there are metrics that specifically capture the value of telepsychiatry. The ATA has identified core mental health care domains and metrics that can help quantify the relative advantage of telepsychiatry as compared with same-room care. A review of these measures shows the range of outcomes that may be improved through the use of telepsychiatry (Shore et al. 2014).

1. First, it is necessary to identify key metrics to demonstrate the *value of care*, with attention added to quantifying the value of telemedicine. Start by using the typical understanding of the value algorithm for value-based care: Value = Outcomes + Patient Experience/Costs. The target domains of patient outcomes, patient experience, and costs are easily identified.
2. *Effectiveness of treatment* would be assessed by targeting symptom measures relevant to the clinical conditions being treated, such as depressive symptom severity assessed through the PHQ-9, or number of days substance free in the treatment of substance abuse. Because well-known standardized outcome measures are available for most mental disorders, providers should be able to rely upon already-developed measures.
3. *Patient experience* is most commonly assessed through patient satisfaction measures and is highly standardized in large health systems through the Survey of Healthcare Experiences of Patients (U.S. Department of Veterans Affairs 2016). Although these measures have been vetted rigorously, patient satisfaction measures often have ceiling effects wherein all patients rate 100% satisfaction, and this is particularly true in telemedicine. Moreover, these measures do not adequately capture the unique benefits of telepsychiatry. Providers may want to adopt or develop more nuanced measures to better cap-

ture patient experience, particularly as their experience relates to telemedicine. Relevant domains to consider include questions about rapport, comfort with technology, and perceived burden of care.

4. There are other aspects of the patient experience that are important to measure in telemedicine. Telepsychiatry leads to ***improved access*** by reducing geographic barriers to care for patients and overcomes other barriers to care, such as physical impairments or competing obligations such as childcare or work. Common metrics reflecting this improved access can include distance to care, travel time to care, and time to first appointment. Providers may also want to track downstream targets that reflect improved access, such as no-show rates, proportion of time-defined treatments received by the patient (such as a standard 10-week psychotherapy protocol), and proportion of first-time patients presenting for follow-up visits within recommended time frames. For example, for patients who started antidepressant treatment in their initial visit, what proportion successfully completed a follow-up visit within 6 weeks of starting therapy?

5. Improved access leads to ***reduced treatment burden*** for patients. Providers can use innovative metrics to demonstrate this. Metrics such as hours of missed work or cost of childcare to attend appointments, travel cost, and patient-perceived inconvenience capture important factors that can influence no-show rates and overall treatment adherence. Older patients and patients with multiple significant morbidities can become quite fatigued by travel to medical appointments. This type of impact could be captured by a question about perceived inconvenience of care.

6. The final component of any value equation is ***cost.*** Detailed cost-based accounting can be prohibitively complex for the average provider. However, some calculation of the cost of staffing, clerical and technical support, and overhead should be within the reach of most providers. Evaluation of costs in telemedicine is particularly important, as it can help demonstrate a relative strength of telemedicine. Metrics for travel costs, gas costs, costs of technology, and any additional staffing costs related to conducting telemedicine will help to quantify the patient, organizational, and societal costs of the care provided.

Patient-centered care focuses on the provision of high-quality health care that is affordable, is delivered in a timely manner, and takes into account patient preferences. Although this care model already aligns to some degree with the outcomes-focused approach of value-based care and reimbursement, in the future clinicians, accountable care organizations, and others will need to increase their efforts to bring their assessment and reporting practices into conformance with the ACA (Figure 10–1).

How Should the Field Approach the Task of Developing Core Competencies for Telepsychiatry?

Competencies across fields of medicine are no longer "optional." Training for all parties is now required as well as potentially critical (Callan et al. 2016). We focus on telepsychiatry competencies, but mental health care–related, technology-based services exist on a continuum, as described in other chapters. These comprise a range of services and needs, from self-help/support groups to asynchronous communication with providers and telepsychiatry services with professionals to Internet-based cognitive-behavioral therapy. The competencies for many of these approaches are not yet defined, and "guidelines" are not grounded in consensus or the evidence base; they are more like suggestions on how to proceed with caution.

While competencies are the consensus for moving forward with education, there are different ways to organize them. The main framework (Dreyfus and Dreyfus 1980) for clinical communication can be applied to telepsychiatry as follows:

- Level 1—novice (medical student)
- Level 2—advanced beginner (first-year resident)
- Level 3—competent (senior resident)
- Level 4—proficient (graduating resident)
- Level 5—expert (e.g., telepsychiatry)

At the level of medical students, the Association of American Medical Colleges (2015) outcome measures are evidence based and include the domains of medical knowledge, patient care skills and attitudes, interpersonal and communication skills and attitudes, ethical judgment, professionalism, lifelong learning and experience-based improvement, and community and systems-based practice. The ACGME competencies include the domains of patient care, medical knowledge, practice-based learning and improvement, interpersonal and communication skills,

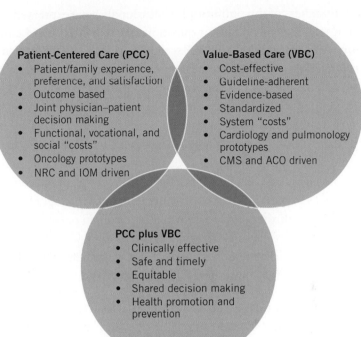

FIGURE 10–1. The integration of patient-centered care (PCC) and value-based care (VBC) has the potential to yield improved outcome targets in telepsychiatry.

ACO=accountable care organization; CMS=Centers for Medicare & Medicaid Services; IOM=Institute of Medicine; NRC=National Research Council.

professionalism, and systems-based practice (Accreditation Council on Graduate Medical Education et al. 2016).

Perhaps the best potential approach to telepsychiatry competencies for all clinicians, including those in training, is the milestone approach from ACGME. The Canadian Medical Educational Directives for Specialists (CanMEDS) framework is also evidence-based (Royal College of Physicians and Surgeons 2015) and directs clinicians toward roles and/or behaviors. Indeed, CanMEDS categorizes the knowledge, skills, and abilities that specialist physicians need for better patient outcomes into seven roles that all physicians play: medical expert, communicator, collaborator, manager, health advocate, scholar, and professional.

Both members of the public and professionals have expressed curiosity about telepsychiatry, asking questions such as "Is it good care?" or "Does it really work?" or "Is it similar to in-person care?" An early model for competencies was introduced in psychology (Maheu 2003), but to date (as of July 2017) no standards for initial and/or follow-up training have been put forward. Technology training in psychology internships is rare, and no certification is in place in any area of clinical medicine or health care. Although psychologists have identified guidelines for, models of, and challenges to the process of assessing competencies, there continues to be a lack of feasible strategies for assessment of telepractice competencies for psychologists and other clinicians throughout their careers, much less during their training (Hilty et al., in press; Kaslow et al. 2007).

The only currently published telepsychiatry competencies (Hilty et al. 2015a) are based on a combination of ACGME and CanMEDS but were simplified into three levels that better fit learner levels and are valid across disciplines (Table 10–1):

- Novice or advanced beginner (e.g., advanced medical student, early resident, other trainees)
- Competent/proficient (e.g., advanced resident; graduating resident; faculty, attending, or interdisciplinary team member)
- Expert (e.g., advanced faculty, attending, or interdisciplinary team member)

The most important area described in telepsychiatry competencies is *patient care.* It is divided into two parts:

1. Clinical—history, interviewing, assessment, and treatment
2. Administrative-based issues related to care—documentation, EHR, medicolegal, billing, and privacy/confidentiality

The *systems-based practice* competencies include outreach, interprofessional education, providers at the medicine–psychiatric interface, geography, models of care, and safety. Attitude, integrity, ethics, scope of practice, and cultural and diversity issues were grouped within *professionalism.* A domain called *technology* was added to include some behavioral, communication, and operational aspects. *Medical knowledge, practice-based learning and improvement,* and *interpersonal and communication*

TABLE 10–1. Telepsychiatry (TP) competencies for clinicians and trainees

Area/Topic	Novice/Advanced Beginner	Competent/Proficient	Expert
Patient Care			
History taking	Take a standard history	Obtain informed consent for telehealth (check state to see if form needed; option not to do telehealth is discussed) Obtain a contextualized history (e.g., aware of geographic and cultural specificity)	Resolve problems with informed consent (e.g., patient lacks capacity), as done in in-person care) Conduct an in-depth, well-paced, and concise interview
Engagement and interpersonal skills	Establish therapeutic alliance Build trust and rapport	Identify and manage problem(s) with alliance, trust, rapport Adjust interview to technological and patient needs, preferences	Determine best appropriate assessment adjustments based on the setting (in-person vs. TP)

TABLE 10–1. Telepsychiatry (TP) competencies for clinicians and trainees *(continued)*

Area/Topic	Novice/Advanced Beginner	Competent/Proficient	Expert
Patient Care *(continued)*			
Assessment and physical examination	Stratify risk and protective factors based on epidemiology (e.g., suicide, homicide risk) Administer tools (e.g., MMSE) from a distance[a] Ascertain need for actual PE	Assess risks for suicide/harm to others and develop follow-up plan Ensure identification of significant exam findings (e.g., movement disorders; intoxication, withdrawal) Examine and administer tools with adjustments (e.g., use staff to complete or perform part of PE)	Synthesize information (including risk vs. protective factors and collateral information) Administer tools contextually (e.g., substitute score item for nonreproducible task at distance) Teach staff and others how to perform parts of PE and trouble-shoot PE problems at the far end

TABLE 10–1. Telepsychiatry (TP) competencies for clinicians and trainees *(continued)*

Area/Topic	Novice/Advanced Beginner	Competent/Proficient	Expert
Patient Care *(continued)*			
Management and treatment planning	Biopsychosocial (BPS) outline Participate in providing summary and recommendations Make medical decisions regarding safety, need for treatment, and other interventions Follow up with PCP or telepsychiatrist by note Follow up with others as necessary	BPS outline with depth and identification of safety and risk factors Be able to provide summary and recommendations to patient and interprofessional team Demonstrate awareness of treatment continuum (levels of care) Follow in-person medication recommendations (i.e., review options, side effects, and alternatives if applicable; provide specific instructions for PCP to initiate, titrate, and augment) Formulate plan for calls, prescriptions, etc. Follow up with PCP by TP or phone	BPS outline with prioritization, with emergency plan execution, and with obstacles anticipated Tailor recommendations to available resources, specific culture, and patient preference Engage patient, referring doctor, or other providers succinctly Select best mode for clinical communication: e-mail, telephone, or other For medication recommendations: consider safety and adherence factors; plan for follow-up and monitoring; be aware of legal and jurisdictional issues related to prescribing

TABLE 10–1. Telepsychiatry (TP) competencies for clinicians and trainees *(continued)*

Area/Topic	Novice/Advanced Beginner	Competent/Proficient	Expert
Patient Care *(continued)*			
Documentation	Draft TP note as hard copy or rudimentary EHR	Create initial/revised draft for primary or other specialty care with modification for TP consultation Complex EHR (e.g., Cerner, Epic)	Provide sufficient detail to allow implementation of plan over time and within local context, resources Phone, e-mail, and asynchronous notes
Billing	Learn why billing is important and how it is configured	Identify diagnoses for billing	Final time spent, diagnosis, and codes Consider health advocacy issues related to billing; access to care
Privacy and confidentiality (medico-legal issues[a])	Learn in-person basic regulations	Be aware of regulations and learn how principles translate to video and adjunct regulations, if applicable Be aware that technologies are encrypted differently	Practice within in-person and telemedicine standards Be aware of pitfalls with technologies (e.g., cellular phones are not private; Gmail is not HIPAA compliant)

TABLE 10–1. Telepsychiatry (TP) competencies for clinicians and trainees *(continued)*

Area/Topic	Novice/Advanced Beginner	Competent/Proficient	Expert
Interpersonal and Communication Skills			
Cultural diversity and social determinants of health	Consider diversity of patients, families, and communities: language fluency, customs Consider one's own cultural values, behaviors, and preferences[a] Learn how social determinants affect in-person care[a]	Adjust in consideration of patient culture and preference Language fluency: double-check, confirm Ways to elicit cultural meaning of illness, wellness Be aware that social determinants may affect interest in, use of, and experience with telemedicine	Follow cultural formulation frameworks Ask if culture affects use of TP (general exploration) or explanation of illness Consider patient–doctor relationship in context of cultural values, behaviors, and preferences Adjust interview, assessment, and treatment per social determinants; consider in-person care if critical need
Language, interpreter ability	Use an interpreter	Time management and preferred types (e.g., professional preferable to family member)	Verbal and nonverbal dimensions
Communication	Clear communication with patient, family, and health care professionals	Clarify and amplify communication	Trouble-shoot communication difficulties

TABLE 10–1. Telepsychiatry (TP) competencies for clinicians and trainees *(continued)*

Area/Topic	Novice/Advanced Beginner	Competent/Proficient	Expert
Systems-Based Practice			
Outreach to community	Participate in and engage with community	Visit community in person before initiating TP Identify relevant resources and needs within community	Establish and maintain relationships with community Use thoughtful integration of in-person and TP care, if applicable
Interprofessional education (IPE) and teamwork[a]; [b] (IPCS)	Participate in and experience different roles; work effectively	Work with interprofessional team and be familiar with IPE Begin to teach within IPE framework	Serve as IPE provider and teacher Support interdisciplinary team care (e.g., PCPs; therapists; care coordinators [Master's degree or RN degree—PAs, NPs])
Collaborative primary care	Consider consults from the perspective of the referring provider's needs	Understand the referring provider's needs and adapt consult and notes appropriately	Engage with providers to clarify unclear needs Use individual consult as an opportunity for building ongoing relationship Integrate indirect care (e.g., case or chart review) into practice

TABLE 10–1. Telepsychiatry (TP) competencies for clinicians and trainees *(continued)*

Area/Topic	Novice/Advanced Beginner	Competent/Proficient	Expert
Systems-Based Practice *(continued)*			
Rural health	Learn about rural access, epidemiology, costs, and other issues	Learn basics of rural health	Practice and serve as role model
Special populations	Learn differences among populations (e.g., veteran, child, adolescent, parent, family, geriatric)	Recognize differences and adapt assessment and management approaches accordingly	Practice and serve as role model
Safety	Learn systematic assessment	Identify problems and stratify risk	Adjust risk and its management to TP system practice
Care models	Learn what in-person care, TP care, and consulting TP care consist of	Demonstrate facility with traditional referral to psychiatry, consultation care, and TP Begin to learn collaborative care	Demonstrate facility with models of consultation, integrated, stepped, and hybrid care; practice with model that fits context

TABLE 10–1. Telepsychiatry (TP) competencies for clinicians and trainees *(continued)*

Area/Topic	Novice/Advanced Beginner	Competent/Proficient	Expert
Systems-Based Practice *(continued)*			
Licensure regulations as applied to telemedicine care model (medico-legal issues[a])	Learn regulations for in-person care and understand that regulations differ by state	Be aware that in-person and telemedicine regulations may or not differ	Practice within telemedicine regulations between states or within a unique system (e.g., VA)
Evaluation	Understand patient satisfaction	Know basic evaluation strategies for TP outcomes	Consider range of evaluation approaches and use results for QI or to inform practice
Health advocacy	Identify issues related to access and health equity	Consider how technology can address and also contribute to health equity gaps	Consider ways that the physician role can impact policy and advocacy through technology

TABLE 10–1. Telepsychiatry (TP) competencies for clinicians and trainees *(continued)*

Area/Topic	Novice/Advanced Beginner	Competent/Proficient	Expert
Professionalism			
Attitude	Learn and be open to technology	Interprofessional clinical practice and teaching, learning	Leadership in groups, teams
Integrity and ethical behavior	Demonstrate behavior consistent with ethical standards	Serve as role model	Serve as role model and provide feedback
Scope	Become aware of scope issues related to in-person care, TP care, and TP consultation	Practice within scope(s)	Provide feedback on scope and boundary issues; trouble-shoot problems
Practice-Based Learning			
Administration	Learn basics of in-person care	Be aware that in-person and telemedicine care have differences	Practice with adjustments to telemedicine care
Quality improvement	Learn how to participate in QI	Apply QI information to cases and systems	Analyze, select, and evaluate QI options
Teaching and learning	Participate in and contribute to teaching/learning	Organize and further the aims of teaching/learning	Provide context and next steps for teaching/learning

TABLE 10–1. Telepsychiatry (TP) competencies for clinicians and trainees *(continued)*

Area/Topic	Novice/Advanced Beginner	Competent/Proficient	Expert
Practice-Based Learning *(continued)*			
Knowledge	Relevance History	Relevance History Evidence base	History Evidence base Clinical guidelines
Technology			
Adaptation to technology	Identify differences between TP and in-person care Try to project self 15% more (voice, animation) Realize that TP has some nonverbal limitations (e.g., offering a tissue, shaking hands)	Take steps to engage and put patient at ease Expect and plan for differences Identify technology-related barriers and implement compensatory behaviors Add a third party by phone	Use humor or self-deprecatory remarks to set patient at ease Analyze what actually happened and make adjustments for next time Additional ways to express empathy
Remote site design	Observe	Identify problems and formulate possible solutions Modification (e.g., toys for a child to play with; furniture)	Pre-planning: continuous, iterative improvement Modification: use professional staff for remote play therapy

TABLE 10–1. Telepsychiatry (TP) competencies for clinicians and trainees *(continued)*

Area/Topic	Novice/Advanced Beginner	Competent/Proficient	Expert
Technology *(continued)*			
Technology operation[a]	Become familiar with use of microphone, camera, and (as needed) second camera Observe how multiple technologies (e.g., primary and secondary cameras) are used simultaneously	Operate hardware, software, and accessories Perform basic troubleshooting (e.g., reboot system, call for assistance) Operate and use multiple technologies	Optimize hardware, software, and accessories based on context (for enhancement and for avoidance of distraction) Manage all troubleshooting operations on near end and provide advice on far end as needed Optimize use of multiple technologies

Note. EHR=electronic health record; EMR=electronic medical record; HIPAA=Health Insurance Portability and Accountability Act; IPE=interprofessional education; IPCS=interpersonal and communication skills (U.S. Milestones); MMSE=Mini-Mental Status Examination; NP=nurse practitioner; PA=physician assistant; PE=physical examination; PCP=primary care provider; QI=quality improvement; RN=registered nurse; VA=U.S. Department of Veterans Affairs.

[a]Based on submission for CanMEDS eHealth competencies (Ho et al. 2014).

[b]U.S. milestones; consistent with non-TP-specific (regular) competencies of the Accreditation Council of Graduate Medical Education (ACGME; 2016): patient care, medical knowledge, practice-based learning and improvement, systems-based practice, professionalism, and interpersonal and communication skills.

Source. Based on Hilty DM, Crawford A, Teshima J, et al.: "A Framework for Telepsychiatric Training and E-Health: Competency-Based Education, Evaluation and Implications." *International Review of Psychiatry* 27(6):569–592. 2015a.

skills are included for completeness, although many skills in these domains are similar to skills needed for in-person care.

Expert-level competencies have also been suggested for telepsychiatry based on clinical complexity, reasoning needed to make adjustments at a distance, and systems-based practice. Examples include the following:

- Completion of a Mini-Mental Status Examination (MMSE) via telepsychiatry—Requires preservation of MMSE testing integrity, ensuring optimal communication, and other clinical reasoning for substituting an item.
- A child/adolescent patient evaluation involving the patient, parent, siblings, and teacher who may telephone in—Requires extra time management, toys on site, the sequencing participation, and technology combinations.
- An evaluation of a Latino teenager, a parent, and a pediatrician in a rural setting—Requires management of language needs (e.g., teenager fluent in English and a parent who needs an interpreter), cultural needs, and primary care/pediatrician needs.

Competencies for clinical practice in the e-mental health spectrum of care—defined as "mental health services and information delivered or enhanced through the Internet and related technologies" (Eysenbach 2001, p. e20)—are in development (Hilty et al. 2015b).

WHICH TEACHING, ASSESSMENT, AND EVALUATION METHODS FIT BEST WITH TELEPSYCHIATRY?

Andragogical adult learning (i.e., pedagogical) methods are suggested for assessment of telepsychiatry competencies in clinical care, seminar, and other educational contexts. These include cross-sectional and longitudinal evaluation using both quantitative and qualitative measures. For clinical care, feedback from patients, trainees, and faculty is useful. For continuing education/continuing medical education (CE/CME) events, pre- and postassessment and interactive methods are suggested. Individual clinicians, programs, agencies, and other institutions may need to consider adjusted approaches to patient care, education, faculty development, and funding. Telepsychiatry skill competencies can be developed in training programs, seminars for agencies, and local/regional/national CE/CME events, as well as through leading organizations such as the ATA.

There is no shortcut for observation, feedback, and evaluation in measuring the progressive acquisition of skills. The evaluation process includes adoption of standardized measures and use of measures with specificity, timeliness, accuracy, and brief completion, with collection of data prospectively rather than retrospectively (Hilty et al. 2015a). Kirkpatrick and Kirkpatrick (2009) stressed that evaluation should include four different levels: reaction, learning, behavior, and results.

- *Level one* of evaluation assesses a participant's reactions to the setting, materials, and learning activities so as to ensure learning and subsequent application of program content. Reactions can be captured through satisfaction ratings.
- *Level two* of evaluation involves determining the extent to which learning has occurred, often employing performance testing, simulations, case studies, plays, and knowledge exercises (e.g., pre- and posttest).
- *Level three* of evaluation attempts to determine the extent to which new skills and knowledge have been applied "on the job," such as in the health care setting.
- *Level four* of evaluation involves measuring the systemwide or organizational impact of training.

CASE EXAMPLE: RESIDENT EXPERIENCE: TELEPSYCHIATRY IN PRIMARY CARE ELECTIVE[1]

In my third year of residency training, I provided psychiatric consultations and continuity treatment to primary care clinics using telehealth technology. Patients lived in rural regions 50–150 miles from the University of California Davis (UCD). As a combined trained resident in family medicine and psychiatry, I had an interest in psychiatric collaboration with primary care specialties. Telepsychiatry appealed to me as a means to increase access and further collaboration. In addition, no matter the future clinical setting I envisioned practicing after residency, telepsychiatry could likely fit into my schedule. Lastly, I wanted to experience for myself the therapeutic alliance potential using telehealth technology. During my month-long elective, I was surprised to find that telepsychiatry proved superior to traditional models in several important ways. First, I was impressed by the seamless workflow. Patients were *physically* roomed at their local clinic, and then *virtually* roomed by staff

---

[1]Case provided by Danielle Alexander, M.D.

from the UCD Center for Health and Technology. A simple click on my part was all that was needed when I was ready to greet the patient. As a result of the technology, I actually had more time to devote to patient care (notes, chart review, etc.) without the delay of my physically traveling to and from clinic rooms or clinic sites. Second, in traditional consultation models, a written note is my only means to communicate or receive specialty recommendations, but in this collaborative model of telepsychiatry consultation within the primary care clinic, I was routinely able to talk directly to the primary care provider (PCP) when, at the end of my visit with the patient, the PCP joined the patient in the examination room. I often asked patients to explain our collaborative treatment plan to their PCPs. This process served multiple purposes, not least of which was confirming the patient's understanding of my recommendations as well as providing the PCP with the opportunity to ask clarifying questions—an unheard-of advantage in the busy primary care clinic. From both the psychiatric and the primary care side, this collaboration and improved communication felt ideal.

▌ KEY CONCEPT

Telepsychiatry within the primary care clinic offers unique opportunities for physician-to-physician communication.

HOW SHOULD PROVIDERS BUILD AND MAINTAIN TELEMEDICINE COMPETENCIES?

Several strategies help providers to build and maintain competencies. Providers and trainees may complete self-study (Myers and Turvey 2013). There is a range of online resources that provide dynamic information on the changing telemedicine landscape: 1) professional organizations; 2) telemedicine resource center resources; 3) federal resources; 4) grant-supported resources; and 5) private companies. Potential telepsychiatry providers may "shadow" an established provider to help consolidate interest and skills, while participation in telepsychiatry committees and professional work groups, as well as in ongoing peer-to-peer support, also builds knowledge and skills. Increasingly, training programs are starting to incorporate telepsychiatry rotations and seminars to teach technological approaches to health care as well as to provide experience with improving access to care for diverse patient populations (e.g., rural families, Native Americans).

Clinical experience and supervision with telepsychiatry is important, given the workforce shortages. Most find it appealing to work with health care trainees in order to expose them early in their training to telepsychiatry best practices. These experiences range from shadowing a telepsychiatry provider to formal telepsychiatry training rotations. In addition, videoconferencing-based supervision, or "telesupervision," offers innovative ways to extend supervision opportunities.

SHOULD PROVIDERS SEEK OR BE REQUIRED TO HAVE CERTIFICATION IN TECHNOLOGY COMPETENCIES?

There is ongoing discussion and debate on whether training or certification is indicated and needed for telepsychiatry and applications of technology in mental health care. The movement toward patient-centered care brings with it more explicit demands for competency for physicians (and other clinicians). At the institutional level, some are requiring 2–4 hours of training in telepsychiatry by CME, watching videos, and/or proctoring observation. The downside to this is that it requires additional time and places a burden on those without telepsychiatry experience (e.g., a clinician in practice who initiates telepsychiatry; a graduating resident whose program did not offer it as a training experience). At the association level (e.g., ATA or American Psychological Association), it is well-intentioned to offer and perhaps advocate for training as a role for the organization and support to the field. Existing CME may be able to meet training needs and provide additional in-person and/or online skills-based training. The tension does exist between supporting standardized training and credentialing compared with creating additional barriers to those wanting to begin the practice of telepsychiatry. Training or certification does provide the practitioner with validation of extra effort and skill. If training or certification were required, it would probably be best to be consistent with American Board of Psychiatry and Neurology philosophy for reasonable skills rather than shooting for all to be "experts."

WHAT ARE THE INTANGIBLES IN THE PRACTICE OF MEDICINE THAT ARE NOT ALWAYS WELL DEFINED IN "EVIDENCE-BASED" PRACTICE?

Psychiatrists and other mental health care professionals explore more than a standard history (symptoms, presentation, past treatments) in order to better understand their patients' concerns (Hilty et al. 2013b). They also explore beliefs, norms, and values, and—to a greater degree than most in medicine—the ethnicity-, culture-, and language-related issues that affect health. The cultural issues for a patient include symptoms, presentation, meaning, causation, family factors, coping styles, treatment seeking, mistrust, stigma, immigration, and overall health status. In order to better understand a patient's perspective, the patient's story is solicited in their own words. The role of such stories in healing has been well described. Stories can convey abstract meaning (myths), move people to change, and teach learners to apply knowledge and learn skills.

Several processes are taken for granted in clinical care, one of which is the biopsychosocial model, which places the presenting problem in the context of the patient's life and identifying determinants of the symptoms/psychopathology. The traditional case (psychodynamic) formulation focuses on central conflicts, anticipates problems, and helps guide treatment. Complex clinical circumstances require partnership with patients to reach the best outcome. Shared decision making, in which both parties share information and develop consensus on a decision, equalizes the informational and power symmetry between doctor and patient.

Learning is a complex neurobiological and social phenomenon based on personal experience and professional training, both formal and informal. Learning is enhanced when attention is paid to learner engagement, centeredness, adaptability, and self-reflection. Discussing what is known, what is not, and how to learn more is a key step. Evaluating our strengths and weaknesses is essential. Using our "best" learning styles and improving others gives us different ways to approach problems. Careful reflection can help educators and learners develop strategies for tolerating ambiguity and dealing with the unexpected.

How Can Providers Keep Up to Date With Evidence and Guidelines in a Rapidly Changing Field?

Change is difficult, and frequently resisted, but the science of how to bring about change when introducing technology innovations is well understood. In 1962, Everett Rogers outlined four elements in the diffusion of innovations: the innovation itself, communication channels, time, and the social system (Rogers 1962). Much of that work had to do with the promise of an innovation, with influential individuals ("innovators"; 2.5%) excitedly sharing it with a group of "early adopters" (13.5%). Early adopters are typically younger in age and of higher social status, have greater financial lucidity and more advanced education, and are more socially forward than late adopters. Once enough individuals join in utilizing an innovative process, the group reaches a "tipping point" where adoption of the innovation evolves rapidly. The early majority (34%) who adopt an innovation tend to be slower in the adoption process, have above-average social status, are in contact with early adopters, and seldom hold positions of opinion leadership in a system. The late majority (34%) will adopt an innovation after the average member of the society, as they are skeptical; interestingly, they have below-average social status and typically little financial lucidity. The laggards (16%) are simply aversive to change.

There is some variation in technology adoption between providers that can be influenced by organizational stances of support or caution. First, clinicians should focus on the expected outcome of how a technology will help rather than simply adopting it to see what happens. Second, being prudent and strategic (i.e., adopt one change at a time for a given patient's care to have time to process it; a clinician may want to try out a single technological change in 5–10 patients to get a feel for the issues and apply the evidence base and/or consensus opinion if available). Third, once an organization supports use or implementation of a technology, significant time has often passed, with many review processes; this is not in the early innovator phase. Once a technology is more widely adopted by an organization, providers have the security of that endorsement leading to more widespread adoption. Some providers will get frustrated with the slow pace of organizational adoption, feeling delays as unnecessary, and will proceed with individual technology adoption and incorporation as possible.

Clinicians and organizations must keep up to date on the evidence base, guidelines, and other resources coming out. There are many ways to do this, and most clinicians use a few:

- Regular journal reading, grand rounds, practice group meetings, and case review
- Search engines connected with large databases (e.g., PubMed) to carefully select new developments on a topic

- Membership in an organization (e.g., ATA, APA): there are special conferences, extensive materials online (e.g., APA Toolkit for Telepsychiatry), listservs, and special interest groups
- Attending meetings with a technology focus (e.g., ATA, APA, American Association for Technology in Psychiatry)
- Journal membership (e.g., *Telemedicine and e-Health, Journal of Telemedicine and Telecare, Journal of Technology in Behavioral Sciences, Journal of Health and Medical Informatics*)
- Online training (e.g., *Focus* has modules consistent with the American Board of Psychiatry and Neurology's certification process)

What Is a "Guideline"?

A key issue to be aware of is the differing levels of evidence and consensus, and the other is the generous overuse of the word "guideline." The gold standard for guidelines comes from medicine, specifically, the Institute of Medicine (2011), which defined clinical practice guidelines as "statements that include recommendations intended to optimize patient care that are informed by a systematic review of evidence and an assessment of the benefits and harms of alternative care options" (p. 1). The standard for guidelines set by the Institute of Medicine and partnering medical organizations usually employs strategies from the Agency for Healthcare Research and Quality (AHRQ) and capitalizes on the Cochrane Database of Systematic Reviews. AHRQ provides a systematic literature review to an interdisciplinary guideline writing group to determine recommendations (and the strength of these recommendations) based on the evidence and on consensus expert opinion. This approach also includes identification and management of financial conflicts.

Guidelines tangibly help by providing clinical criteria, protocols, algorithms, review criteria, and other components, all aimed at supporting clinicians to make the best clinical decisions, avoid bad outcomes, and suggest an approach in uncharted circumstances. The available general telemedicine guidelines for videoconferencing-based telemental health care (e.g., American Telemedicine Association 2013) provide overarching strategies for best practices in telepsychiatry. However, the ultimate judgment regarding the care of a particular patient and how closely to adhere to a guideline must be made by the clinician in light of all circumstances surrounding the patient and his or her family. Providers need to take into account the diagnostic and treatment options available, resources, and all pertinent clinical, administrative, and regulatory circumstances.

How Are Technologies Best Integrated Into Clinical Practice?

The application of new telemedicine modalities to one's practice must be carefully selected, discussed with patients, and adaptable to the rapidly changing literature. When first selecting which modalities to add to or subtract from one's practices, recommendations should be considered, as is the case with the addition or change of any medical protocol. The Cochrane Database of Systematic Reviews is considered the highest standard in evidence-based health care resources, consisting of systematic reviews of primary research that result in recommendations on specifically formulated health questions for providers (Tables 10–2 and 10–3). Expert consensus recommendation of Levels I/II or Grades A/B should be regarded as the standard of care and should be integrated into all practices. Recommendations of Levels III/IV or Grades C/D may be more suited for practitioners and patients who may receive the most benefit from the application of that recommendation, keeping in mind whether the reason for the lower recommendation is lack of evidence or additional conferred risks to the patient. Considerations when applying a new model or technology include the following:

1. *The patient.* Depending on comfort, familiarity with technology, and the provider, individual patients may have varying degrees of receptiveness to the telemedicine model. A patient's willingness to engage and favorable opinion are key factors to the success of implementation and efficacy of a particular treatment. In addition, we must consider the patient's familiarity with technology or the availability of a social support system that can assist the patient in navigating the new technology. The patient's familiarity may also play into his or her view of the professionalism of telemedicine. While some may prefer in-person interactions, others may feel they are receiving a higher quality of care through additional adjuncts.
2. *The disease.* The telemedicine modality chosen must be appropriate and effective for the natural history of the disease. For example, a

TABLE 10–2. Standard criteria for evidence base (levels I–IV) of expert consensus recommendations

Level	Description
I	High-quality randomized trial or prospective study; testing of previously developed diagnostic criteria on consecutive patients; sensible costs and alternatives; values obtained from many studies with multi-way sensitivity analyses; systematic review of Level I RCTs and Level I studies.
II	Lesser-quality RCT; prospective comparative study; retrospective study; untreated controls from an RCT; lesser-quality prospective study; development of diagnostic criteria on consecutive patients; sensible costs and alternatives; values obtained from limited studies; with multiway sensitivity analyses; systematic review of Level II studies or Level I studies with inconsistent results.
III	Case–control study (therapeutic and prognostic studies); retrospective comparative study; study of nonconsecutive patients without consistently applied reference "gold standard"; analyses based on limited alternatives and costs and on poor estimates; systematic review of Level III studies.
IV	Case series; case–control study (diagnostic studies); poor reference standard; analyses with no sensitivity analyses; may or may not include evidence from a panel of experts.

Note. RCT = randomized controlled trial. Author's portrayal and description of evidence-based levels and recommendations (rating/grading of evidence and consensus of experts) is based on Institute of Medicine 2011, Cochrane Library 2017, and Agency for Healthcare Research and Quality 2014.

TABLE 10–3. Grades/ratings of expert consensus recommendations

Grade	Descriptor	Qualifying evidence	Implications for practice
A	Strong recommendation	Level I evidence or consistent findings from multiple studies of Levels II, III, or IV	Clinicians should follow a strong recommendation unless a clear and compelling rationale for an alternative approach is present.
B	Recommendation	Levels II, III, or IV evidence and findings are generally consistent	Generally, clinicians should follow a recommendation but should remain alert to new information and sensitive to patient preferences.
C	Option	Levels II, III, or IV evidence but findings are inconsistent	Clinicians should be flexible in their decision making regarding appropriate practice, although they may set bounds on alternatives; patient preference should have a substantial influencing role.
D	Option	Less than Level IV evidence: little or no systematic empirical evidence	Clinicians should consider all options in their decision making and be alert to new published evidence that clarifies the balance of benefit versus harm; patient preference should have a substantial influencing role.

Note. Author's portrayal and description of evidence-based levels and recommendations (rating/grading of evidence and consensus of experts) is based on Institute of Medicine 2011, Cochrane Library 2017, and Agency for Healthcare Research and Quality 2014.

condition that requires in-clinic examinations and procedures (e.g., rheumatoid arthritis requiring constant steroid joint injections, or schizophrenia requiring regular long-acting antipsychotic injections) may be less suited to at-home monitoring using synchronous technology. At the same time, these diseases may have a severe impact on quality of life that may benefit from the support of an online chat group. Chronic medical conditions requiring constant monitoring that is not feasible through in-person visits, such as diabetes mellitus or hypertension, could benefit from wearable devices and/or the submission of data to the practitioner. For all diseases, patient understanding of pathophysiology and/or treatment regimens may be improved by the adjunct of at-home reading done by the patient through online portals. Thus, the appropriate telemedicine modality should be applied fitted to the needs of the patient and maximizing benefit.

3. *The provider.* Before offering telemedicine services, the provider must ensure that he or she has the time and resources to provide quality and consistent care as expected through the new modality. If the telemedicine modality is offered in replacement of some in-person services (i.e., synchronous technology, at-home reading rather than in-person educational sessions), time constraints may not be an issue and may actually be relieved; however, if the telemedicine modality is offered as an additional adjunct, time may become the limiting factor in offering care, either in availability or in quality, neither of which should be sacrificed. Other points to consider are whether the provider him- or herself is familiar with the technology he or she is undertaking and whether all of the providers within the practice are able to offer the same standard of telemedicine care.

There can be different goals in the integration of telemedicine into one's practice; these goals include providing *continuity of care* between scheduled patient visits; *triaging patients* if they need to be seen between regular appointments; providing *adjunctive support; improving access* to care in terms of geography, time, and transportation; *providing privacy/confidentiality* for patients seeking care; and *improving efficiency* of care for both patients and physicians. The first two of these goals require that the physician be actively involved and that telemedicine acts as a mode of communication between physicians and patient (e.g., e-mail check-ins, monitoring of wearable device data, posts on support chat groups). For adjunctive support, this may be in the form of patient self-directed monitoring applications or Web-available informational handouts. The benefits of increased access to care, privacy, and efficiency accompany the use of telemedicine and do not require additional physician activity. Selecting how one wants to use telemedicine in their practice, and to what outcome, should direct which modalities to incorporate.

As with many "new" fields, telemedicine is rapidly changing, with a growing literature; the question will be how fast is too fast to apply changes to one's practice in order to avoid hasty changes and manage newly established protocols. The best way to protect your patients is to be thorough in patient education, explaining new methods and protocols to the patient and allowing him or her to be part of the decision as to whether or not to adopt a specific change. When patients are empowered with shared decision making, they gain the ability to better understand changes to protocols as well as the power to raise concerns when they feel that something is not working well in their care.

SUMMARY

The central aim of this chapter has been to inform providers regarding how best to evaluate technology options and use them in practice to set goals, achieve quality outcomes, and maintain good clinical care through focused, skilled development in telepsychiatry.

- Patient-centered care—defined as the provision of high-quality health care that is affordable and delivered in a timely manner— aligns to a degree with the outcomes-focused approach of value-based reimbursement, and clinicians, accountable care organizations, and others are intensifying their efforts to align with the ACA.
- The evidence base for telepsychiatry is growing, and its effectiveness is clearer, although its cost effectiveness needs further evaluation.
- Clinicians are faced with balancing the results of formal research projects against day-to-day clinical judgment and practical concerns. There are some low-intensity, high-quality evaluation methods that providers can adopt to demonstrate the value of their care.
- Competencies for telepsychiatry across fields of medicine are no longer optional and are now skills- and attitude-based rather than knowledge-focused. A key issue for clinicians adapting to changes in

health care is integration of new findings into their practices. The available general telemedicine guidelines for videoconferencing-based telemental health care provide overarching strategies for best practices in telepsychiatry.

• More caution is indicated for other newer technologies, because services exist on a continuum across a wide range of technologies and clinical practices and workflows.

The ultimate judgment regarding the care of a particular patient must be made by the clinician in light of all circumstances presented by the patient, the diagnostic and treatment options available, resources, and in light of all pertinent clinical, administrative, and regulatory circumstances.

REFERENCES

Accreditation Council on Graduate Medical Education; Holmboe ES, Edgar L, Hamstra S: The Milestones Guidebook, Version 2016. Available at: https://www.acgme.org/Portals/0/MilestonesGuidebook.pdf. Accessed August 17, 2017.

Agency for Healthcare Research and Quality: Clinical Guidelines and Recommendations. Rockville, MD, Agency for Healthcare Research and Quality, content last reviewed November 2014. Available at: http://www.ahrq.gov/professionals/clinicians-providers/guidelines-recommendations/index.html. Accessed September 1, 2016.

American Telemedicine Association: Practice Guidelines for Video-Based Online Mental Health, 2013. Available at: http://www.americantelemed.org/resources/telemedicine-practice-guidelines/telemedicine-practice-guidelines/practice-guidelines-for-video-based-online-mental-health-services#.V6DgyVe1eoI. Accessed July 31, 2016.

Association of American Medical Colleges: 2015 AAMC Annual Report. 2015. Available at: https://www.aamc.org/about/451624/annual-report-2015.html. Accessed September 21, 2017.

Callan JE, Maheu MM, Bucky SF: Crisis in the behavioral health classroom: enhancing knowledge, skills, and attitudes in telehealth training, in Field Guide to Evidence-Based, Technology Careers in Behavioral Health: Professional Opportunities for the 21st Century. Edited by Maheu M, Drude K, Wright S. New York, Springer, 2016, pp 63–80. Available at: https://link.springer.com/chapter/10.1007/978-3-319-23736-7_5. Accessed April 6, 2017.

Centers for Medicare & Medicaid Services: Additional Information Regarding Electronic Clinical Quality Measures (eCQMs) for CMS Reporting Programs for Eligible Professionals and Eligible Clinicians. Baltimore, MD, Centers for Medicare & Medicaid Services, March 2017. Available at:

https://www.cms.gov/Regulations-and-Guidance/Legislation/EHR IncentivePrograms/Downloads/eCQM_2016EPEC_MeasuresTable.pdf. Accessed June 22, 2017.

Cochrane Library: Cochrane Database of Systematic Reviews (CDSR). Available at: http://www.cochranelibrary.com/cochrane-database-of-systematic-reviews/. Accessed April 21, 2017.

Dreyfus SE, Dreyfus HL: A Five-Stage Model of the Mental Activities Involved in Directed Skill Acquisition. Berkeley, CA, University of California, Operations Research Center, 1980. Available at: http://www.dtic.mil/cgi-bin/GetTRDoc?AD=ADA084551. Accessed October 1, 2016.

Eysenbach G: What is e-health? J Med Internet Res 3(2):E20, 2001 11720962

Hilty DM, Ferrer DC, Parish MB, et al: The effectiveness of telemental health: a 2013 review. Telemed J E Health 19(6):444–454, 2013a 23697504

Hilty DM, Srinivasan M, Xiong GL, et al: Lessons from psychiatry and psychiatric education for medical learners and teachers. Int Rev Psychiatry 25(3):329–337, 2013b 23859096

Hilty DM, Crawford A, Teshima J, et al: A framework for telepsychiatric training and e-health: competency-based education, evaluation and implications. Int Rev Psychiatry 27(6):569–592, 2015a 26540642

Hilty DM, Chan S, Torous J, et al: New frontiers in healthcare and technology: Internet- and web-based mental options emerge to complement in-person and telepsychiatric care options. J Health Med Informat 6(4):1–14, 2015b. Available at: https://www.omicsonline.org/open-access/new-frontiers-in-health-care-and-technology-internetand-webbasedmental-options-emerge-to-complement-inperson-and-telepsychiatriccare-options-2157-7420-1000200.php?aid=58390. Accessed April 6, 2017.

Hilty DM, Maheu M, Hertlein K, et al: The need for e-behavioral health competencies: an approach based on competency frameworks and common themes across fields. Journal of Technology in Behavioral Science (in press)

Ho K, Ellaway R, Littleford J: The CanMEDS 2015 eHealth Expert Working Group Report. Ottawa, ON, The Royal College of Physicians and Surgeons of Canada, February 2014. Available at: http://www.royalcollege.ca/portal/page/portal/rc/common/documents/canmeds/framework/ehealth_ewg_report_e.pdf. Accessed September 7, 2017.

Institute of Medicine, Committee on Quality of Health Care in America: Crossing the Quality Chasm: A New Health System for the 21st Century. Washington, DC, National Academy Press, 2001. 25057539

Institute of Medicine, Committee on Standards for Developing Trustworthy Clinical Practice Guidelines: Clinical Practice Guidelines We Can Trust. Washington, DC, National Academies Press, 2011. Available at: https://www.ncbi.nlm.nih.gov/pubmedhealth/PMH0079468/. Accessed April 6, 2017.

Kaslow NJ, Rubin NJ, Bebeau M, et al: Guiding principles and recommendations for the assessment of competence. Professional Psychology: Research and Practice 38(5):441–451, 2007. Available at: http://psycnet.apa.org/index.cfm?fa=buy.optionToBuy&id=2007-14485-001. Accessed April 6, 2017.

Kirkpatrick J, Kirkpatrick W: The Kirkpatrick Four Levels: A Fresh Look After 50 Years, 1959–2009. Newnan, GA, Kirkpatrick Partners, 2009. Available at: http://www.kirkpatrickpartners.com/Portals/0/Resources/Kirkpatrick%20Four%20Levels%20white%20paper.pdf. Accessed October 1, 2016.

Krägeloh CU, Czuba KJ, Billington DR, et al: Using feedback from patient-reported outcome measures in mental health services: a scoping study and typology. Psychiatr Serv 66(3):224–241, 2015 25727110

Maheu M: The online clinical practice model. Psychotherapy: Theory, Research, Practice, Training 40(1–2):20–32, 2003. Available at: http://psycnet.apa.org/doiLanding?doi=10.1037%2F0033-3204.40.1-2.20. Accessed April 6, 2017.

Myers K, Turvey C (eds): Telemental Health: Clinical, Technical and Administrative Foundation for Evidence-Based Practice. London, Elsevier Insights, 2013

Rogers EM: Diffusion of Innovations, 4th Edition. New York, Free Press, 1962

Royal College of Physicians and Surgeons: CanMEDS 2015 Physician Competency Framework. Edited by Frank JR, Snell L, Sherbino J. Ottawa, Royal College of Physicians and Surgeons of Canada, 2015. Available at: www.royalcollege.ca/rcsite/documents/canmeds/canmeds-full-framework-e.pdf. Accessed August 27, 2017.

Shore JH, Mishkind MC, Bernard J, et al: A lexicon of assessment and outcome measures for telemental health. Telemed J E Health 20(3):282–292, 2014 24476192

U.S. Department of Veterans Affairs: Survey of Healthcare Experiences of Patients: Recently Discharged Inpatient 2016. Washington, DC, U.S. Department of Veterans Affairs, 2016. Available at: https://www.reginfo.gov/public/do/DownloadDocument?objectID=64954701. Accessed October 1, 2016.

Index

*Page numbers printed in **boldface** type refer to tables or figures.*